Lyme Disease and Other Infections Transmitted by *Ixodes scapularis*

Editor

PAUL G. AUWAERTER

INFECTIOUS DISEASE CLINICS OF NORTH AMERICA

www.id.theclinics.com

Consulting Editor
HELEN W. BOUCHER

June 2015 • Volume 29 • Number 2

ELSEVIER

1600 John F. Kennedy Boulevard • Suite 1800 • Philadelphia, Pennsylvania, 19103-2899.

http://www.theclinics.com

INFECTIOUS DISEASE CLINICS OF NORTH AMERICA Volume 29, Number 2
June 2015 ISSN 0891-5520, ISBN-13: 978-0-323-38892-4

Editor: Jessica McCool
Developmental Editor: Donald Mumford

Infectious Disease Clinics of North America (ISSN 0891-5520) is published in March, June, September, and December by Elsevier Inc., 360 Park Avenue South, New York, NY 10010-1710. Periodicals postage paid at New York, NY and additional mailing offices. Subscription prices are $295.00 per year for US individuals, $510.00 per year for US institutions, $145.00 per year for US students, $350.00 per year for Canadian individuals, $638.00 per year for Canadian institutions, $420.00 per year for international individuals, $638.00 per year for international institutions, and $200.00 per year for Canadian and international students. To receive student rate, orders must be accompanied by name of affiliated institution, date of term, and the *signature* of program/residency coordinator on institution letterhead. Orders will be billed at individual rate until proof of status is received. Foreign air speed delivery is included in all *Clinics* subscription prices. All prices are subject to change without notice. **POSTMASTER**: Send address changes to *Infectious Disease Clinics of North America*, Elsevier Health Sciences Division, Subcription Customer Service, 3251 Riverport Lane, Maryland Heights, MO 63043. **Customer Service: 1-800-654-2452 (US). From outside of the US and Canada, call 1-314-447-8871. Fax: 1-314-447-8029. E-mail: JournalsCustomerService-usa@elsevier.com (print support) or JournalsOnlineSupport-usa@elsevier.com (online support).**

Infectious Disease Clinics of North America is also published in Spanish by Editorial Inter-Médica, Junin 917, 1er A 1113, Buenos Aires, Argentina.

Reprints. For copies of 100 or more, of articles in this publication, please contact the Commercial Reprints Department, Elsevier Inc., 360 Park Avenue South, New York, New York 10010-1710. Tel. 212-633-3874, Fax: 212-633-3820, E-mail: reprints@elsevier.com.

Infectious Disease Clinics of North America is covered in *MEDLINE/PubMed (Index Medicus), Current Contents/Clinical Medicine, Science Citation Alert, SCISEARCH,* and *Research Alert.*

Contributors

CONSULTING EDITOR

HELEN W. BOUCHER, MD, FIDSA, FACP
Director, Infectious Diseases Fellowship Program, Division of Geographic Medicine and
Infectious Diseases, Tufts Medical Center; Associate Professor of Medicine, Tufts
University School of Medicine, Boston, Massachusetts

EDITOR

PAUL G. AUWAERTER, MD
Sherrilyn and Ken Fisher Professor of Medicine, Sherrilyn and Ken Fisher Center for
Environmental Infectious Diseases, Division of Infectious Diseases, Johns Hopkins
University School of Medicine, Baltimore, Maryland

AUTHORS

SHEILA L. ARVIKAR, MD
Instructor in Medicine, Center for Immunology and Inflammatory Diseases, Division of
Rheumatology, Allergy, and Immunology, Massachusetts General Hospital, Harvard
Medical School, Charlestown, Massachusetts

JOHN N. AUCOTT, MD
Assistant Professor of Medicine, Division of Rheumatology, Department of Medicine,
Johns Hopkins University School of Medicine, Baltimore, Maryland

JOHAN S. BAKKEN, MD, PhD
Associate Professor of Medicine, Department of Family Medicine, University of Minnesota
School of Medicine; St. Luke's Infectious Disease Associates, Duluth, Minnesota

CHOUKRI BEN MAMOUN, PhD
Yale School of Medicine, New Haven, Connecticut

HUGH CALKINS, MD, FACC, FHRS, FAHA
Professor of Medicine and Pediatrics; Director, Cardiac Arrhythmia Service, Division of
Cardiology, Department of Medicine, Johns Hopkins University, Baltimore, Maryland

MARIA A. DIUK-WASSER, PhD
Columbia University, New York, New York

J. STEPHEN DUMLER, MD
Professor, Division of Medical Microbiology, Departments of Pathology and Microbiology
& Immunology, University of Maryland School of Medicine, Baltimore, Maryland

JOHN J. HALPERIN, MD
Chair, Department of Neurosciences, Overlook Medical Center, Summit, New Jersey;
Professor of Neurology and Medicine, Icahn School of Medicine at Mount Sinai, New York,
New York

YVONNE HIGGINS, PA, MAS, MS/ITS
The Sherrilyn and Ken Fisher Center for Environmental Infectious Diseases, Division of Infectious Diseases, Department of Medicine, Johns Hopkins University, Baltimore, Maryland

TAKAAKI KOBAYASHI, MD
The Sherrilyn and Ken Fisher Center for Environmental Infectious Diseases, Division of Infectious Diseases, Department of Medicine, Johns Hopkins University, Baltimore, Maryland

PETER J. KRAUSE, MD
Yale School of Public Health, Yale School of Medicine, New Haven, Connecticut

PAUL M. LANTOS, MD
Instructor in Internal Medicine and Pediatrics, Divisions of Pediatric Infectious Diseases and General Internal Medicine, Duke University School of Medicine, Durham, North Carolina

ADRIANA R. MARQUES, MD
Laboratory of Clinical Infectious Diseases, National Institute of Allergy and Infectious Diseases, National Institutes of Health, Bethesda, Maryland

PAUL S. MEAD, MD, MPH
Chief, Epidemiology and Surveillance Activity, Bacterial Diseases Branch, Division of Vector-Borne Diseases, National Center for Emerging and Zoonotic Infectious Diseases, Centers for Disease Control and Prevention (CDC), Fort Collins, Colorado

MICHAEL T. MELIA, MD
Assistant Professor of Medicine, Division of Infectious Diseases, Department of Medicine, Johns Hopkins University, Baltimore, Maryland

ROBERT B. NADELMAN, MD
Professor, Division of Infectious Diseases, Department of Medicine, New York Medical College, Valhalla, New York

BOBBI PRITT, MD, MSc, DTM&H
Associate Professor, Department of Laboratory Medicine and Pathology, Division of Clinical Microbiology, Mayo Clinic, Rochester, Minnesota

MATTHEW L. ROBINSON, MD
Post-Graduate Fellow, Division of Infectious Diseases, Department of Medicine, Johns Hopkins University, Baltimore, Maryland

SUNIL K. SOOD, MBBS, DCH, MD
Professor of Pediatrics and Family Medicine, Hofstra North Shore-LIJ School of Medicine, Hempstead, New York; Chairman of Pediatrics, Southside Hospital, North Shore-LIJ Health System, Bay Shore, New York; Attending, Pediatric Infectious Diseases, Cohen Children's Medical Center, New Hyde Park, New York

ALLEN C. STEERE, MD
Professor of Medicine, Center for Immunology and Inflammatory Diseases, Division of Rheumatology, Allergy, and Immunology, Massachusetts General Hospital, Harvard Medical School, Charlestown, Massachusetts

EDOUARD G. VANNIER, PhD
Tufts Medical Center, Tufts University School of Medicine, Boston, Massachusetts

GARY P. WORMSER, MD
Professor of Medicine, Microbiology and Immunology, and Pharmacology, Division of Infectious Diseases, New York Medical College, Valhalla, New York

Contents

Lyme disease is the most common vector-borne illness in North America and Europe. The etiologic agent, *Borrelia burgdorferi* sensu lato, is transmitted to humans by certain species of *Ixodes* ticks, which are found widely in temperate regions of the Northern hemisphere. Clinical features are diverse, but death is rare. The risk of human infection is determined by the geographic distribution of vector tick species, ecologic factors that influence tick infection rates, and human behaviors that promote tick bite. Rates of infection are highest among children 5 to 15 years old and adults older than 50 years.

Erythema migrans (EM) is the most common objective manifestation of *Borrelia burgdorferi* infection. Systemic symptoms are usually present. Most patients do not recall a preceding tick bite. Despite a characteristic appearance, EM is not pathognomonic for Lyme disease and must be distinguished from other similar appearing skin lesions. EM is a clinical diagnosis; serologic and PCR assays are unnecessary. Leukopenia and thrombocytopenia are indicative of either an alternative diagnosis, or coinfection with another tick-borne pathogen. When EM is promptly treated with appropriate antimicrobial agents, the prognosis is excellent. Persons in endemic areas should take measures to prevent tick bites.

Lymphocytic meningitis, cranial neuritis or radiculoneuritis occur in up to 15% of patients with untreated *Borrelia burgdorferi* infection. Presentations of multifocal PNS involvement can range from painful monoradiculitis to confluent mononeuropathy multiplex. Serologic testing is highly accurate after 4 to 6 weeks of infection. In CNS infection, production of anti-*B burgdorferi* antibody is often demonstrable in CSF. Oral antimicrobials are microbiologically curative in virtually all patients, including acute European neuroborreliosis. Severe cases may require parenteral treatment. The fatigue and cognitive symptoms seen in some patients with extra-neurological disease are neither evidence of CNS infection nor specific to Lyme disease.

Lyme disease is a common disease that uncommonly affects the heart. Because of the rarity of this diagnosis and the frequent absence of other concurrent clinical manifestations of early Lyme disease, consideration of Lyme carditis demands a high level of suspicion when patients in endemic areas come to attention with cardiovascular symptoms and evidence of higher-order heart block. A majority of cases manifest as atrioventricular block. A minority of Lyme carditis cases are associated with myopericarditis. Like other manifestations of Lyme disease, carditis can readily be managed with antibiotic therapy and supportive care measures, such that affected patients almost always completely recover.

In the United States, Lyme arthritis is the most common feature of late-stage *Borrelia burgdorferi* infection, usually beginning months after the initial bite. In some, earlier phases are asymptomatic and arthritis is the presenting manifestation. Patients with Lyme arthritis have intermittent or persistent attacks of joint swelling and pain in 1 or a few large joints. Serologic testing is the mainstay of diagnosis. Synovial fluid polymerase chain reaction for *B burgdorferi* DNA is often positive before treatment, but is not a reliable marker of spirochetal eradication after therapy. This article reviews the clinical manifestations, diagnosis, and management of Lyme arthritis.

The diagnosis and management of Lyme disease in children is similar to that in adults with a few clinically relevant exceptions. The use of doxycycline as an initial empiric choice is to be avoided for children 8 years old and younger. Children may present with insidious onset of elevated intracranial pressure during acute disseminated Lyme disease; prompt diagnosis and treatment of this condition is important to prevent loss of vision. Children who acquire Lyme disease have an excellent prognosis even when they present with the late disseminated manifestation of Lyme arthritis. Guidance on the judicious use of serologic tests is provided. Pediatricians and family practitioners should be familiar with the prevention and management of tick bites, which are common in children.

The majority of laboratory tests performed for the diagnosis of Lyme disease are based on detection of the antibody responses against *B burgdorferi* in serum. The sensitivity of antibody-based tests increases with the duration of the infection. Patients early in their illness are more likely to have a negative result. There is a need to simplify the testing algorithm for Lyme disease, improving sensitivity in early disease while still maintaining high specificity and providing information about the stage of infection. The development of a point of care assay and biomarkers for active infection would be major advances for the field.

The prognosis following appropriate antibiotic treatment of early or late Lyme disease is favorable but can be complicated by persistent symptoms of unknown cause termed posttreatment Lyme disease syndrome (PTLDS), characterized by fatigue, musculoskeletal pain, and cognitive complaints that persist for 6 months or longer after completion of antibiotic therapy. Risk factors include delayed diagnosis, increased severity of symptoms, and presence of neurologic symptoms at time of initial treatment. Two-tier serologic testing is neither sensitive nor specific for diagnosis of PTLDS because of variability in convalescent serologic responses after treatment of early Lyme disease. Optimal treatment of PTLDS awaits more precise understanding of the pathophysiologic mechanisms involved in this illness and future treatment trials.

Chronic Lyme disease is a poorly defined diagnosis that is usually given to patients with prolonged, unexplained symptoms or with alternative medical diagnoses. Data do not support the proposition that chronic, treatment-refractory infection with *Borrelia burgdorferi* is responsible for the many conditions that get labeled as chronic Lyme disease. Prolonged symptoms after successful treatment of Lyme disease are uncommon, but in rare cases may be severe. Prolonged courses of antibiotics neither prevent nor ameliorate these symptoms and are associated with considerable harm.

Human granulocytic anaplasmosis, a deer tick–transmitted rickettsial infection caused by *Anaplasma phagocytophilum*, is a common cause of undifferentiated fever in the northeast and upper Midwest United States. Patients are often initially diagnosed with a mild viral infection, and illness readily resolves in most cases. However, as many as 3% develop life-threatening complications and nearly 1% die from the infection. Although coinfections with *Borrelia burgdorferi* and *Babesia microti* occur, there is little evidence to suggest synergism of disease or a role for *A phagocytophilum* in chronic illness. No vaccine is available.

Babesiosis is caused by intraerythrocytic protozoan parasites that are transmitted by ticks, or less commonly through blood transfusion or trans-placentally. Human babesiosis was first recognized in a splenectomized

INFECTIOUS DISEASE CLINICS
OF NORTH AMERICA

RELATED INTEREST

Clinics in Laboratory Medicine, June 2014 (Volume 34, Issue 2)
Respiratory Infections
Michael J. Loeffelholz, *Editor*
Available at: http://www.labmed.theclinics.com/

THE CLINICS ARE AVAILABLE ONLINE!
Access your subscription at:
www.theclinics.com

Preface

Lyme Disease: Knowing Good Evidence to Help Inform Practice

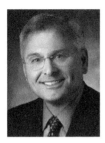

Paul G. Auwaerter, MD
Editor

Depending on the clinical situation and presence or absence of preconceived notions, evaluations for Lyme disease can range from efficient visits solved with a short course of antibiotic therapy to involved encounters that include a review of long-standing, nonspecific symptoms such as fatigue and pain that are less likely to represent an active infection. While the majority of patients with authentic Lyme disease improve with treatment, some have a slower resolution of symptoms and still others appear to have problems persisting beyond 6 months, which is called posttreatment Lyme disease syndrome (PTLDS). Those who have true *Borrelia burgdorferi* infection are relatively easily to determine; however, others may be well complicated by confusion regarding test result interpretation as well as competing ideas about Lyme disease from Internet sources or alternative practitioners who often use the term "chronic Lyme disease" or diagnose concomitant tick-borne coinfections. As Lyme disease is the most common vector-borne infection in North America, clinicians who diagnose and treat Lyme disease need to be aware of not only evidenced-based recommendations but also opposing ideas and theories that may be part of an office-based evaluation and discussion.

A PERSONAL PERSPECTIVE

As a young faculty member in the mid-1990s, I was asked to see patients in a newly established outpatient clinic in suburban Baltimore County, Maryland. Having just completed my infectious diseases fellowship, Lyme disease was a bit of a novelty

Disclosures: The author has provided medical-legal expert testimony related to Lyme disease. The author has received support from the Sherrilyn and Ken Fisher Center for Environmental Infectious Diseases, Johns Hopkins University School of Medicine.

Infect Dis Clin N Am 29 (2015) xi–xvi
http://dx.doi.org/10.1016/j.idc.2015.03.001   **id.theclinics.com**
0891-5520/15/$ – see front matter © 2015 Published by Elsevier Inc.

diagnosis during my training at Johns Hopkins Hospital, located deep as it is in urban Baltimore City, a locale decidedly free of ticks. On occasion, a patient referred from the suburbs would be hospitalized with advanced heart block deemed due to *B burgdorferi* that an antibiotic appeared to solve rather quickly for expeditious discharge. Otherwise, my experience with this tick-borne pathogen was minimal. The 1995 publication of codified serologic testing to assist in the diagnosis of patients with Lyme disease was not something mentioned or discussed by my teachers during training.[1] My clearest recollection of a useful quote from that time was that Lyme disease "hadn't crossed the Potomac and doesn't occur in the mountains," a seemingly useful phrase that seemed to have geographically appropriate Civil War–based overtones backed up by early serologic studies.[2,3] When treatment for Lyme disease was discussed, most experts recommended 2 or 3 weeks of antibiotics such as doxycycline or amoxicillin with resulting success.[4,5] So, armed with this perspective, I found myself underprepared for what soon became the most common reason for outpatient infectious diseases consultation: to assist in the diagnosis and the treatment of Lyme disease. More often than not, these evaluations were often neither easy nor quick for me or many of my patients. These experiences soon prompted an in-depth education and fascination for this infection, which even in my first few years often seemed to be diagnosed more liberally in Maryland than suggested criteria.[6]

EPIDEMIOLOGY

From the initial 1976 clinical description by Steere and colleagues[7,8] of Lyme arthritis among a cohort of children afflicted with an apparently epidemic form of joint disease to the final isolation of the causative spirochete by Willy Burgdorfer and colleagues[9] in 1981 from ticks from Shelter Island, New York, the range of potential problems caused by this infection grew to include the characteristic erythema migrans rash as well as cardiac and neurologic problems. From this New England and Mid-Atlantic base, Lyme disease has expanded geographically over the past decades, but remains an infection for which key clinical questions depend on the epidemiology of whether a given patient may have had a tick bite by an *Ixodes scapularis* tick potentially carrying *B burgdorferi*. From my perspective, more than 20 years after seeing my first patients for Lyme disease consultation, Northern Virginia is now clearly endemic for Lyme disease (so the Potomac has been breached!), and patients routinely acquire the infection in hilly western Maryland (Feldman K, personal communication, 2015).[10] This slow but not glacial expansion bodes a challenge for those practicing medicine on the borders of known endemic regions. Those seeking up-to-date and comprehensive perspective on the epidemiology of Lyme disease would be well-served by Mead's article examining trends in the United States as well as the potential for acquisition of infection in other endemic regions such as Eurasia (See article by Mead, "Epidemiology of Lyme disease", in this issue). Perhaps just as important is knowing where Lyme disease is improbably acquired to avoid misdiagnosis or inappropriate antibiotic therapy.[11]

LYME DISEASE OR NOT?

An accurate diagnosis best informs treatment. This simple statement, if applied to Lyme disease, vexes many a patient and clinician alike. Much of this confusion arises from improper interpretation of serologic tests for Lyme disease, most notably, reliance on IgM immunoblots for symptoms of beyond 4 weeks' duration despite admonition otherwise due to high rates of inaccuracy, or application of such testing in nonendemic regions where acquisition of true infection is improbable and therefore false positive findings are highly likely.[11–13] Objective and evidence-based diagnostics are widely available and their use and interpretation are well represented by the review of Marques (See article by Marques, "Laboratory Diagnosis of Lyme Disease Advances and Challenges", in this issue), which is highly important for diagnostic accuracy when less characteristic findings such as an erythema migrans rash are lacking.[14] Infection present for only a week or two often results in negative serologic tests; this is not unexpected given the time required for immunologic responses to be mounted, but is partly the reason Lyme disease serology has a reputation as an inaccurate test. On the other hand, it is not uncommon to encounter patients who have tests in hand "proving" they have Lyme disease from so-called Lyme specialty labs that offer assays that have not been well-characterized or have a questionable basis.[15,16] Savviness must extend beyond the customary to include good knowledge of potential pitfalls and a well-measured pause before taking diagnostic information for granted. Quite frequently, I am e-mailed or otherwise curbsided by colleagues in other specialties, such as general medicine, neurology, and rheumatology, asking whether a certain test for Lyme disease is a valid or truly secures the diagnosis.

Clinicians who may not consider Lyme disease frequently or who wish to review in-depth information on the spectrum of *B burgdorferi* infection would be well served by reading the excellent treatises (See article by Nadelman, "Erythema Migrans", in this issue), Halperin on neurologic consequences of infection (See article by Halperin, "Nervous System Lyme Disease", in this issue), Melia and colleagues on Lyme carditis (See article by Melia and colleagues, "Lyme Carditis", in this issue), Arvikar and Steere addressing Lyme arthritis (See article by Arvikar and Steere, "Diagnosis and Treatment of Lyme Arthritis", in this issue), and Lyme disease in children by Sood (See article by Sood, "Lyme disease in children", in this issue). Though many areas, such as treatment for an erythema migrans rash, appear well settled, others are not yet well studied in rigorous fashion, such as how to handle antibiotic-refractory Lyme arthritis. These expert clinicians offer valuable insights and approaches for many scenarios that may arise. These articles also help catalog the conditions that either are extraordinarily rare or have no clearly defined association with Lyme disease but are tenuously grasped by some based perhaps on chance coincidence, such as "congenital" Lyme disease, cardiomyopathy, hearing loss, optic neuritis, multiple sclerosis, Alzheimer disease, Parkinson disease, or amyotrophic lateral sclerosis.[17–22]

Knowledge regarding Lyme disease is only a part of what clinicians should know regarding illnesses that could represent other potential infections transmitted by the black-legged deer tick. Excellent reviews covering these aspects include human granulocytic anaplasmosis by Dumler and Bakken (See article by Dumler and Bakken, "Human Granulocytic Anaplasmosis", in this issue) and babesiosis by Krause and colleagues (See article by Krause and colleagues, "Babesiosis", in this issue). Several emerging infections borne by the deer tick that are less familiar but capable of posing serious disease include Powassan virus, *Ehrlichia muris*-like agent and *Borrelia miyamotoi*; these entities are well recounted by Wormser and Pritt (See article by Wormser and Pritt, "Update and Commentary on Four Emerging Tick-Borne Infections: Ehrlichia muris–like Agent, Borrelia miyamotoi, Deer Tick Virus, Heartland Virus, and Whether Ticks Play a Role in Transmission of Bartonella henselae", in this issue). These infections may cause flulike illness with fever as well as cytopenias that should raise the specter of tick-borne disease, and in the case of Powassan virus, acute neurologic disease. On the other hand, some patients are told that these coinfections are responsible for chronic symptoms, such as fatigue or pain, that had not responded to antibiotics targeting Lyme disease. A recent systematic review of the literature did not find convincing evidence that anaplasmosis, babesiosis, or bartonellosis is present in such patients or that their nonspecific symptoms respond to antimicrobial therapy.[23]

Although coinfections are at times invoked for chronic conditions, Lyme disease is more frequently considered a convenient or default explanation when evident explanations are not in hand. One such patient who presented to a number of specialists at Johns Hopkins was a 62-year-old man from the Eastern shore of Maryland who developed decreased hearing, joint pains, numbness, fatigue, and low-grade fever. Doxycycline treatment prior to his evaluation did not yield durable benefit but concern existed by his referring provider and the patient for antibiotic-unresponsive Lyme disease; the patient was ultimately diagnosed with granulomatosis with polyangitis, an uncommon and difficult-to-diagnose disorder.[24] As Lyme disease remains a clinically diagnosed infection based on appropriate epidemiology plus either symptoms with history of erythema migrans rash or objective symptoms and serology, it is both underdiagnosed and overdiagnosed. Yet, a worrisome aspect began soon after the description of Lyme disease, as some physicians advocated for both a wider role for the infection as a cause of numerous problems and a long-term antibiotic therapy for those who had slow resolution of symptoms.[25,26] Physicians practicing evidence-based medicine began to see numerous patients who were labeled with Lyme disease but had no evidence of infection.[27,28] For patients who do seem to be troubled by long-term symptoms after treatment for Lyme disease, trials to date have not demonstrated benefit of additional antibiotic therapy.[29] This has evolved as one of the major aspects of what is often referred to as the debate or the controversy regarding Lyme disease. While I am empathetic to patients who are suffering, many patients have medically unexplained symptoms not due to Lyme disease.

Some find Lyme disease or "chronic Lyme disease" to be more plausible explanations for complex constellations of symptoms than syndromic diagnoses, such as chronic fatigue or fibromyalgia.[30] Many patients are confused by the apparently polar sets of diagnostic and therapeutic advice voiced by most established professional societies as compared with those articulated by advocates of chronic Lyme disease. For providers who are sorting out patients who might have PTLDS or who bring up concerns of "chronic Lyme disease," two helpful reviews help bring perspective and highlight educational points for patients (See article by Aucott, "Post-treatment Lyme Disease syndrome"; See article by Lantos "Chronic Lyme disease", in this issue). Regardless of the cause, patients who do suffer from long-term fatigue, musculoskeletal pains, and subjective neurocognitive disorders usually appreciate thoughtful evaluations and discussions of what may be their diagnoses; they often readily engage in dialogs regarding the limits of current medical science, and they welcome advice on interventions that may lead to functional improvements. Practically, however, this is rarely accomplished with one visit or even two.

Many questions remain about *B burgdorferi*, an organism that harbors a complex genome and provokes host immune responses that remain to be more fully characterized. I have learned considerably from the experts who have authored these articles, and who have clearly put heart and soul into providing the best information currently known about Lyme disease and potential coinfections in this issue of *Infectious Diseases Clinics of North America* (Auwaerter, ed, "Lyme disease" IDCA, Volume 29, Issue 2, June 2015). With some apology, I have taken more space directed toward what is not Lyme disease or coinfections, but it is the reality that at least for a specialist at a referral center, this is now more often the case in consultation than management of true *B burgdorferi* infection. I admire the dedication and persistence of all who are working to help advance the field and provide the better care for our patients.

ACKNOWLEDGMENTS

I wish to thank Michael Melia, MD and Paul Lantos, MD for their gracious review and comments.

Paul G. Auwaerter, MD
Johns Hopkins University School of Medicine
Sherrilyn and Ken Fisher Professor of Medicine
Sherrilyn and Ken Fisher Center for Environmental Infectious Diseases
725 North Wolfe Street, Room # 231
Baltimore, MD 21205, USA

E-mail address:
pauwaert@jhmi.edu

REFERENCES

1. Centers for Disease Control and Prevention (CDC). Recommendations for test performance and interpretation from the Second National Conference on Serologic Diagnosis of Lyme Disease. MMWR Morb Mortal Wkly Rep 1995;44: 590–1.
2. Frank C, Fix AD, Peña CA, et al. Mapping Lyme disease incidence for diagnostic and preventive decisions, Maryland. Emerg Infect Dis 2002;8(4):427–9.
3. Peña CA, Strickland GT. Incidence rates of Lyme disease in Maryland: 1993 through 1996. Md Med J 1999;48(2):68–73.
4. Rahn DW, Malawista SE. Lyme disease: recommendations for diagnosis and treatment. Ann Intern Med 1991;114(6):472–81.
5. Strickland GT, Caisley I, Woubeshet M, et al. Antibiotic therapy for Lyme disease in Maryland. Public Health Rep 1994;109(6):745–9.
6. Peña CA, Mathews AA, Siddiqi NH, et al. Antibiotic therapy for Lyme disease in a population-based cohort. Clin Infect Dis 1999;29(3):694–5.
7. Steere AC, Malawista SE, Snydman DR, et al. Lyme arthritis: an epidemic of oligoarticular arthritis in children and adults in three connecticut communities. Arthritis Rheum 1977;20(1):7–17.
8. Steere AC, Malawista SE, Hardin JA, et al. Erythema chronicum migrans and Lyme arthritis. The enlarging clinical spectrum. Ann Intern Med 1977;86(6): 685–98.
9. Burgdorfer W, Barbour AG, Hayes SF, et al. Lyme disease—a tick-borne spiro-chetosis? Science 1982;216(4552):1317–9.
10. Brinkerhoff RJ, Gilliam WF, Gaines D. Lyme disease, Virginia, USA, 2000-2011. Emerg Infect Dis 2014;20(10):1661–8.
11. Lantos PM, Brinkerhoff RJ, Wormser GP, et al. Empiric antibiotic treatment of er-ythema migrans-like skin lesions as a function of geography: a clinical and cost effectiveness modeling study. Vector Borne Zoonotic Dis 2013;13(12):877–83.
12. Barclay SS, Melia MT, Auwaerter PG. Misdiagnosis of late-onset Lyme arthritis by inappropriate use of Borrelia burgdorferi immunoblot testing with synovial fluid. Clin Vaccine Immunol 2012;19(11):1806–9.
13. Seriburi V, Ndukwe N, Chang Z, et al. High frequency of false positive IgM immu-noblots for Borrelia burgdorferi in clinical practice. Clin Microbiol Infect 2012; 18(12):1236–40.
14. Klempner MS, Halperin JJ, Baker PJ, et al. Lyme borreliosis: the challenge of ac-curacy. Neth J Med 2012;70(1):3–5.

15. Centers for Disease Control and Prevention. Notice to Readers: Caution regarding testing for lyme disease. MMWR Morb Mortal Wkly Rep 2005;54(05):125.
16. Nelson C, Hojvat S, Johnson B, et al. Concerns regarding a new culture method for Borrelia burgdorferi not approved for the diagnosis of Lyme disease. MMWR Morb Mortal Wkly Rep 2014;63(15):333.
17. Lakos A, Solymosi N. Maternal Lyme borreliosis and pregnancy outcome. Int J Infect Dis 2010;14(6):e494–8.
18. Halperin JJ. Nervous system lyme disease: is there a controversy? Semin Neurol 2011;31(3):317–24.
19. Traisk F, Lindquist L. Optic nerve involvement in Lyme disease. Curr Opin Ophthalmol 2012;23(6):485–90.
20. Bakker R, Aarts MC, van der Heijden GJ, et al. No evidence for the diagnostic value of Borrelia serology in patients with sudden hearing loss. Otolaryngol Head Neck Surg 2012;146(4):539–43.
21. Rees DH, Keeling PJ, McKenna WJ, et al. No evidence to implicate Borrelia burgdorferi in the pathogenesis of dilated cardiomyopathy in the United Kingdom. Br Heart J 1994;71(5):459–61.
22. Piccirillo BJ, Pride YB. Reading between the Lyme: is Borrelia burgdorferi a cause of dilated cardiomyopathy? The debate continues. Eur J Heart Fail 2012; 14(6):567–8.
23. Lantos PM, Wormser GP. Chronic coinfections in patients diagnosed with chronic lyme disease: a systematic review. Am J Med 2014;127(11):1105–10.
24. Marinopoulos SS, Coylewright M, Auwaerter PG, et al. Clinical problem-solving. More than meets the ear. N Engl J Med 2010;362(13):1228–33.
25. Burrascano J. Lyme disease. In: Rakel R, editor. Conn's current therapy. 97th edition. Philadelphia: WB Saunders Co; 1997. p. 140–3.
26. Cameron D, Gaito A, Harris N, et al. Evidence-based guidelines for the management of Lyme disease. Expert Rev Anti Infect Ther 2004;2(Suppl 1):S1–13.
27. Steere AC, Taylor E, McHugh GL, et al. The overdiagnosis of Lyme disease. JAMA 1993;269(14):1812–6.
28. Sigal LH. Overdiagnosis and overtreatment of Lyme disease leads to inappropriate health service use. Clin Exp Rheumatol 1999;17(1):41.
29. Klempner MS, Baker PJ, Shapiro ED, et al. Treatment trials for post-Lyme disease symptoms revisited. Am J Med 2013;126(8):665–9.
30. Feder HM Jr, Johnson BJ, O'Connell S, et al. A critical appraisal of "chronic Lyme disease". N Engl J Med 2007;357(14):1422–30.

Epidemiology of Lyme Disease

Paul S. Mead, MD, MPH

KEYWORDS

- Lyme disease • Epidemiology • Incidence • *Borrelia burgdorferi*
- Tick-borne diseases • Human • Zoonosis • *Ixodes*

KEY POINTS

- More than 36,000 confirmed and probable Lyme disease cases were reported in the United States in 2013. The true number of cases is estimated to be approximately 300,000 per year.
- Cases are focused in 14 high-incidence states located in the Northeast and North Central United States; discrete areas of risk exist in Pacific Coast states. The number and geographic distribution of cases has been increasing steadily.
- Epidemiologic factors including local incidence should factor heavily when evaluating patients with signs and symptoms consistent with Lyme disease.
- Health care providers can prevent Lyme disease by educating their patients about personal protective measures, including repellent use, daily ticks, and prompt bathing after exposure.

INTRODUCTION

Lyme disease is a tick-borne zoonosis caused by several genospecies of the spirochete *Borrelia burgdorferi* sensu lato.[1] The organism normally cycles among small mammals and birds, transmitted by ticks of the *Ixodes ricinus* complex.[2] Human illness is characterized by diverse dermatologic, neurologic, rheumatologic, or cardiac abnormalities.[3–6] Also called *Lyme borreliosis*, the disease was named in the mid-1970s for a small town in Connecticut.[7] In retrospect, illness consistent with Lyme disease was reported in Europe as early as 1883.[8–10] Lyme disease is now recognized as the most common vector-borne disease in both Europe and North America.

Disclaimer: The findings and conclusions in this article are those of the author and do not necessarily represent the views of the Centers for Disease Control and Prevention.

Epidemiology and Surveillance Activity, Bacterial Diseases Branch, Division of Vector-Borne Diseases, National Center for Emerging and Zoonotic Infectious Diseases, Centers for Disease Control and Prevention (CDC), 3156 Rampart Road, Fort Collins, CO 80521, USA

E-mail address: pfm0@CDC.GOV

Infect Dis Clin N Am 29 (2015) 187–210
http://dx.doi.org/10.1016/j.idc.2015.02.010
0891-5520/15/$ – see front matter Published by Elsevier Inc.

id.theclinics.com

Etiologic Agent

At least 18 distinct genospecies of *Borrelia burgdorferi* sensu lato have been described based on isolates obtained from small vertebrates or ticks (**Box 1**).[11] Most human infections are caused by 3 genospecies: *B afzelii*, *B garinii*, and *B burgdorferi* sensu stricto (hereafter referred to as *B burgdorferi*). Among these, only *B burgdorferi* causes Lyme disease in North America. Other genospecies occasionally isolated from humans include *B spielmanii*, *B bavariensis*, *B valaisiana*, *B lusitaniae*, and *B bissetii*.[12–16] The public health importance of these other agents remains unclear. Additional genospecies will likely be identified as advanced molecular techniques are applied more broadly.

Tick Vectors

Although multiple species of *Ixodes* ticks are capable of transmitting *B burgdorferi* sensu lato among animals, only 4 commonly bite humans. Two of these, *I ricinus* and *I persulcatus*, are the principal vectors in Europe and Asia, respectively. In the United States, the principal vector is the black-legged or deer tick, *I scapularis*. These ticks are abundant in areas in the Northeastern, Mid-Atlantic, and North Central states; up to 40% are infected with *B burgdorferi*. In the Western United States, the principal human-biting vector is *I pacificus*, the western black-legged tick. Foci of *I pacificus* ticks occur from the central California coast northward into southern British Columbia. Western transmission cycles are such that *I pacificus* are rarely infected and, therefore, account for relatively few human infections.[2]

The life cycle of *I scapularis* generally lasts 2 years, during which the tick takes 3 blood meals, one each as a larvae, nymph, and adult (**Fig. 1**). Ticks are uninfected when they hatch from eggs; they acquire *B burgdorferi* by feeding on infected reservoir hosts, principally mice, shrews, other small mammals and various species of birds. Infected ticks are able to transmit the pathogen during subsequent feedings to new reservoir hosts, thereby perpetuating the natural cycle. Unlike reservoir hosts, humans are incidental or dead-end hosts that do not sustain large numbers of spirochetes in their tissues. Adult ticks feed preferentially on deer, which are immune to *B burgdorferi* but play an important role in the ecology of disease by transporting ticks and supporting tick populations.[2,17]

Although *I scapularis* ticks are also present in the Southeastern United States, questing ticks are much less abundant and are rarely infected with *B burgdorferi*.[18–20] These differences seem to be driven by genetic, phenotypic, and local ecologic

---

Box 1
Named genospecies of *Borrelia burgdorferi* sensu lato

North America	Europe	Asia
B americana	*B afzelii*[a]	*B afzelii*[a]
B andersonii	*B bavariensis*	*B bissettii*
B bissettii	*B bissettii*	*B garinii*[a]
B burgdorferi[a]	*B burgdorferi*[a]	*B japonica*
B californiensis	*B garinii*[a]	*B sinica*
B carolinensis	*B lusitaniae*	*B tanukii*
B kurtenbachii	*B spielmanii*	*B turdii*
	B valaisiana	*B valaisiana*
		B yangtze

[a] Established human pathogens.

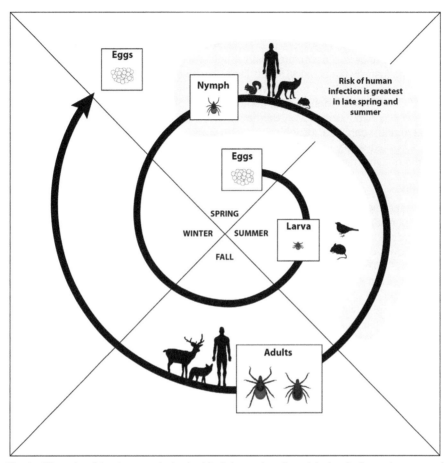

Fig. 1. Life cycle of *Ixodes scapularis*, the black-legged or deer tick that is the main vector of *Borrelia burgdorferi* in the United States.

factors.[2,21,22] Although immature ticks in the Northeast feed primarily on small rodents, ticks in the Southeast feed primarily on lizards.[20,23] Questing habits differ, and southern *Ixodes scapularis* seem less prone to biting humans.[24] The few *B burgdorferi* sensu stricto isolates that have been identified in the Southeast have all been collected from animals within a few miles of the Atlantic Coast.[25,26] This distribution is notable in that the coastline is an important landmark for migratory birds, which may play a role in long-distance dispersal of infected ticks.[27]

Clinical Features

Clinical features of Lyme disease are diverse and vary with the stage and duration of infection. Erythema migrans (EM) is universally the most common feature, occurring in 60% to 90% of cases in North America. EM reflects localized reproduction of spirochetes within the skin and typically begins 3 to 14 days after the tick bite. A gradually expanding erythematous rash, EM is often accompanied by symptoms of fatigue, fever, headache, mild stiff neck, arthralgia, or myalgia. If not treated promptly, infection can disseminate to other parts of the body causing neurologic defects (eg, facial palsy, meningitis, radiculopathy), cardiac abnormalities (eg, carditis with atrioventricular heart block), and monoarticular or oligoarticular arthritis. In the United States where human infection is limited to *B burgdorferi*, 32% of cases reported through national surveillance are associated with arthritis, whereas only 12% have neurologic symptoms (usually facial palsy).[28] It is likely, however, that routine surveillance favors reporting of cases that are more severe and more likely to have positive laboratory results.[29] Carditis is universally rare, generally accounting for less than 1% in most series.[3,5,30,31] Two distinctive dermatologic manifestations of Lyme disease, acrodermatitis chronica atrophicans (ACA) and lymphocytoma, are well known in Europe but extremely rare in the United States.[32] Detailed descriptions of the clinical features of Lyme disease are available elsewhere.[3,5,33–37]

Mortality

Despite the high frequency of infection, few deaths caused by Lyme disease have been reported in the medical literature.[38–41] A review of US death certificates identified 23 records during 1999 to 2003 that listed Lyme disease as the underlying cause of death; however, 11 were improperly coded, and only one listed a consistent causal sequence.[42] The potential for occult death caused by Lyme carditis was demonstrated by a recent report of fatal Lyme carditis cases discovered through postmortem examination of donated tissues.[43] Nevertheless, a follow-up study of more than 120,000 patients with Lyme disease during 1995 to 2013 found that only 0.6% died of all causes within a year of diagnosis, a rate less than the expected, age-adjusted, all-cause mortality for this population.[31]

RISK FACTORS

The risk of human infection with *B burgdorferi* is determined by the geographic distribution of vector tick species, local factors that increase or decrease tick abundance and rates of infection, and human behaviors that affect the likelihood of being bitten. In the Northeast where homes are often situated in heavily tick-infested areas, exposure is thought to occur primarily in the peridomestic environment immediately around the home.[44–47] In the North Central states, areas of highest risk are often lightly populated[48]; infection in these areas is more often related to weekend travel and recreation. Specific peridomestic risk factors include the presence of a suitable tick habitat, landscaping practices that enhance tick survival (eg, failure to clear leaf litter), deer density, and outdoor activities, such as gardening.[49–53] Certain occupations and hobbies also increase the risk of infection. Forestry workers, farmers, soldiers, hunters, hikers, and orienteers have higher rates of infection in studies from the United States,[54] Asia,[55,56] and throughout Europe.[57–61] Animal studies and clinical observations indicate that *I scapularis* ticks require at least 36 hours of attachment in order to transmit *B burgdorferi*,[62] supporting a possible preventive role for daily tick checks and showering after potential exposure.[53,63] Unfortunately, similar studies have demonstrated that *I ricinus* ticks, especially when infected with *B afzelii*, can transmit infection efficiently after much shorter periods of attachment.[2]

Although the epidemiology of Lyme disease is consistent with the well-established mechanism of transmission by *Ixodes* ticks, alternate modes of transmission have been investigated. Inoculation of blood with laboratory-adapted strains of *B burgdorferi* has demonstrated the organism's ability to survive under blood banking conditions.[64] Nevertheless, transmission by transfusion has never been documented. Meanwhile, transfusion-associated transmission of less common *Ixodes*-transmitted pathogens (*Babesia, Anaplasma*) has been demonstrated repeatedly.[65,66] There is also no credible evidence of transmission through sexual contact, semen, urine, or breast milk, despite a series of studies in animals.[67,68] As described in the next section, the epidemiology of Lyme disease is the exact opposite of most sexually transmitted diseases, which are most common among persons aged 18 to 30 years. Intrauterine infection has been documented in rare reports of miscarriage and stillbirth in women infected during pregnancy.[69] A causal relationship to miscarriage has not been established; however, as *B burgdorferi* has also been identified in placentas of women with normal pregnancy outcomes.[70] Larger epidemiologic studies have identified no definable pattern of teratogenicity,[71,72] and pregnant women who develop Lyme disease generally have good outcomes when they receive appropriate antimicrobial therapy.[72]

UNITED STATES INCIDENCE

Lyme disease has been a nationally notifiable condition in the United States since 1991. Health care providers report cases to state or local health officials, who categorize reports according to standardized surveillance case definitions developed by the Council of State and Territorial Epidemiologists.[73] Case definitions are revised periodically, as in 1996 to clarify laboratory criteria and again in 2008 to allow reporting of probable cases.[74] Data for each state are shared with the Centers for Disease Control and Prevention (CDC) for publication; provisional data are published weekly and finalized data annually. Although some states reported cases to the CDC before 1991, comparisons with data collected later are limited by variable case definitions and reporting practices. It is important to note that surveillance data are captured by county of residence, not county of exposure. Consequently, occasional case reports from a state are not necessarily evidence of local transmission.

During 1992 to 2013, US states and territories reported 430,540 confirmed Lyme disease cases to the CDC.[28,75,76] Annual case counts increased approximately 3-fold during the period, from 9908 confirmed cases in 1992 to 27,203 confirmed and 9104 probable cases in 2013 (**Fig. 2**).[28,75,76] Some of this increase can be attributed to greater recognition and enhanced surveillance. In Connecticut, for example, total cases increased 3-fold following implementation of laboratory-based reporting, even while the number ascertained through physician reporting remained stable.[77] There is also evidence, however, of true increases in disease incidence and geographic expansion, as described later.

Geographic Distribution

Within North America, Lyme disease incidence is highest in the Northeastern, Mid-Atlantic, and North Central United States. In 2013, 14 states (Connecticut, Delaware, Maine, Massachusetts, Maryland, Minnesota, New Hampshire, New Jersey, New York, Pennsylvania, Rhode Island, Vermont, Virginia, and Wisconsin) accounted for more than 96% of confirmed US cases (**Fig. 3**).[76] Verified cases reported from other US states are usually associated with travel to states with high rates of infection.[28] Exceptions occur along the West Coast in California, Oregon, and Washington where *I pacificus* is an established though rarely infected vector.[2] In Canada, populations of *I scapularis* have been identified along the US border in Manitoba, Ontario, and Nova Scotia; *I pacificus* ticks are established in coastal areas of southern British Columbia.[78] During 2009 to 2012, a total of 833 Lyme disease cases were reported to the Public Health Agency of Canada.[79] *Ixodes* ticks are found in Northeastern Mexico and in Baja[2,80]; however, evidence for human Lyme borreliosis in Mexico is limited to a few case reports.[81]

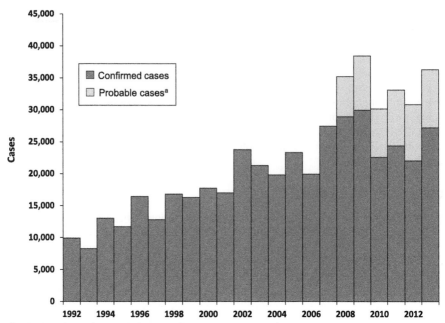

Fig. 2. Number of reported Lyme disease cases, United States, 1992 to 2013. [a] National surveillance case definition revised in 2008 to include probable cases.

Although *I scapularis* ticks are found in the Southeastern and South Central United States, human surveillance data indicate that *B burgdorferi* transmission is rare to nonexistent in these areas. This conclusion is corroborated by a nationwide seroprevalence study in which nearly 1 million dogs were tested for antibodies to *B burgdorferi* (**Fig. 4**).[82] In 14 states with a high incidence of reported human illness, 7% to nearly 20% of dogs statewide were seropositive.[83] These values underscore the sensitivity of dogs as sentinels for the presence of *B burgdorferi* in the environment. In contrast, less than 0.5% of dogs in the southeastern and south central states were seropositive. This value is consistent with the false positivity rate for the assay[84] and the occasional immigration of dogs from high-risk areas.[85] Notably, the assay used in this study is based on a generally conserved C6 oligopeptide and is, therefore, capable of detecting infection with multiple genospecies of *B burgdorferi* sensu lato.

Incidence of human Lyme disease typically ranges from 10 to 100 per 100,000 population in endemic states (**Table 1**). The highest recorded statewide incidence was 134 per 100,000, reported in Connecticut in 2002 following implementation of mandatory laboratory-based reporting.[28,77] Areas of hyperendemicity with county-level rates in excess of 200 per 100,000 population include Windham County in Connecticut; Dukes and Nantucket counties in Massachusetts; Hunterdon County in New Jersey; Columbia, Dutchess, Putnam, and Greene counties in New York; and Washburn County in Wisconsin.[28]

As the number of reported Lyme disease cases has increased over the last 2 decades, the geographic distribution of cases has also expanded, moving outward from the 2 major foci in the Northeastern and North Central United States (see **Fig. 3**). Comparing the time periods of 1993 to 1997 to 2008 to 2012, the number of statistically defined high-incidence counties increased from 43 to 182 in the

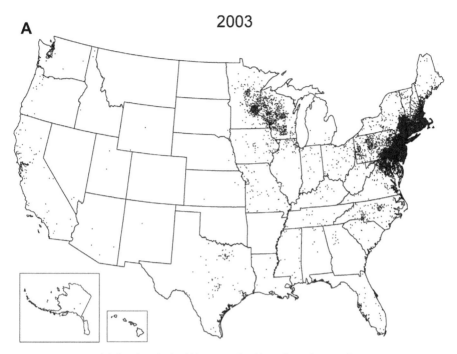

1 dot placed randomly within county of residence for each reported case

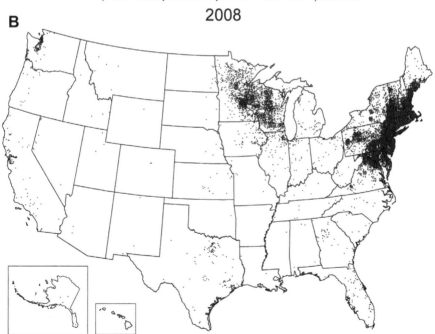

1 dot placed randomly within county of residence for each confirmed case

Fig. 3. Geographic distribution of confirmed Lyme disease cases, United States, 2003 (*A*), 2008 (*B*), and 2013 (*C*). One dot placed randomly within county of patient residence.

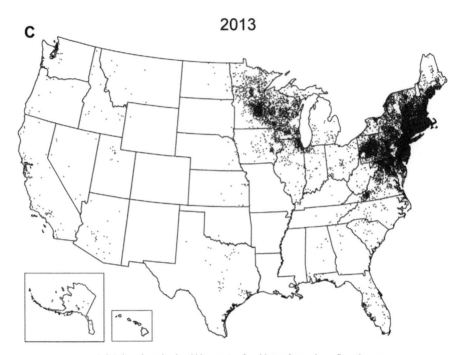

C   **2013**

1 dot placed randomly within county of residence for each confirmed case

Fig. 3. (*continued*)

northeastern states and from 22 to 78 in the north central states (K. Kugeler, personal communication, 2014). The effect has been most pronounced in the states of New Hampshire, Vermont, and Maine. The incidence in these states has increased 5- to 10-fold over the last 10 years to become among the highest nationwide (see **Table 1**). Locally, the incidence rates have increased disproportionately northward along the upper Hudson River Valley in New York and southward into Fairfax County Virginia.[28]

Patient Characteristics

As shown for the years 2010 to 2013, Lyme disease incidence is bimodal with respect to age, with highest rates among children aged 5 to 15 years and adults older than 50 years (**Fig. 5**). In the United States, the incidence is higher among males in all age groups. In contrast, females account for 51% to 60% of identified cases in many European series, yielding an incidence higher than males in at least some series.[28,61,86,87] Although these patterns likely reflect behavior-related differences in exposure across populations, age and sex-specific differences in susceptibility and care-seeking behavior may also contribute. Over time, the US incidence has increased disproportionately among males, shifting the overall sex ratio from 51% male in 1992 to 53% male in 2006.[28] This sex-specific increase has been most pronounced among children. In a separate analysis of US data for 2001 to 2002, age and sex distribution were found to vary among cases reported in endemic and nonendemic areas.[88] In 12 high-incidence states, the modal age for cases was 6 years, and 54% were among males. In contrast, in nonendemic states, the modal age was 44 years, and 47% were among males. Barring fundamental differences in risk factors for infection, this

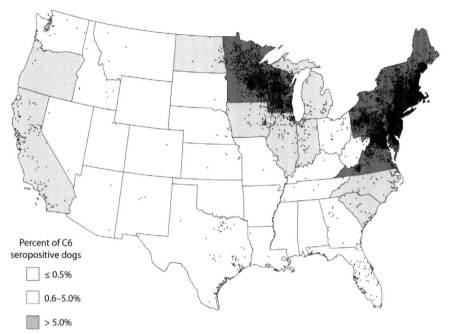

Percent of C6
seropositive dogs

☐ ≤ 0.5%

☐ 0.6–5.0%

■ > 5.0%

Fig. 4. Seroprevalence of C6 anti–*Borrelia burgdorferi* antibody among dogs, 2001-2007, and reported human Lyme disease cases, 2010, United States. No canine data for Nevada and Montana. (*Data from* Bowman D, Little SE, Lorentzen L, et al. Prevalence and geographic distribution of *Dirofilaria immitis, Borrelia burgdorferi, Ehrlichia canis,* and *Anaplasma phagocytophilum* in dogs in the United States: results of a national clinic-based serologic survey. Vet Parasitol 2009;160:138–48.)

discrepancy suggests misclassification (ie, that a substantial proportion of illnesses reported in nonendemic areas are actually caused by other conditions). This finding is consistent with a higher risk of misdiagnosis in nonendemic areas, a consequence of the effect of prior probability on the predictive value of clinical and laboratory findings.[89]

Seasonality

Lyme borreliosis occurs most often in the warmer months, influenced by the questing habits of ticks and the recreational tendencies of humans.[2,28,90] Nymphal ticks are thought to play a particularly important role in transmission because of their small size and relative abundance. Questing by nymphs usually peaks in spring or early summer; this is followed by a similar peak in the onset of acute cases in humans.[91] In the United States, more than 50% of human cases have an onset in June and July (**Fig. 6**).[28] A slightly later peak in August has been reported in Estonia[92] and Sweden,[87] perhaps because of their more northern latitude. Questing behavior is sensitive to meteorologic factors,[93,94] and onset of human illness can vary from year to year based on climatic conditions.[95] Because of the longer and more variable incubation periods, later stages of disease tend to peak slightly later in the calendar year[87,96] and show less seasonal fluctuation.[28,96,97] For example, during 1992 to 2006, 67% of US EM cases had an onset in June and July, as compared with only 37% of arthritis cases.[28]

Table 1
Lyme disease incidence by state and year (United States 2004–2013)

State	2004	2005	2006	2007	2008	2009	2010	2011	2012	2013
Alabama	0.1	0.1	0.2	0.3	0.1	0.1	0.0	0.2	0.3	0.2
Alaska	0.5	0.6	0.4	1.5	0.9	1.0	1.0	1.2	0.5	1.9
Arizona	0.2	0.2	0.2	0.0	0.0	0.0	0.0	0.1	0.1	0.3
Arkansas	0.0	0.0	0.0	0.0	0.0	0.0	0.0	0.0	0.0	0.0
California	0.1	0.3	0.2	0.2	0.2	0.3	0.4	0.0	0.2	0.2
Colorado	0.0	0.0	0.0	0.0	0.0	0.0	0.0	0.0	0.0	0.0
Connecticut	38.5	51.7	51.0	87.3	78.2	78.2	55.0	56.0	46.0	58.7
Delaware	40.8	76.7	56.5	82.7	88.4	111.2	73.1	84.6	55.3	43.2
Florida	0.3	0.3	0.2	0.2	0.4	0.4	0.3	0.4	0.3	0.4
Georgia	0.1	0.1	0.1	0.1	0.4	0.4	0.1	0.3	0.3	0.1
Hawaii	0.0	0.0	0.0	0.0	0.0	0.0	0.0	0.0	0.0	0.0
Idaho	0.4	0.1	0.5	0.6	0.3	0.3	0.4	0.2	0.0	0.9
Illinois	0.7	1.0	0.9	1.2	0.8	1.1	1.1	1.5	1.6	2.6
Indiana	0.5	0.5	0.4	0.9	0.7	0.9	1.0	1.2	1.0	1.5
Iowa	1.7	3.0	3.3	4.1	2.8	2.6	2.2	2.4	3.0	5.0
Kansas	0.1	0.1	0.1	0.3	0.6	0.6	0.2	0.4	0.3	0.6
Kentucky	0.4	0.1	0.2	0.1	0.1	0.0	0.1	0.1	0.2	0.4
Louisiana	0.0	0.1	0.0	0.0	0.1	0.0	0.0	0.0	0.1	0.0
Maine	17.1	18.7	25.6	40.2	59.2	60.0	42.1	60.3	66.6	84.8
Maryland	16.0	22.1	22.2	45.8	31.0	25.7	20.1	16.1	18.9	13.5
Massachusetts	23.9	36.3	22.2	46.3	60.9	61.0	36.3	27.3	51.1	57.0
Michigan	0.3	0.6	0.5	0.5	0.8	0.8	0.8	0.9	0.8	1.2
Minnesota	20.1	17.9	17.7	23.8	20.0	20.2	24.4	22.2	16.9	26.4
Mississippi	0.0	0.0	0.1	0.0	0.0	0.0	0.0	0.1	0.0	0.0
Missouri	0.4	0.3	0.1	0.2	0.1	0.1	0.1	0.1	0.0	0.0
Montana	0.0	0.0	0.1	0.4	0.6	0.3	0.3	0.9	0.6	1.6
Nebraska	0.1	0.1	0.6	0.4	0.4	0.2	0.4	0.4	0.3	0.4
Nevada	0.0	0.1	0.2	0.6	0.3	0.4	0.1	0.1	0.4	0.4
New Hampshire	17.4	20.3	46.9	68.1	92.0	75.2	63.0	67.3	75.9	100.0
New Jersey	31.0	38.6	27.9	36.1	37.0	52.8	37.8	38.5	30.8	31.3
New Mexico	0.1	0.2	0.2	0.3	0.2	0.0	0.1	0.1	0.0	0.0
New York	26.5	28.8	23.1	21.6	29.5	21.2	12.3	16.0	10.4	17.9
North Carolina	1.4	0.6	0.4	0.6	0.2	0.2	0.2	0.2	0.3	0.4
North Dakota	0.0	0.5	1.1	1.9	1.2	1.5	3.1	3.2	1.4	1.7
Ohio	0.4	0.5	0.4	0.3	0.3	0.4	0.2	0.3	0.4	0.6
Oklahoma	0.1	0.0	0.0	0.0	0.0	0.1	0.0	0.1	0.0	0.0
Oregon	0.3	0.1	0.2	0.2	0.5	0.3	0.2	0.2	0.1	0.3
Pennsylvania	32.1	34.6	26.1	32.1	30.7	39.3	26.0	37.2	32.5	39.0
Rhode Island	23.0	3.6	28.8	16.7	17.7	14.2	10.9	10.6	12.7	42.2
South Carolina	0.5	0.4	0.5	0.7	0.3	0.5	0.4	0.5	0.7	0.7
South Dakota	0.1	0.3	0.1	0.0	0.4	0.1	0.1	0.2	0.5	0.4
Tennessee	0.3	0.1	0.2	0.5	0.1	0.2	0.1	0.1	0.0	0.2

(continued on next page)

Table 1
(continued)

State	2004	2005	2006	2007	2008	2009	2010	2011	2012	2013
Texas	0.4	0.3	0.1	0.4	0.4	0.4	0.2	0.1	0.1	0.2
Utah	0.0	0.1	0.2	0.3	0.1	0.2	0.1	0.2	0.1	0.3
Vermont	8.0	8.7	16.8	22.2	53.1	51.9	43.3	76.0	61.7	107.6
Virginia	2.9	3.6	4.7	12.4	11.4	8.9	11.4	9.3	9.8	11.2
Washington	0.2	0.2	0.1	0.2	0.3	0.2	0.2	0.2	0.2	0.2
West Virginia	2.1	3.4	1.5	4.6	6.6	7.9	6.9	5.8	4.4	6.3
Wisconsin	20.8	26.4	26.4	32.4	26.5	34.5	44.0	42.2	23.9	25.2
Wyoming	0.8	0.6	0.2	0.6	0.2	0.2	0.0	0.2	0.5	0.2
US incidence	**6.7**	**7.9**	**8.2**	**9.1**	**9.4**	**9.8**	**7.3**	**7.8**	**7.0**	**8.6**

Reports based on state of residence, which is not always state of exposure.
Cases per 100,000 population per year.

Underreporting and Disease Burden

As with other notifiable conditions, not every case of Lyme disease is reported to the CDC; some reported cases may result from other causes. Underreporting is more likely in highly endemic areas, whereas misclassification (overreporting) is more likely in nonendemic areas.

Studies conducted in the 1990s yielded estimates of 3- to 12-fold underreporting for Lyme disease.[98–101] These studies were limited to specific states and are not generalizable to national reporting. More recently, a survey of laboratory testing practices found that 7 large commercial laboratories tested approximately 2.4 million clinical

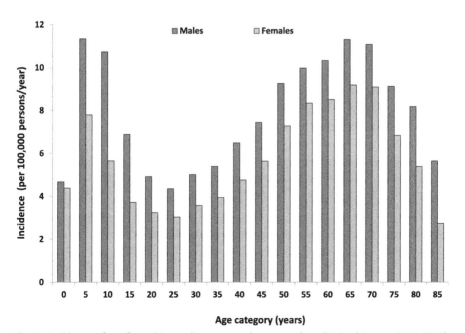

Fig. 5. Incidence of confirmed Lyme disease cases by age and sex (United States, 2010–2013).

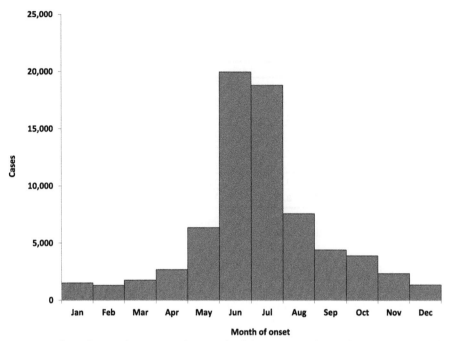

Fig. 6. Confirmed Lyme disease cases by month of disease onset (United States, 2010–2013).

specimens for Lyme disease in 2008, at a total estimated cost of $492,000,000. When applied to the estimated percentage of true infections within the source population (12%), this yielded an estimate of 288,000 (range 240,000–444,000) infected source patients in the United States in 2008. Approximately 35,000 Lyme disease cases were reported to the CDC during this same year, suggesting approximately 8-fold underreporting by this measure. Although this value likely represents a slight underestimate because it excludes patients for whom a laboratory testing was not conducted, it is comparable with estimates of underreporting for other nationally notifiable conditions.[102]

WORLDWIDE/REGIONAL INCIDENCE
Europe

Lyme borreliosis is widespread in Europe (**Table 2**). *I ricinus* is the principal vector and transmits all 3 major pathogenic genospecies. Populations of *I ricinus* are found throughout Western, Central, and Eastern Europe, generally at elevations less than 1300 m^2. Rates of infection in adult ticks tend to be higher in Eastern as compared with Western Europe, and the relative frequency of infection with the different genospecies seems to vary across regions. Ticks collected in the northern and eastern regions of Europe (eg, Scandinavia, Baltic states, Czech Republic, Slovakia, Croatia, Bulgaria) are most likely to carry *B afzelii*, whereas those from Western European countries (eg, Austria, Switzerland, United Kingdom) are more likely to be infected with *B garinii*.[103] The distribution of *I ricinus* also extends into the northern reaches of Morocco, Algeria, and Tunisia, where they are most often infected with *B lusitaniae*.[2]

Endemic foci are found from Portugal and the British Isles east to Turkey and north into Scandinavia and Russia. Reporting practices vary widely, and Lyme borreliosis is

Table 2
Reported or estimated incidence of Lyme borreliosis for selected countries

Country/Region	Cases/100,000 pop/y	Period/y	Reference
Austria	135.0[a]	2005	[106]
Belarus	10.8	2013	[105]
Belgium	16.0	2005	[106]
Bulgaria	13.0	2005	[106]
Canada	<0.1	1995–2006	[144]
Croatia	5.9	1993–2000	[61]
Czech Republic	36.0	2005	[106]
Denmark	1.2	2012	[105]
Estonia	84.5	2013	[105]
Finland	29.4	2013	[105]
France	42.0	2009–2012	[145]
Germany	36.5	2006	[86]
Great Britain			
England and Wales	1.7	2008–2009	[146]
Scotland	1.7	2002–2005	[61]
Hungary	12.8	2001–2005	[61]
Iceland	7.0	2011	[105]
Ireland	0.6	1995	[61]
Italy	<0.1	2001–2005	[61]
Japan	<0.1	2000–2005	[116]
Latvia	22.4	2013	[105]
Lithuania	86.8	2013	[105]
Moldova	0.7	2003–2005	[61]
The Netherlands	103.0[a]	2005	[107]
Norway	5.1	2012	[105]
Poland	22.8	2012	[105]
Portugal	0.1	1999–2004	[61]
Russia			
Central okrug	3.4	1999–2006	[61]
Northwest okrug	9.2	1999–2006	[61]
Urals okrug	8.3	1999–2006	[61]
Siberian okrug	9.8	1999–2006	[61]
Far Eastern okrug	4.3	1999–2006	[61]
Sverdlovsk/Jekaterinburg	14.7	1999–2006	[61]
Tomsk	28.0	1993–1994	[61]
Serbia and Montenegro	2.4	1988–1994	[61]
Slovakia	19.2	2008	[147]
Slovenia	206.0	2005	[106]
Spain[b]	3–5[a]	n/a	[148]
Sweden (southern)	69.0	1992	[149]
Switzerland	25.1	1988–1998	[61]
Turkey	<0.1	1990–2002	[61]
Ukraine	3.6	2012	[105]
United States	8.6	2013	[75]

Surveillance methods vary widely, and values may not be directly comparable.

Abbreviation: Pop, population.

[a] Estimated.
[b] La Rioja.

not a notifiable condition in many countries.[104] Nevertheless, available data suggest that transmission is most intense in Central and Northeastern Europe. Reported incidence ranges from 20 to 80 per 100,000 in the Czech Republic, Germany, Latvia, the Netherlands, Poland, Switzerland, and Sweden.[61,86,92,104] In Austria, Estonia, Lithuania, and Slovenia, rates in excess of 100 per 100,000 have been reported.[61,105] Reported incidence generally decreases moving northward in Scandinavia, from east to west in central Europe, and southward in Spain, France, Italy, and Greece.[92] In the British Isles, rates average approximately 1 case per 100,000 population. Over the last decade, the incidence of reported cases has increased in Poland, Eastern Germany, Slovenia, Bulgaria, Norway, Finland, Belgium, Britain (England, Wales, and Scotland), and the Netherlands.[86,106,107] As in North America, this increase may reflect a combination of both improved awareness and a true increase in transmission in some areas.[106–108]

Asia

The distribution of *I persulcatus*, the principal vector in Asia, extends from Western Russia, where it overlaps with *I ricinus*, eastward through Mongolia and China to the Pacific Ocean and Japan. This species transmits *B afzelii* as well as Asian and Eurasian variants of *B garinii*; it is not known to transmit *B burgdorferi*.[109–111]

Risk of Lyme borreliosis extends in a large swath across Eurasia, reaching from Japan to the western border of Russia. In Russia, official records on Lyme borreliosis have been kept since 1992.[109] Reported incidence in endemic areas generally ranges from 5 to 10 per 100,000 population. However, considerably higher rates are reported in areas northeast of Moscow in Vologda oblast, in the Sverdlovsk (Urals) region, and Western Siberia.[105,112] Infected ticks are found through much of Mongolia, although information on human cases seems scarce. *B burgdorferi* sensu lato strains have been isolated from rodents and ticks in at least 20 provinces in China, including Heilongjiang in the northeast, Xinjiang in the northwest, and Guizhou, Hunan, and Zhejiang provinces in Southern China.[90,113–115] *B garinii* and *B afzelii* are among the isolated strains, and human illness has been detailed among forestry workers in Heilongjiang Province.[30,115] Both *B garinii* and *B afzelii* have been isolated from patients in Japan; however, the overall incidence is less than 0.1 per 100,000. Most cases occur on Hokkaido Island in Northern Japan or, less commonly, from exposures in subalpine-forested areas in central Japan.[56,116] Enzootic cycles are established in Korea and Taiwan, and *B garinii* has been isolated in culture from at least one patient from northern Taiwan.[117]

Tropics and Southern Hemisphere

Lyme disease–like illness has been reported periodically in tropical and southern hemisphere countries, including Australia,[118] Brazil,[119] and South Africa.[120] In addition, serosurveys and diagnostic testing have occasionally detected antibodies reactive to *B burgdorferi* sensu lato antigens among residents of tropical areas.[121,122] Although the possibility of *Borrelia*-related illness with distinct enzootic cycles in these areas cannot be excluded, a great deal more information will be needed to determine the relationship, if any, between these reports and Lyme borreliosis as currently defined.

CLINICAL CORRELATION

Given the diverse and sometimes nonspecific clinical manifestations of *B burgdorferi* infection, clinicians must consider epidemiologic clues when evaluating patients with compatible signs or symptoms. In particular, the potential for exposure to infected ticks should be considered. As with other vector-borne diseases, Lyme disease is a disease of place, whose risk is geographically focal and curtailed by environmental factors. A patient's whereabouts strongly influence the prior probability of disease, which in turn influences to predictive value of diagnostic tests and clinical signs. In general, serologic testing is only considered useful when the prior probability of disease is between 20% and 80%.[89] In circumstances when the risk is lower, positive laboratory results are more likely to reflect a false-positive result than actual infection. Although not as well quantified, the same principle applies to clinical signs and symptoms. Unfortunately, misinformation about Lyme disease is widespread, and patients may misinterpret their level of risk.[123]

Clinical features of Lyme disease are potentially influenced by patient age and sex, although this is more apparent in European series. In the United States, the frequency of clinical features is generally consistent across age groups, with the exception of arthritis, which is more common among children aged 5 to 15 years,[28] and carditis, which seems to be disproportionately common among younger adults.[31] A higher rate of arthritis among children has also been noted in some European studies,[124] perhaps suggesting a particular susceptibility during this period of rapid bone growth. A retrospective study of 125 US patients found no difference in clinical presentation by sex.[125]

In Europe, children are more likely than adults to present with lymphocytoma or neuroborreliosis, especially facial palsy.[61,87,96,124,126] Conversely, ACA is a condition of adults, particularly women, who outnumber men among patients with this manifestation.[61,96,112,127] As a general rule, cutaneous involvement seems to be more common in Europe among women, whereas males predominate among patients with neuroborreliosis.[61,86] In a series of more than 10,000 patients with Lyme disease seen at a single medical center in Slovenia, those with cutaneous manifestations (EM and ACA) were significantly more likely to be female, whereas those with arthritis were more likely to be male.[128] This difference persisted even after correcting for the age and sex structure of the underlying population.

Along with host factors, the genospecies of the infecting organism is also thought to influence clinical features. This influence is primarily a concern in Europe and Asia where multiple genospecies commonly infect humans. All 3 genospecies can cause cutaneous, neurologic, and rheumatologic illness; however, isolates from patients with neuroborreliosis are most commonly *B garinii*,[129] whereas those from patients with EM and ACA are predominantly *B afzelii*.[32,130–132] Conversely, *B burgdorferi* is thought to have a propensity for causing arthritis.[3,133] In series from Europe, arthritis is generally reported less commonly than neuroborreliosis, sometimes markedly so.[87,96,134] Among 1471 Swedish patients, 16% had manifestations of neuroborreliosis, whereas only 7% had arthritis[87]; among 873 Austrian patients, 24% had neurologic manifestations, as compared with only 2% with arthritis.[96]

DISCUSSION

Many factors interact to determine the epidemiology of Lyme disease in humans. These factors include the genospecies of *B burgdorferi* and its distribution in nature, the abundance and feeding habits of the vector tick species, and the demographic and behavioral characteristics of the exposed human population. Etiologic agents, principal vectors, and clinical manifestations vary by region, as does the underlying risk of infection. A detailed knowledge of Lyme disease epidemiology is clinically useful,[135] allowing the provider to know when, and when not, to suspect the disease. Despite enormous gains in knowledge over the last 2 decades, a great deal remains to be learned about the risk factors for infection, enzootic cycles, and the potential role of other *B burgdorferi* genospecies.

Lyme disease poses special challenges for clinicians and public health alike. Diagnostic testing generally relies on serologic assays that are relatively insensitive for early forms of the disease.[136] Furthermore, once a patient is seropositive, elevated antibody titers can persist for years. In a follow-up study of patients treated 10 to 20 years earlier, 28% to 63% of patients still had a positive immunoglobulin G response as determined by 2-tiered testing.[137] The inability to distinguish acute from previous infection all but excludes laboratory-based reporting as an efficient mode of public health surveillance. Perhaps the most concerning challenge, however, is the ever-increasing number and distribution of cases. The ongoing emergence of Lyme disease underscores the urgent need for new and more effective interventions.

By educating patients at risk, heath care providers can play an important role in preventing Lyme disease.[138] Unfortunately, the only vaccine for Lyme disease licensed in the United States was removed from the market in 2003 amid poor sales and unsubstantiated complaints of increased adverse events.[139] Alternate approaches include both personal protective measures and environmental mitigation. Personal protective measures include regular use of insect repellents containing 20% to 30% DEET (N,N-diethyl-m-toluamide), wearing protective clothing (long-sleeved shirts, long pants), and performing daily tick checks.[138,140] A large case-control study in Connecticut found that bathing within 2 hours of spending time in the yard was strongly protective, as was performing tick checks within 36 hours of time spent in the yard.[53] The risk may be reduced further by treating clothing with permetherin.[141] Tick abundance around homes and in recreational areas can be reduced by removing brush and leaf litter, creating buffer zones of wood chips or gravel between forests and lawn, and excluding deers.[140,142] Pesticide barrier sprays are also effective at reducing ticks but have not been proven to reduce tick-borne diseases in humans.[138,142] When these measures fail, a single dose of doxycycline may be considered for prophylaxis following a high-risk tick bite in persons aged greater than 8 years.[143] For patients with symptoms, prompt diagnosis and proper treatment of early Lyme disease are essential to preventing more serious complications.[62,143]

ACKNOWLEDGMENTS

The author thanks Anna Perea, Kiersten Kugeler, Alison Hinckley, Sarah Hook, and Mary Baxter for their comments and assistance.

REFERENCES

1. Steere AC, Coburn J, Glickstein L. The emergence of Lyme disease. J Clin Invest 2004;113:1093–101.
2. Piesman J, Gern L. Lyme borreliosis in Europe and North America. Parasitology 2004;129(Suppl):S191–220.
3. Steere AC. Lyme disease. N Engl J Med 2001;345:115–25.
4. Strle F, Stantic-Pavlinic M. Lyme disease in Europe. N Engl J Med 1996;334:803.
5. Stanek G, Strle F. Lyme borreliosis. Lancet 2003;362:1639–47.
6. Nau R, Christen HJ, Eiffert H. Lyme disease–current state of knowledge. Dtsch Arztebl Int 2009;106:72–81, I.
7. Steere AC, Malawista SE, Snydman DR, et al. Lyme arthritis: an epidemic of oligoarticular arthritis in children and adults in three Connecticut communities. Arthritis Rheum 1977;20:7–17.

8. Steere AC, Malawista SE, Hardin JA, et al. Erythema chronicum migrans and Lyme arthritis. The enlarging clinical spectrum. Ann Intern Med 1977;86:685–98.
9. Matuschka FR, Ohlenbusch A, Eiffert H, et al. Antiquity of the Lyme-disease spirochaete in Europe. Lancet 1995;346:1367.
10. Edlow JA. Bull's eye. Unraveling the medical mystery of Lyme disease. New Haven (CT): Yale University Press; 2003.
11. Rudenko N, Golovchenko M, Grubhoffer L, et al. Borrelia carolinensis sp. nov., a novel species of the Borrelia burgdorferi sensu lato complex isolated from rodents and a tick from the south-eastern USA. Int J Syst Evol Microbiol 2011; 61:381–3.
12. Maraspin V, Ruzic-Sabljic E, Strle F. Lyme borreliosis and Borrelia spielmanii. Emerg Infect Dis 2006;12:1177.
13. Diza E, Papa A, Vezyri E, et al. Borrelia valaisiana in cerebrospinal fluid. Emerg Infect Dis 2004;10:1692–3.
14. de Carvalho IL, Fonseca JE, Marques JG, et al. Vasculitis-like syndrome associated with Borrelia lusitaniae infection. Clin Rheumatol 2008;27:1587–91.
15. Rudenko N, Golovchenko M, Mokracek A, et al. Detection of Borrelia bissettii in cardiac valve tissue of a patient with endocarditis and aortic valve stenosis in the Czech Republic. J Clin Microbiol 2008;46:3540–3.
16. Rudenko N, Golovchenko M, Ruzek D, et al. Molecular detection of Borrelia bissettii DNA in serum samples from patients in the Czech Republic with suspected borreliosis. FEMS Microbiol Lett 2009;292:274–81.
17. Telford SR 3rd, Mather TN, Moore SI, et al. Incompetence of deer as reservoirs of the Lyme disease spirochete. Am J Trop Med Hyg 1988;39:105–9.
18. Diuk-Wasser MA, Gatewood AG, Cortinas MR, et al. Spatiotemporal patterns of host-seeking Ixodes scapularis nymphs (Acari: Ixodidae) in the United States. J Med Entomol 2006;43:166–76.
19. Maggi RG, Reichelt S, Toliver M, et al. Borrelia species in Ixodes affinis and Ixodes scapularis ticks collected from the coastal plain of North Carolina. Ticks Tick Borne Dis 2010;1:168–71.
20. Oliver JH Jr, Lin T, Gao L, et al. An enzootic transmission cycle of Lyme borreliosis spirochetes in the southeastern United States. Proc Natl Acad Sci U S A 2003;100:11642–5.
21. Ginsberg HS, Rulison EL, Azevedo A, et al. Comparison of survival patterns of northern and southern genotypes of the North American tick Ixodes scapularis (Acari: Ixodidae) under northern and southern conditions. Parasit Vectors 2014;7:394.
22. Sakamoto JM, Goddard J, Rasgon JL. Population and demographic structure of Ixodes scapularis Say in the eastern United States. PLoS One 2014;9:e101389.
23. Spielman A, Wilson ML, Levine JF, et al. Ecology of Ixodes dammini-borne human babesiosis and Lyme disease. Annu Rev Entomol 1985;30:439–60.
24. Goddard J. A ten-year study of tick biting in Mississippi: implications for human disease transmission. J Agromedicine 2002;8:25–32.
25. Lin T, Oliver JH Jr, Gao L. Comparative analysis of Borrelia isolates from southeastern USA based on randomly amplified polymorphic DNA fingerprint and 16S ribosomal gene sequence analyses. FEMS Microbiol Lett 2003;228:249–57.
26. Oliver JH, Gao L, Lin T. Comparison of the spirochete Borrelia burgdorferi s.l. isolated from the tick Ixodes scapularis in southeastern and northeastern United States. J Parasitol 2008;94:1351–6.
27. Smith RP Jr, Rand PW, Lacombe EH, et al. Role of bird migration in the long-distance dispersal of Ixodes dammini, the vector of Lyme disease. J Infect Dis 1996;174:221–4.

28. Bacon RM, Kugeler KJ, Mead PS. Surveillance for Lyme disease–United States, 1992-2006. MMWR Surveill Summ 2008;57:1–9.
29. Ertel SH, Nelson RS, Cartter ML. Effect of surveillance method on reported characteristics of Lyme disease, Connecticut, 1996-2007. Emerg Infect Dis 2012;18:242–7.
30. Ai CX, Wen YX, Zhang YG, et al. Clinical manifestations and epidemiological characteristics of Lyme disease in Hailin county, Heilongjiang Province, China. Ann N Y Acad Sci 1988;539:302–13.
31. Forrester JD, Meiman J, Mullins J, et al. Notes from the field: update on Lyme carditis, groups at high risk, and frequency of associated sudden cardiac death–United States. MMWR Morb Mortal Wkly Rep 2014;63:982–3.
32. Busch U, Hizo-Teufel C, Bohmer R, et al. *Borrelia burgdorferi* sensu lato strains isolated from cutaneous Lyme borreliosis biopsies differentiated by pulsed-field gel electrophoresis. Scand J Infect Dis 1996;28:583–9.
33. Nadelman R, Auwaerter P, Mumford D. Early Lyme disease: erythema migrans. Infect Dis Clin North Am 2015.
34. Halperin J, Auwaerter PG, Mumford D. Neuroborreliosis. Infect Dis Clin North Am 2015.
35. Melia M, Auwaerter P, Mumford D, et al. Lyme carditis. Infect Dis Clin North Am 2015.
36. Steere A, Auwaerter P, Mumford D. Lyme arthritis. Infect Dis Clin North Am 2015.
37. Sood S. Pediatric Lyme disease. Infect Dis Clin North Am 2015.
38. Marcus LC, Steere AC, Duray PH, et al. Fatal pancarditis in a patient with coexistent Lyme disease and babesiosis. Demonstration of spirochetes in the myocardium. Ann Intern Med 1985;103:374–6.
39. Kirsch M, Ruben FL, Steere AC, et al. Fatal adult respiratory distress syndrome in a patient with Lyme disease. J Am Med Assoc 1988;259:2737–9.
40. Waniek C, Prohovnik I, Kaufman MA, et al. Rapidly progressive frontal-type dementia associated with Lyme disease. J Neuropsychiatry Clin Neurosci 1995;7:345–7.
41. Tavora F, Burke A, Li L, et al. Postmortem confirmation of Lyme carditis with polymerase chain reaction. Cardiovasc Pathol 2008;17:103–7.
42. Kugeler KJ, Griffith KS, Gould LH, et al. A review of death certificates listing Lyme disease as a cause of death in the United States. Clin Infect Dis 2011;52:364–7.
43. CDC. Three sudden cardiac deaths associated with Lyme carditis - United States, November 2012-July 2013. Morb Mortal Wkly Rep 2013;62:993–6.
44. Cromley EK, Cartter ML, Mrozinski RD, et al. Residential setting as a risk factor for Lyme disease in a hyperendemic region. Am J Epidemiol 1998;147:472–7.
45. Falco RC, Fish D. Prevalence of *Ixodes dammini* near the homes of Lyme disease patients in Westchester County, New York. Am J Epidemiol 1988;127:826–30.
46. Klein JD, Eppes SC, Hunt P. Environmental and life-style risk factors for Lyme disease in children. Clin Pediatr (Phila) 1996;35:359–63.
47. Maupin GO, Fish D, Zultowsky J, et al. Landscape ecology of Lyme disease in a residential area of Westchester County, New York. Am J Epidemiol 1991;133:1105–13.
48. Neitzel DF, Kemperman MM. Tick-borne diseases in Minnesota: an update. Minn Med 2012;95:41–4.
49. Orloski KA, Campbell GL, Genese CA, et al. Emergence of Lyme disease in Hunterdon County, New Jersey, 1993: a case-control study of risk factors and evaluation of reporting patterns. Am J Epidemiol 1998;147:391–7.

50. Rand PW, Lubelczyk C, Lavigne GR, et al. Deer density and the abundance of *Ixodes scapularis* (Acari: Ixodidae). J Med Entomol 2003;40:179–84.
51. Ley C, Olshen EM, Reingold AL. Case-control study of risk factors for incident Lyme disease in California. Am J Epidemiol 1995;142:S39–47.
52. Smith G, Wileyto EP, Hopkins RB, et al. Risk factors for Lyme disease in Chester County, Pennsylvania. Public Health Rep 2001;116(Suppl 1):146–56.
53. Connally NP, Durante AJ, Yousey-Hindes KM, et al. Peridomestic Lyme disease prevention: results of a population-based case-control study. Am J Prev Med 2009;37:201–6.
54. Schwartz BS, Goldstein MD. Lyme disease in outdoor workers: risk factors, preventive measures, and tick removal methods. Am J Epidemiol 1990;131: 877–85.
55. Ai CX, Zhang WF, Zhao JH. Sero-epidemiology of Lyme disease in an endemic area in China. Microbiol Immunol 1994;38:505–9.
56. Nakama H, Muramatsu K, Uchikama K, et al. Possibility of Lyme disease as an occupational disease– seroepidemiological study of regional residents and forestry workers. Asia Pac J Public Health 1994;7:214–7.
57. Kaya AD, Parlak AH, Ozturk CE, et al. Seroprevalence of *Borrelia burgdorferi* infection among forestry workers and farmers in Duzce, north-western Turkey. New Microbiol 2008;31:203–9.
58. Buczek A, Rudek A, Bartosik K, et al. Seroepidemiological study of Lyme borreliosis among forestry workers in southern Poland. Ann Agric Environ Med 2009; 16:257–61.
59. Bilski B. Occurrence of cases of borreliosis certified as an occupational disease in the province of Wielkopolska (Poland). Ann Agric Environ Med 2009;16: 211–7.
60. Cinco M, Barbone F, Grazia Ciufolini M, et al. Seroprevalence of tick-borne infections in forestry rangers from northeastern Italy. Clin Microbiol Infect 2004;10: 1056–61.
61. Hubalek Z. Epidemiology of Lyme borreliosis. Curr Probl Dermatol 2009;37: 31–50.
62. des Vignes F, Piesman J, Heffernan R, et al. Effect of tick removal on transmission of Borrelia burgdorferi and Ehrlichia phagocytophila by Ixodes scapularis nymphs. J Infect Dis 2001;183:773–8.
63. Vazquez M, Muehlenbein C, Cartter M, et al. Effectiveness of personal protective measures to prevent Lyme disease. Emerg Infect Dis 2008;14:210–6.
64. Johnson SE, Swaminathan B, Moore P, et al. *Borrelia burgdorferi*: survival in experimentally infected human blood processed for transfusion. J Infect Dis 1990;162:557–9.
65. McQuiston JH, Childs JE, Chamberland ME, et al. Transmission of tick-borne agents of disease by blood transfusion: a review of known and potential risks in the United States. Transfusion 2000;40:274–84.
66. CDC. *Anaplasma phagocytophilum* transmitted through blood transfusion–Minnesota, 2007. MMWR Morb Mortal Wkly Rep 2008;57:1145–8.
67. Woodrum JE, Oliver JH Jr. Investigation of venereal, transplacental, and contact transmission of the Lyme disease spirochete, *Borrelia burgdorferi*, in Syrian hamsters. J Parasitol 1999;85:426–30.
68. Moody KD, Barthold SW. Relative infectivity of *Borrelia burgdorferi* in Lewis rats by various routes of inoculation. Am J Trop Med Hyg 1991;44:135–9.
69. Schlesinger PA, Duray PH, Burke BA, et al. Maternal-fetal transmission of the Lyme disease spirochete, *Borrelia burgdorferi*. Ann Intern Med 1985;103:67–8.

70. Figueroa R, Bracero LA, Aguero-Rosenfeld M, et al. Confirmation of *Borrelia burgdorferi* spirochetes by polymerase chain reaction in placentas of women with reactive serology for Lyme antibodies. Gynecol Obstet Invest 1996;41: 240–3.
71. Markowitz LE, Steere AC, Benach JL, et al. Lyme disease during pregnancy. J Am Med Assoc 1986;255:3394–6.
72. Walsh CA, Mayer EW, Baxi LV. Lyme disease in pregnancy: case report and review of the literature. Obstet Gynecol Surv 2007;62:41–50.
73. CDC. Nationally Notifiable Diseases Surveillance System (NNDSS). 2014. Available at: http://wwwn.cdc.gov/NNDSS/script/casedefDefault.aspx. Accessed November 2, 2014.
74. CSTE. Lyme disease surveillance case definition. 2011. Available at: http://wwwn.cdc.gov/NNDSS/script/conditionsummary.aspx?CondID=100. Accessed November 2, 2014.
75. Adams DA, Jajosky RA, Ajani U, et al. Summary of notifiable diseases–United States, 2012. MMWR Morb Mortal Wkly Rep 2014;61:1–121.
76. CDC. Notice to readers: final 2013 reports of nationally notifiable infectious diseases. MMWR Morb Mortal Wkly Rep 2014;63:702–15.
77. Connecticut Department of Public Health. Lyme disease – Connecticut, 2008. Connecticut Epidemiologist 2009;29:14–6.
78. Ogden NH, Lindsay LR, Morshed M, et al. The emergence of Lyme disease in Canada. Can Med Assoc J 2009;180:1221–4.
79. Public Health Agency of Canada. Lyme disease. Surveillance. 2014; Available at: http://www.phac-aspc.gc.ca/id-mi/lyme/surveillance-eng.php. Accessed December 20, 2014.
80. Gordillo-Perez G, Vargas M, Solorzano-Santos F, et al. Demonstration of *Borrelia burgdorferi* sensu stricto infection in ticks from the northeast of Mexico. Clin Microbiol Infect 2009;15:496–8.
81. Gordillo-Perez G, Torres J, Solorzano-Santos F, et al. *Borrelia burgdorferi* infection and cutaneous Lyme disease, Mexico. Emerg Infect Dis 2007;13:1556–8.
82. Mead P, Goel R, Kugeler K. Canine serology as adjunct to human Lyme disease surveillance. Emerg Infect Dis 2011;17:1710–2.
83. Bowman D, Little SE, Lorentzen L, et al. Prevalence and geographic distribution of *Dirofilaria immitis, Borrelia burgdorferi, Ehrlichia canis*, and *Anaplasma phagocytophilum* in dogs in the United States: results of a national clinic-based serologic survey. Vet Parasitol 2009;160:138–48.
84. IDEXX. Sensitivity and specificity of the SNAP® 4Dx® Test 2010. Available at: http://www.idexx.com/view/xhtml/en_us/smallanimal/inhouse/snap/4dx.jsf?selectedTab=Accuracy#tabs. Accessed October 1, 2010.
85. Duncan AW, Correa MT, Levine JF, et al. The dog as a sentinel for human infection: prevalence of *Borrelia burgdorferi* C6 antibodies in dogs from southeastern and mid-Atlantic States. Vector Borne Zoonotic Dis 2005;5:101–9.
86. Fulop B, Poggensee G. Epidemiological situation of Lyme borreliosis in Germany: surveillance data from six Eastern German States, 2002 to 2006. Parasitol Res 2008;103(Suppl 1):S117–20.
87. Berglund J, Eitrem R, Ornstein K, et al. An epidemiologic study of Lyme disease in southern Sweden. N Engl J Med 1995;333:1319–27.
88. Centers for Disease Control and Prevention (CDC). Lyme disease–United States, 2001-2002. MMWR Morb Mortal Wkly Rep 2004;53:365–9.
89. Tugwell P, Dennis DT, Weinstein A, et al. Laboratory evaluation in the diagnosis of Lyme disease. Ann Intern Med 1997;127:1109–23.

90. Ai CX, Hu RJ, Hyland KE, et al. Epidemiological and aetiological evidence for transmission of Lyme disease by adult Ixodes persulcatus in an endemic area in China. Int J Epidemiol 1990;19:1061–5.

91. Falco RC, McKenna DF, Daniels TJ, et al. Temporal relation between *Ixodes scapularis* abundance and risk for Lyme disease associated with erythema migrans. Am J Epidemiol 1999;149:771–6.

92. Lindgren E, Jaenson T. Lyme borreliosis in Europe: influences of climate and climate change, epidemiology, ecology and adaptation measures. 2006; 34. Available at: http://www.euro.who.int/__data/assets/pdf_file/0006/96819/E89522.pdf. Accessed 1 October 2010.

93. Alekseev AN, Dubinina HV. Abiotic parameters and diel and seasonal activity of *Borrelia*-infected and uninfected *Ixodes persulcatus* (Acarina: Ixodidae). J Med Entomol 2000;37:9–15.

94. Eisen L, Eisen RJ, Lane RS. Seasonal activity patterns of *Ixodes pacificus* nymphs in relation to climatic conditions. Med Vet Entomol 2002;16:235–44.

95. Moore SM, Eisen RJ, Monaghan A, et al. Meteorological influences on the seasonality of Lyme disease in the United States. Am J Trop Med Hyg 2014;90:486–96.

96. Stanek G, Flamm H, Groh V, et al. Epidemiology of Borrelia infections in Austria. Zentralbl Bakteriol Mikrobiol Hyg A 1987;263:442–9.

97. Strle F. Lyme borreliosis in Slovenia. Zentralbl Bakteriol Mikrobiol Hyg A 1999; 289:643–52.

98. Coyle BS, Strickland GT, Liang YY, et al. The public health impact of Lyme disease in Maryland. J Infect Dis 1996;173:1260–2.

99. Meek JI, Roberts CL, Smith EV Jr, et al. Underreporting of Lyme disease by Connecticut physicians, 1992. J Public Health Manag Pract 1996;2:61–5.

100. Campbell GL, Fritz CL, Fish D, et al. Estimation of the incidence of Lyme disease. Am J Epidemiol 1998;148:1018–26.

101. Naleway AL, Belongia EA, Kazmierczak JJ, et al. Lyme disease incidence in Wisconsin: a comparison of state-reported rates and rates from a population-based cohort. Am J Epidemiol 2002;155:1120–7.

102. Doyle TJ, Glynn MK, Groseclose SL. Completeness of notifiable infectious disease reporting in the United States: an analytical literature review. Am J Epidemiol 2002;155:866–74.

103. Rauter C, Hartung T. Prevalence of *Borrelia burgdorferi* sensu lato genospecies in *Ixodes ricinus* ticks in Europe: a meta-analysis. Appl Environ Microbiol 2005; 71:7203–16.

104. EUCALB. European Union Concerted Action on Lyme Borreliosis. 2014. Available at: http://www.eucalb.com. Accessed October 1, 2014.

105. EpiNorth. A co-operation project for communicable disease control in Northern Europe. EpiNorth Data: Lyme borreliosis. 2014. Available at: http://www.epinorth.org. Accessed July 10, 2014.

106. Smith R, Takkinen J. Lyme borreliosis: Europe-wide coordinated surveillance and action needed? Euro Surveill 2006;11:E060622.1.

107. Hofhuis A, van der Giessen JW, Borgsteede FH, et al. Lyme borreliosis in the Netherlands: strong increase in GP consultations and hospital admissions in past 10 years. Euro Surveill 2006;11:E060622.2.

108. Kampen H, Rotzel DC, Kurtenbach K, et al. Substantial rise in the prevalence of Lyme borreliosis spirochetes in a region of western Germany over a 10-year period. Appl Environ Microbiol 2004;70:1576–82.

109. Korenberg E. Comparative ecology and epidemiology of Lyme disease and tick-borne encephalitis in the former Soviet Union. Parasitol Today 1994;4:157–60.

110. Korenberg E, Gorelova N, Kovalevskii Y. Ecology of *Borrelia burgdorferi* sensu lato in Russia. In: Gray JS, Kahl O, Lane RS, et al, editors. Lyme borreliosis: biology, epidemiology and control. New York: CABI Publishing; 2002. p. 175–200.

111. Masuzawa T. Terrestrial distribution of the Lyme borreliosis agent *Borrelia burgdorferi* sensu lato in East Asia. Jpn J Infect Dis 2004;57:229–35.

112. WHO workshop on Lyme borreliosis diagnosis and surveillance, Warsaw, Poland, 20-22 June 1995 (who/cds/vph/95141-1). Geneva (Switzerland): World Health Organization; 1995.

113. Chu CY, Jiang BG, Liu W, et al. Presence of pathogenic *Borrelia burgdorferi* sensu lato in ticks and rodents in Zhejiang, south-east China. J Med Microbiol 2008;57:980–5.

114. Zhang F, Gong Z, Zhang J, et al. Prevalence of *Borrelia burgdorferi* sensu lato in rodents from Gansu, northwestern China. BMC Microbiol 2010;10:157.

115. Hao Q, Hou X, Geng Z, et al. Distribution of *Borrelia burgdorferi* sensu lato in China. J Clin Microbiol 2010;49(2):647–50.

116. Hashimoto S, Kawado M, Murakami Y, et al. Epidemics of vector-borne diseases observed in infectious disease surveillance in Japan, 2000-2005. J Epidemiol 2007;17(Suppl):S48–55.

117. Chao LL, Chen YJ, Shih CM. First detection and molecular identification of *Borrelia garinii* isolated from human skin in Taiwan. J Med Microbiol 2010;59:254–7.

118. Russell RC. Lyme disease in Australia-still to be proven! Emerg Infect Dis 1995; 1:29–31.

119. Mantovani E, Costa IP, Gauditano G, et al. Description of Lyme disease-like syndrome in Brazil. Is it a new tick borne disease or Lyme disease variation? Braz J Med Biol Res 2007;40:443–56.

120. Stanek G, Hirschl A, Stemberger H, et al. Does Lyme borreliosis also occur in tropical and subtropical areas? Zentralbl Bakteriol Mikrobiol Hyg A 1987;263:491–5.

121. Miranda J, Mattar S, Perdomo K, et al. Seroprevalence of Lyme borreliosis in workers from Cordoba, Colombia. Rev Salud Publica (Bogota) 2009;11:480–9 [in Spanish].

122. Santos M, Ribeiro-Rodrigues R, Lobo R, et al. Antibody reactivity to *Borrelia burgdorferi* sensu stricto antigens in patients from the Brazilian Amazon region with skin diseases not related to Lyme disease. Int J Dermatol 2010;49:552–6.

123. Cooper JD, Feder HM Jr. Inaccurate information about Lyme disease on the internet. Pediatr Infect Dis J 2004;23:1105–8.

124. Huppertz HI, Bohme M, Standaert SM, et al. Incidence of Lyme borreliosis in the Wurzburg region of Germany. Eur J Clin Microbiol Infect Dis 1999;18:697–703.

125. Schwarzwalder A, Schneider MF, Lydecker A, et al. Sex differences in the clinical and serologic presentation of early Lyme disease: results from a retrospective review. Gend Med 2010;7:320–9.

126. Henningsson AJ, Malmvall BE, Ernerudh J, et al. Neuroborreliosis–an epidemiological, clinical and healthcare cost study from an endemic area in the southeast of Sweden. Clin Microbiol Infect 2010;16:1245–51.

127. Asbrink E, Brehmer-Andersson E, Hovmark A. Acrodermatitis chronica atrophicans–a spirochetosis. Clinical and histopathological picture based on 32 patients; course and relationship to erythema chronicum migrans Afzelius. Am J Dermatopathol 1986;8:209–19.

128. Strle F, Wormser GP, Mead P, et al. Gender disparity between cutaneous and non-cutaneous manifestations of Lyme borreliosis. PLoS One 2013;8: e64110.

129. Ruzic-Sabljic E, Lotric-Furlan S, Maraspin V, et al. Analysis of *Borrelia burgdorferi* sensu lato isolated from cerebrospinal fluid. APMIS 2001;109: 707–13.
130. Ruzic-Sabljic E, Arnez M, Lotric-Furlan S, et al. Genotypic and phenotypic characterisation of *Borrelia burgdorferi* sensu lato strains isolated from human blood. J Med Microbiol 2001;50:896–901.
131. van Dam A, Kuiper H, Vos K, et al. Different genospecies of *Borrelia burgdorferi* are associated with distinct clinical manifestations of Lyme borreliosis. Clin Infect Dis 1993;17:708–17.
132. Ornstein K, Berglund J, Nilsson I, et al. Characterization of Lyme borreliosis isolates from patients with erythema migrans and neuroborreliosis in southern Sweden. J Clin Microbiol 2001;39:1294–8.
133. Steere AC, Glickstein L. Elucidation of Lyme arthritis. Nat Rev Immunol 2004;4: 143–52.
134. Letrilliart L, Ragon B, Hanslik T, et al. Lyme disease in France: a primary care-based prospective study. Epidemiol Infect 2005;133:935–42.
135. Makhani N, Morris SK, Page AV, et al. A twist on Lyme: the challenge of diagnosing European Lyme neuroborreliosis. J Clin Microbiol 2010;49(1):455–7.
136. Bacon RM, Biggerstaff BJ, Schriefer ME, et al. Serodiagnosis of Lyme disease by kinetic enzyme-linked immunosorbent assay using recombinant VlsE1 or peptide antigens of *Borrelia burgdorferi* compared with 2-tiered testing using whole-cell lysates. J Infect Dis 2003;187:1187–99.
137. Kalish RA, Kaplan RF, Taylor E, et al. Evaluation of study patients with Lyme disease, 10-20-year follow-up. J Infect Dis 2001;183:453–60.
138. Hayes EB, Piesman J. How can we prevent Lyme disease? N Engl J Med 2003; 348:2424–30.
139. Plotkin SA. Correcting a public health fiasco: the need for a new vaccine against Lyme disease. Clin Infect Dis 2011;52(Suppl 3):s271–5.
140. Piesman J, Eisen L. Prevention of tick-borne diseases. Annu Rev Entomol 2008; 53:323–43.
141. Vaughn MF, Meshnick SR. Pilot study assessing the effectiveness of long-lasting permethrin-impregnated clothing for the prevention of tick bites. Vector Borne Zoonotic Dis 2011;11:869–75.
142. Stafford K. The tick management handbook: an integrated guide for homeowners, pest control operators, and public health officials for the prevention of tick-associated disease. New Haven (CT): Connecticut Agricultural Experiment Station; 2004.
143. Wormser GP, Dattwyler RJ, Shapiro ED, et al. The clinical assessment, treatment, and prevention of Lyme disease, human granulocytic anaplasmosis, and babesiosis: clinical practice guidelines by the Infectious Diseases Society of America. Clin Infect Dis 2006;43:1089–134.
144. Ogden NH, Lindsay LR, Morshed M, et al. The rising challenge of Lyme borreliosis in Canada. Can Commun Dis Rep 2008;34:1–19.
145. Vandenesch A, Turbelin C, Couturier E, et al. Incidence and hospitalisation rates of Lyme borreliosis, France, 2004 to 2012. Euro Surveill 2014;19:34.
146. Smith R, O'Connell S. Lyme borreliosis trends in England and Wales: 2005-2009. 12th International Conference on Lyme Borreliosis and other Tick-borne Diseases. Ljubljana (Slovenia): Austrian Society for Hygiene, Microbiology, and Preventive Medicine; 2010.
147. Svihrova V, Hudeckova H, Jesenak M, et al. Lyme borreliosis–analysis of the trends in Slovakia, 1999-2008. Folia Microbiol (Praha) 2011;56:270–5.

148. Portillo A, Santibanez S, Oteo JA. Lyme disease. Enferm Infecc Microbiol Clin 2014;32(Suppl 1):37–42 [in Spanish].
149. Berglund J, Eitrem R, Norrby SR. Long-term study of Lyme borreliosis in a highly endemic area in Sweden. Scand J Infect Dis 1996;28:473–8.

Erythema Migrans

Robert B. Nadelman, MD

KEYWORDS

- Lyme disease • Erythema migrans • *Borrelia burgdorferi*

KEY POINTS

- Erythema migrans (EM) is the most common objective manifestation of *Borrelia burgdorferi* infection. It is associated with systemic symptoms in most but not all cases. Despite a characteristic appearance, EM should not be considered pathognomonic for Lyme disease because it must be distinguished from other similar-appearing skin lesions, including local reactions to uninfected arthropod bites in endemic areas, and southern tick-associated rash illness in nonendemic areas.
- An evaluation for early Lyme disease by health care practitioners should include a complete skin examination with all patient clothes removed, in order to uncover EM skin lesions that may otherwise go unrecognized.
- EM should be considered a clinical diagnosis, and serologic and polymerase chain reaction assays are not necessary.
- Leukopenia and thrombocytopenia are not characteristic of Lyme disease and should be considered to indicate either an alternative diagnosis or a coinfection with the agents of human granulocytic anaplasmosis or babesiosis.
- EM has an excellent prognosis when appropriate antimicrobial treatment is initiated promptly.

INTRODUCTION

Erythema migrans (EM; previously known as erythema chronicum migrans), the distinctive skin lesion of early Lyme disease, has a unique appearance, so early investigators were able to describe the clinical manifestations of Lyme disease years before the discovery of the causative pathogen, *Borrelia burgdorferi*, or the development of the first diagnostic laboratory assays. Transmission by an *Ixodes* tick vector was recognized after noting that EM develops at the exact site of a tick bite that occurred days to weeks earlier.[1–5] EM is the most common objective manifestation of Lyme disease, accounting for about 90% of cases.[1,6–8]

Historical Perspective

Two Connecticut mothers, Polly Smith and Judith Mensch, can be credited with spurring the investigations that eventually led to the recognition of the clinical manifestations and,

Division of Infectious Diseases, Department of Medicine, New York Medical College, Skyline Office #2NC20, 40 Sunshine Cottage Road, Valhalla, NY 10595, USA
E-mail address: robert_nadelman@nymc.edu

Infect Dis Clin N Am 29 (2015) 211–239
http://dx.doi.org/10.1016/j.idc.2015.02.001   id.theclinics.com

ultimately, the pathogenesis and treatment of Lyme disease. They were skeptical of the diagnosis of juvenile rheumatoid arthritis given to their children and many others by physicians in October 1975, and requested a formal investigation from Connecticut health authorities and the US Centers for Disease Control and Prevention (CDC).[3] As a result, it was found that, in Old Lyme, Connecticut, an inflammatory joint syndrome occurred at a frequency more than 100 times that of juvenile rheumatoid arthritis. It was preceded in many cases by a characteristic skin rash that was noted by some patients to follow an arthropod bite after a median of 12 days. A team of researchers led by Dr Allen Steere realized that this skin lesion was reminiscent of the European erythema chronicum migrans (ECM) lesion, initially described in 1909,[3,4] which had been associated with the bite of the *Ixodes ricinus* tick. A quarter of a century before Dr Steere's investigation, some European physicians had observed a favorable response of ECM to penicillin treatment, as might be expected with a bacterial illness.[9] By 1982, a previously unrecognized spirochete, subsequently named *B burgdorferi*, was isolated from *Ixodes dammini* (now known as *Ixodes scapularis*) ticks from Shelter Island, New York, and also from the blood, skin, and cerebrospinal fluid of human patients with Lyme disease, finally establishing the cause and vector.[3] Treatment studies soon confirmed the efficacy of certain antimicrobial medications in improving patient outcomes.[10]

CLINICAL DIAGNOSIS

Primary EM is an expanding erythematous skin lesion, usually round or oval, that develops at a site where ticks belonging to certain *Ixodes* species have inoculated the spirochete *B burgdorferi*, 7 to 14 days (range, 1–36 days) earlier.[2,5,11–13] Secondary EM lesions may develop after *B burgdorferi* spreads from the site of the tick bite through the blood and back to other areas of skin (discussed later). In order to increase the specificity of the diagnosis, the CDC and others have designated 5 cm in largest diameter as a minimum size for primary EM lesions.[14] Use of this cutoff is helpful in differentiating EM from other lesions; in particular, a localized and transient inflammatory reaction to the bite of an arthropod that is not associated with infection and, in contrast with EM, resolves spontaneously within a day or two.[2,15–17] The 5-cm size limitation is useful for increasing accuracy in the clinical diagnosis of Lyme disease and, in particular, in clinical and epidemiologic studies, but should not be used alone to exclude the diagnosis of EM in individual patients with otherwise suggestive clinical and epidemiologic features.[2,6,14,16]

Tick Bite

Only about 25% (range, 14%–32%) of US patients with EM recalled the preceding tick bite that transmitted the infection.[12,16,18] One explanation for this is that the nymphal stage of *I scapularis*, the principal vector for Lyme disease in the United States, is only about the size of a poppy seed, and most tick bites are unassociated with pruritus or pain.[2,16,19] In addition, tick bites that result in infection occur at body sites such as the back or posterior thigh in adults or the hairline of children, where the tick can feed for days without being noticed.[2,12,20] The reason for this is that the transmission of *B burgdorferi* takes at least 36 hours, during which time the spirochete must move from the tick midgut to the salivary glands before it can be transmitted to the skin of the human host.[21] The locations of primary EM lesions in one study of 79 adult patients whose EM was culture confirmed are listed in **Table 1**.[12]

Evolution of Erythema Migrans and Central Clearing

EM begins as a small macule or papule at the tick bite site and progresses into a slowly enlarging erythematous patch over days.[5,11,13,22] A depressed or raised area (punctum)

Table 1 Body location of EM in 79 patients with culture-confirmed infection	
Location	No. (%)
Thigh	14 (18)
Back	12 (15)
Shoulder	11 (14)
Calf	8 (10)
Groin	6 (8)
Popliteal	5 (6)
Flank	5 (6)
Axilla	4 (5)
Buttock	4 (5)
Upper arm	4 (5)
Other[a]	6 (8)

[a] Chest, 2 (2.5%); abdomen, 2 (2.5%); neck, 1 (1%); ankle, 1 (1%).

From Nadelman RB, Nowakowski J, Forseter G, et al. The clinical spectrum of early Lyme borreliosis in patients with culture-confirmed erythema migrans. Am J Med 1996;100(5):502–8; with permission.

may remain at the center of the lesion at the site where the tick had previously detached (**Fig. 1**).[11,13,23,24] As the lesion expands over days to weeks, it may take on an annular or targetlike appearance as clearing develops in or around the center. The EM lesion remains flat, blanches with pressure, and usually does not desquamate or vesiculate at the periphery, although these changes may occur centrally.[2,5,12,13,18,22] The median diameter in each of 5 studies involving more than 500 US patients was between 10 and 16 cm but lesions may exceed 70 cm.[5,12,13,18,25,26] EM size is a function of its duration,[4,11,12,26] varying in a linear fashion with a correlation coefficient of 0.7.[12] Spirochetes migrate in an outward direction from the inoculation site, resulting in a growth rate of 20 cm^2/d for early EM lesions.[11] European patients with infection caused by *Borrelia garinii* may have even more rapid expansion of EM.[27]

Using special culture media, *B burgdorferi* can regularly be isolated from the leading margin of the lesions and even from adjacent normal-appearing skin external to the lesion.[2,12,18,27–29] The organism may also be isolated from the center of the lesion.[26,27] As with EM size, central clearing is a function of duration of EM.[4,11,26] Thus, an annular

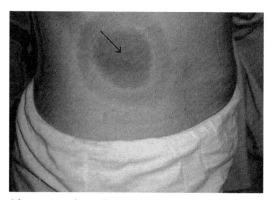

Fig. 1. EM lesion with punctum (*arrow*).

appearance was emphasized in the early descriptions of the long-standing rashes (ie, then known as ECM) that were most commonly observed before the recognition of effective antimicrobial treatment. In addition, the first descriptions of EM were in Europe, where most cases have been shown to be associated with *Borrelia afzelii*, and EM has a different clinical course and appearance than that associated with *B burgdorferi* sensu stricto in the United States.[4,26,29–31] Although 80% of cases had central clearing in one early Swedish study in which lesions had been present for 5 to 6 weeks,[4] central clearing occurred in only 37% and 9% of cases respectively in 2 large studies conducted in the northeastern United States, involving nearly 200 patients with culture-confirmed EM.[12,18] Central clearing was also much more likely to occur in Slovenian patients with infection caused by *B garinii* than in American patients in Westchester County, New York, caused by *B burgdorferi* sensu stricto (61.2% compared with 35.3%; *P*<.0001), despite similar duration of EM.[27] Aside from the variations in rash morphology attributed to the distinctly separate genospecies causing illness in the two continents, the lack of central or paracentral clearing at the time of presentation in US patients is also likely partly related to the more rapid diagnosis and treatment (within 1–2 weeks of onset) of EM in the United States during the last 25 years.[2,6,12,18]

Local Characteristics of Erythema Migrans

EM lesions are warmer than surrounding normal-appearing skin and usually have regular margins. The periphery is not raised compared with the interior. Lesions are usually oval or circular, with the shape partly determined by lines of skin tension.[2,11,13,23] For instance, groin lesions tend to be oval along the horizontal axis (**Fig. 2**).[2,13,23] Unusual configurations such as triangles may appear when spirochetes migrate over skin folds (**Fig. 3**).[11] Central vesicles were observed in 8% of lesions in one study and may be clear, cloudy, or hemorrhagic (**Fig. 4**).[32] Vesicular EM lesions may be difficult to differentiate from bacterial cellulitis, arthropod bite, contact dermatitis, or even herpes simplex and varicella zoster virus infection.

Scaling is uncommon in EM lesions, occurring primarily at the tick bite site (punctum), in fading rashes of long duration, or after antimicrobial treatment.[2] Use of topical steroids may also lead to scaling, in addition to giving EM an uncharacteristic pallor.[2] Although EM lesions characteristically display a shade of erythema from faint pink to dark red, lesions on the lower extremities may develop a bluish color.[11,13] Lesions in dark-skinned persons may be difficult to recognize (**Fig. 5**). Pruritus or pain may be noted at the site of EM but is almost always mild in severity.[4,12,13,31,33] A minority of patients, most often in Europe, complain of transient numbness or tingling at the site of EM.[4,5,12,13,18,29,31] Spirochetemia may result in secondary skin lesions (discussed later). The characteristics of EM from 79 patients from Westchester County, New York, with culture-proven EM are summarized in **Table 2**.[12]

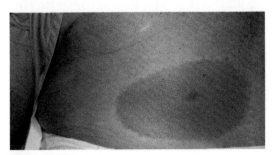

Fig. 2. Oval EM lesion.

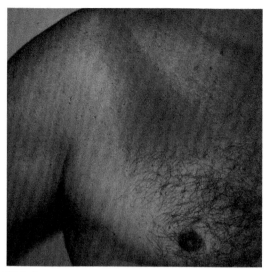

Fig. 3. Triangular EM lesion.

Associated Systemic Symptoms

As many as 80% of patients in the United States with EM have simultaneous systemic symptoms.[5] These symptoms are often experienced together with the EM but may precede the onset or develop after resolution of skin lesions.[2,11] The most common systemic symptoms in more than 600 US patients enrolled in 4 large prospective

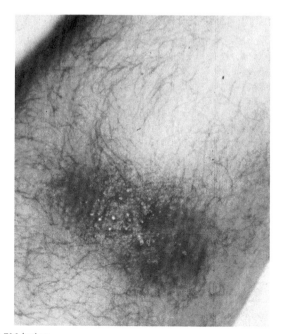

Fig. 4. Vesicular EM lesion.

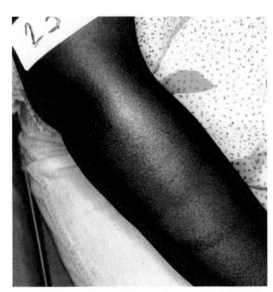

Fig. 5. EM lesion in a patient from the Caribbean who acquired the infection in Westchester County, New York.

studies were malaise (10%–80%), headache (28%–64%), fever and chills (31%–59%), and myalgias and arthralgias (35%–48%), with nausea, anorexia, dizziness, and difficulty concentrating reported less frequently.[5,11,12,18] Respiratory symptoms (ie, cough or rhinorrhea) and diarrhea are not characteristic of Lyme disease and should raise the possibility of an alternative or concurrent process.

European patients are less likely than US patients to experience systemic symptoms (23%–50% of more than 800 patients in representative prospective studies in 6 different European countries).[4,26,27,29–31,33–35] This finding is likely attributable to the lower virulence of *B afzelii* (the major cause of EM in Europe) compared with *B burgdorferi* sensu stricto, the only genospecies that has been implicated as causing human disease in the United States.[1,26,31] *B afzelii* also seems to be less virulent than *B garinii*, another European genospecies.[31] However, European patients with *B garinii* infection also seem to have fewer systemic symptoms and less dissemination to multiple skin sites (secondary EM) than patients from the United States with *B burgdorferi* sensu stricto infection.[27] These differences may be partially caused by the greater ability of *B burgdorferi* sensu stricto to stimulate macrophages to secrete

Table 2	
Selected characteristics of EM in 79 patients with culture-confirmed infection	
Feature	**No. (%)**
Central clearing	22 of 59 (37)
Uniform color	16 of 59 (27)
Fading rash at presentation	12 of 59 (20)
Vesicular	4 of 59 (7)
Multiple EM	14 of 79 (18)

From Nadelman RB, Nowakowski J, Forseter G, et al. The clinical spectrum of early Lyme borreliosis in patients with culture-confirmed erythema migrans. Am J Med 1996;100(5):502–8; with permission.

higher levels of chemokines and cytokines and to activate both innate and adaptive immune responses compared with *B afzelii* and *B garinii*.[36]

Associated Physical Findings

Regional lymphadenopathy (23%–41%), fever (14%–31%), and pain on neck flexion (5%–20%) are the most common objective physical findings at the time of diagnosis of EM in patients in the United States.[5,12,18,25] Concurrent cranial nerve palsies (usually facial nerve) are reported in 1% to 6% of patients.[5,12,18,25] Patients with associated heart block may have bradycardia or irregular heart beats.

Patients with EM from New York State with infection caused by *B burgdorferi* sensu stricto were significantly more likely than those from Slovenia with either *B afzelii* or *B garinii* infection to have more physical findings, including regional lymphadenopathy and fever.[26,27] Regional lymphadenopathy was the most common finding in European patients, found in 7.2% of 316 patients from 2 prospective studies from Slovenia.[26,33]

Multiple Erythema Migrans and Spirochetemia

Half of a cohort of 314 patients in an observational study in Connecticut conducted from 1976 to 1982 developed multiple annular secondary lesions,[5] with 40 of the 314 (13%) patients having more than 20 secondary lesions, and 2 patients having more than 100 (**Fig. 6**). Secondary lesions were similar in morphology to the initial solitary (ie, primary) lesion with which most patients presented, but tended to be smaller (usually 2–3 cm) and did not have an indurated center (ie, punctum).[5,13,23] Neither secondary nor primary lesions are present on mucous membranes, palms,

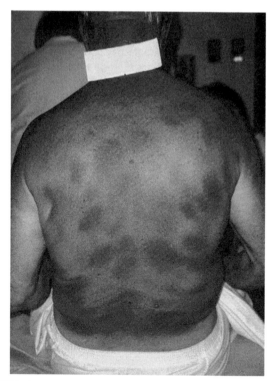

Fig. 6. Multiple EM lesions.

or soles. Secondary lesions are the result of hematogenous spread from the original tick bite and contain viable spirochetes.[23,37] However, secondary lesions lack a punctum because they do not occur at the site of tick inoculation; they also are not associated with local pruritus, tenderness, or vesiculation. Some secondary lesions may be transient, appearing and disappearing suddenly during examination.[5] These evanescent lesions may be observed for several weeks in untreated patients, even after resolution of primary and secondary lesions.[5]

Using high-volume (≥9 mL) blood culture samples, using special media, it can be shown that as many as 50% of patients with EM from the United States have spirochetemia; multiple EM lesions are observed in more than 40% of patients with detectable spirochetemia (**Table 3**).[37] Spirochetemic patients are significantly more likely than those with negative blood cultures to have systemic symptoms, to have more symptoms, and to have a higher cumulative symptom severity score.[37] The presence of multiple EM lesions, regional lymphadenopathy, headaches, stiff neck, and chills (but not fever) are also significantly more likely to be associated with positive blood cultures.[37] However, no single characteristic or combination of variables had enough specificity and sensitivity (>80%) to predict spirochetemia.[37]

Influence of Strain Differences on Manifestations of Erythema Migrans

Hematogenous dissemination of B burgdorferi from the initial focus of infection at the site of tick bite and primary EM lesion is thought to account not only for multiple EM lesions but for objective extracutaneous manifestations of Lyme disease (eg, facial nerve palsy, meningitis, carditis, and arthritis). B burgdorferi can be classified into subtypes based on RNA intergenic spacer type (RST; also referred to as restriction fragment length polymorphism) at the 16S-23S ribosome of B burgdorferi,[38] genotyping of the outer surface protein (Osp) C gene,[39,40] or multilocus sequence typing.[41] Some subtypes of B burgdorferi are less likely to be associated with spirochetemia,[37–39,42] perhaps explaining why 20% of 55 untreated patients with EM remained symptom free after a mean of 6 years in one study.[43] In general, patients with RST types 1 and 2 and OspC types A, B, I, and K are more likely to have multiple EM lesions and spirochetemia.[37,38,42] In contrast, some patients with solitary EM lesions and less invasive subtypes have significant systemic symptoms, implying that other factors (eg, host factors or cytokines) may contribute to these symptoms.[44] In one report, patients with EM infected with RST 1 strains had more symptoms than those infected with other strains and greater cytokine levels, including interferon-gamma (IFN-γ), IFN-γ–inducible chemokines, CCL2, CXCL9, and CXCL10.[42] In addition, in

Table 3
Comparison of selected clinical and laboratory characteristics of 213 patients with EM with and without spirochetemia

Variable	Spirochetemia (93 Patients) No. (%)	No Spirochetemia (120 Patients) No. (%)	P Value
Multiple EM lesions	39 (41.9)	18 (15.0)	<.001
Symptomatic	83 (89.2)	89 (74.2)	.006
Regional lymphadenopathy	46 (49.5)	43 (35.8)	.05
Lymphocyte count <1.0 × 10⁹ cells/L	26 of 91[a] (28.6)	10 of 116[a] (8.6)	<.001

[a] Number of patients for whom lymphocyte count was obtained.
From Wormser GP, McKenna D, Carlin J, et al. Brief communication: hematogenous dissemination in early Lyme disease. Ann Intern Med 2005;142(9):751–5; with permission.

this report, RST 1 strains stimulated peripheral blood mononuclear cells from healthy humans to secrete significantly higher levels of interferon-alfa (INF-α), IFN-γ, and CXCL10 than RST 2 or RST 3 strains.[42]

Epidemiology

It has been estimated by the CDC that approximately 300,000 cases of Lyme disease occur annually in the United States.[45] Of the approximately 25,000 confirmed cases reported in 2012, 13 states in New England, the Middle Atlantic (and Virginia), and North Central regions accounted for 95% of cases.[14,46] Although more than 70% of these patients had a reported history of EM, the incidence of EM is likely to be under-estimated because this skin lesion may go unnoticed when it occurs at body sites that are not readily visualized by a patient (or even health care provider), or when minimal or no systemic or local symptoms are present.[1,2,7,8,16] In addition, case reporting is intrin-sically biased toward later manifestations of Lyme disease, such as arthritis, because in many states positive serologic tests are reported (which are usually negative in EM but positive in late disease; discussed later).[15,47–49] There are 2 peaks in the age dis-tribution for EM, at 5 to 14 years old and 45 to 54 years old. Because nymphal *I scap-ularis*, the stage most closely associated with transmission of *B burgdorferi*, are most active from May to July, the overwhelming majority of cases of EM occur in late spring or summer.[50–52] Nymphal ticks are more numerous than adult ticks and are also much smaller and thus less likely to be detected and removed before transmission of infec-tion can occur.[16,19] Ticks are also more likely to be encountered during the warmer months, when people tend to increase outdoor activity.[52]

EM has been reported, and *B burgdorferi* sensu lato has been isolated, from clinical specimens throughout Europe and parts of Asia (eg, Japan) where *B afzelii* and *B garinii* are the most common causal genospecies.[26,29–31,33,53–56] Reports of EM from regions (including in the United States) without prior culture isolation of *B burgdorferi* sensu lato from human specimens or vector ticks should be viewed with skepticism.[57]

Differential Diagnosis

One group of investigators attempted to examine the diagnostic value of clinical his-tory and physical examination in the evaluation of rashes consistent with EM.[20] The investigators were unable to identify a single sign or symptom or any epidemiologic information diagnostic of EM. They commented on the need for an algorithm that com-bines specific signs or symptoms in order to improve diagnostic sensitivity.[20]

The diagnosis of EM should be considered in patients who present with nonspecific illnesses in endemic areas during the late spring and summer, even if a rash is initially not reported.[2,58] Health care providers should perform a complete skin examination with all clothing removed to evaluate areas poorly visualized by the patient. In this way, previously unrecognized EM may be identified. EM should also be considered (and searched for) when examining patients with unexplained atrioventricular heart block because carditis caused by *B burgdorferi* has been reported in 2% to 9% of untreated patients with EM, with the higher incidence seen in early studies before recognition of the value of antimicrobial therapy for this disorder.[5,59,60]

EM can usually be differentiated from other skin disorders. EM occurs infrequently from autumn to midspring (although this may vary with weather patterns and tick den-sity and activity). Arthropod bites unassociated with *B burgdorferi* infection may resemble EM. Because it generally takes days for transmission of *B burgdorferi* to occur after a tick bite,[16,19] an erythematous lesion surrounding the bite site while a tick is still attached, or within 48 hours of detachment, is most likely a hypersensitivity reaction to the tick bite rather than an infection (**Fig. 7, Table 4**).[2,15–17] Such hypersensitivity

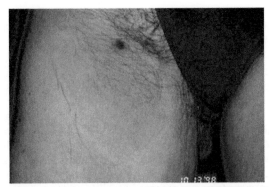

Fig. 7. A probable hypersensitivity reaction to a tick bite, mimicking EM. The rash (more than 5 cm and thus technically fulfilling CDC criteria for a diagnosis of EM) was noted at the time an adult *I scapularis* tick was removed, a few hours before taking this photograph. The patient experienced intense pruritus at the site, which she had noted in the past with tick bites. There were no associated systemic symptoms. The rash resolved within approximately 48 hours without treatment. The patient remained well and serology for antibodies to *B burgdorferi*, performed after approximately 3 months, was negative.

reactions are usually less than 5 cm in the largest diameter, may be associated with significant pruritus (atypical for EM), and tend to fade spontaneously within 24 to 48 hours. In contrast, an EM lesion typically increases progressively in size over days. Most patients with EM seen in the United States also have associated systemic

Table 4
Differentiating EM from hypersensitivity reaction to an arthropod bite

Characteristic	EM	Arthropod Bite Hypersensitivity Reaction
Recall of bite at site	~20%	Variable
Tick present at time of rash	No	Yes (or detached within prior 24 h); also may occur after other arthropod (eg, mosquito) bites
Time interval between bite and rash	Median 7–10 d (range, 1–36 d)[2,5,11,12]	Hours
Location	Intertriginous areas, border of tight-fitting clothing	Same; also can occur on exposed areas such as face or forearm
Local symptoms	Rare; minimal if present	Pruritus
Evolution	Expands over days to weeks	Expands over hours
Resolution	Days to weeks (median 4 wk if untreated[5])	<48 h
Size	≥5 cm (can be smaller)	<5 cm (can be larger)
Systemic symptoms	Up to 80%	Absent
Fever	16% documented, 39% subjective[12]	Absent

See **Fig. 7.**
From Nadelman RB, Wormser GP. Erythema migrans and early Lyme disease. Am J Med 1995;98(4A):15S–23S; with permission.

symptoms, in contrast to those with local tick bite hypersensitivity reactions. It may be helpful in some cases for the health care practitioner to demarcate the lesion with ink and observe evolution over 1 to 2 days without treatment. If the rash expands or systemic symptoms develop, antimicrobial treatment should be initiated, whereas if the rash resolves within 48 hours no treatment is necessary.[2,16] Factors that may be used to distinguish EM from arthropod bite reactions unassociated with B burgdorferi infection are listed in **Table 4**.

In contrast with EM, both staphylococcal and streptococcal cellulitis develop suddenly, evolving over hours with a bandlike rather than oval or circular shape, and are usually painful. Although fever may accompany both EM and pyogenic cellulitis, leukocytosis and a toxic-appearing patient may be observed in staphylococcal and streptococcal cellulitis but are rarely noted in patients with EM. The typical body sites at which skin manifestations occur also differ for these infections. Cellulitis caused by pyogenic organisms usually develops on the distal lower extremities, sometimes after trauma, and often in a person with underlying peripheral vascular disease (eg, venous stasis) or with a history of prior surgery affecting venous or lymphatic flow (eg, saphenous vein harvesting for coronary artery bypass surgery or mastectomy).[2] In contrast, EM tends to occur in the axillae, back, buttocks, popliteal fossae, and other sites where a tick may feed unnoticed for a sufficient period of time (2 days or more) to transmit infection (see **Table 1**).

Herpes simplex and Varicella zoster may usually be distinguished from EM by their dermatomal distribution and tenderness, although vesicular EM lesions tend to be more painful than those without vesiculation. Patients with vesicular EM often present complaining of an unwitnessed spider bite. It is important to recognize that the range of the brown recluse spider (which extends southerly from southeastern Nebraska to southern Ohio) does not include most of the geographic region in which Lyme disease is endemic.[61,62]

An erythematous border and central clearing are characteristic of tinea infection, and thus may resemble EM. However, tinea rashes evolve much more slowly (weeks rather than days) compared with EM and are not associated with systemic symptoms. Scaling and thin, irregular, raised borders should suggest tinea. Characteristics of some skin disorders that may be confused with EM are summarized in **Table 5**.

Southern Tick-associated Rash Infection

An EM-like rash has been identified in many patients residing in regions of the United States (especially the South) where B burgdorferi infection has not been identified in humans.[63–66] This rash has some features reminiscent of EM, including peak summer incidence, similar incubation period after a tick bite, and a similar appearance to EM, including the occasional presence of multiple lesions. However, in contrast with patients with Lyme disease, B burgdorferi has failed to grow in Barbour-Stoenner-Kelly medium from biopsied skin lesions. Acute and convalescent phase serologic assays are almost always negative for antibodies to B burgdorferi.[65,66] In addition, I scapularis ticks, the usual vector for Lyme disease, are rarely infected with B burgdorferi in the southern United States (<0.5%) and infrequently bite humans.[67] The tick vector for this EM-like rash is Amblyomma americanum, which is not thought to be a competent vector for B burgdorferi.[68] Therefore it may be concluded that this rash does not represent Lyme disease; it has come to be known as southern tick-associated rash illness (STARI), or Masters disease (after a key investigator).[63,65,66] At one time, a new Borrelia genospecies, Borrelia lonestarii, was postulated to be the causal agent,[69] but a subsequent study of 19 patients with STARI failed to detect this organism.[66] A prospective clinical evaluation of patients from Missouri with STARI

Table 5
Differential diagnosis of EM

Diagnosis	Appearance	Body Site	Size	Progression	Seasonal Tendency	Miscellaneous
Tinea (ringworm)	Ring shape, with satellite lesions; scaling at periphery	Variable; exposed skin	1–10 cm	Days to weeks	No	Pruritus; pet exposure
Bacterial cellulitis	Homogenous erythema; bandlike appearance; warm and tender, lymphangitic streaking; tender regional lymphadenopathy	Distal extremities; site of prior trauma	Rarely large except on lower extremities	More rapid than EM (hours to days)	No	Pain, fever, leukocytosis; history of prior trauma, vascular disease, or surgery
Contact dermatitis	Shape related to contact; vesicles and bullae may be present	Variable	Variable	Variable (often slow progression)	No	Pruritus often severe; history of contact with inciting substance (eg, poison ivy)
Urticaria	Raised, multiple lesions	Variable	Variable	Waxes and wanes over hours	No	Pruritus
Fixed drug eruption	Deep, well-demarcated, violaceous plaque	Fixed, often involves genitals	Variable	Fixed in size	No	Burning
Brown recluse spider bite	Necrotic; red, white, and blue sign	Extremities	Variable	Spreads centrifugally	Yes (mates May to September)	May be painful; uncommon in northeastern United States
Herpes simplex / Varicella zoster	Vesicles on erythematous base	Dermatomal distribution	Variable	May progress rapidly (days)	No	Prodrome may occur; pain (sometimes severe); pruritus, fever

See **Table 4** for distinguishing EM from a hypersensitivity reaction to an arthropod bite.
Adapted from Feder HM, Whitaker DL. Misdiagnosis of erythema migrans. Am J Med 1995;99(4):412–9, with permission; and Tibbles CD, Edlow JA. Does this patient have erythema migrans? JAMA 2007;297(23):2617–27.

and patients from New York with EM showed distinct differences in the clinical characteristics of patients from the two regions.[65] Missouri patients were significantly more likely to recall a preceding tick bite at the site of the lesion, and had a shorter time to onset of lesions than New York patients. New York patients with EM were more likely to be symptomatic and were more likely to have multiple skin lesions. Missouri patients tended to have skin lesions that were more circular and smaller in size, and were more likely to have central clearing. Missouri patients recovered more rapidly than New York patients after antibiotic treatment.[65]

Coinfection

I scapularis, the vector for *B burgdorferi*, is also known to transmit *Babesia microtia*, causing babesiosis, a malarialike infection,[8,16,70] and *Anaplasma phagocytophilum*, the agent of human granulocytic anaplasmosis (HGA; formerly known as human granulocytic ehrlichiosis).[16,58,70,71] The presence of these two organisms may confound the typical clinical picture of Lyme disease. The occurrence of leukopenia, thrombocytopenia, or anemia in a patient with Lyme disease should suggest coinfection, because cytopenias are not characteristic of Lyme disease.[58,71–73] Abnormal levels of transaminases and other liver enzymes are common in patients with HGA but may occur in patients with Lyme disease alone.[5,12] The lack of rapid response (48 hours) to amoxicillin or cefuroxime axetil, particularly the persistence of fever, should raise consideration of the diagnosis of coinfection.[15,16] A patient with EM who appears toxic or requires intensive care should prompt an evaluation for babesiosis, especially in an immunocompromised or asplenic patient,[74] or HGA.[75] Deer tick virus, a cause of meningoencephalitis, and *Borrelia miyamotoi*, which has been associated with viral-like syndromes as well as meningoencephalitis, are two recently described pathogens that have also been linked to *I scapularis* bites.[76–78]

Laboratory Diagnosis

EM is a clinical diagnosis that is based on the characteristic appearance of the skin lesion in a patient with the appropriate epidemiologic and exposure history. Results of routine laboratory tests, such as complete blood counts, liver enzyme assays, and sedimentation rate, are generally not helpful in the diagnosis of Lyme disease and are usually normal (except in the case of coinfection with *A phagocytophilum* or *B microtia*; discussed earlier). However, the clinical diagnosis can be confirmed through laboratory testing, with isolation of *B burgdorferi* in culture being the gold standard for accurate identification. Laboratory validation is important primarily in the investigational setting (ie, treatment trials or epidemiologic studies). The diagnosis of infection with *B burgdorferi* may be supported by serology (acute and convalescent phase), culture of clinical specimens (skin and blood), and polymerase chain reaction (PCR; nested and quantitative reverse transcription PCR from skin). These tests were compared in 47 patients with EM in Westchester County, New York (**Table 6**).[79] In a more recent report, the sensitivity of quantitative PCR of blood culture and plasma, and nested PCR of plasma and skin, were compared with skin culture (61.5% sensitivity) in Westchester patients with EM.[80] Using quantitative PCR blood culture, 39 of 52 (75%) untreated patients with EM tested positive; 48 of 52 (92.3%) patients tested positive using at least 1 of the 5 methods.[80] Culture methods have in general been restricted to specialty and/or research laboratories; as with PCR (which has recently become more readily available), they are not useful in routine patient care.

The most practical laboratory method available to clinicians is serologic testing for antibodies to *B burgdorferi*. For many years, a 2-tier system has been recommended, usually polyvalent enzyme-linked immunosorbent assay (ELISA) followed by

Table 6
Comparison of diagnostic tests for 47 adult patients with EM

Diagnostic Method	No. (%) Positive Result
Skin culture	24 (51.1)
Blood culture (18 mL)	21 (44.7)
Any culture	31 (66)
Nested PCR	30 (63.8)
Quantitative PCR	38 (80.9)
Any PCR	38 (80.9)
Acute phase serology	19 (40.4)
Convalescent phase serology	31 (66)
Any serology	32 (68.1)
Any test positive	44 (93.6)
All tests negative	3 (6.4)

From Nowakowski J, Schwartz I, Liveris D, et al. Laboratory diagnostic techniques for patients with early Lyme disease associated with erythema migrans: a comparison of different techniques. Clin Infect Dis 2001;33(12):2023–7; with permission.

immunoglobulin (Ig) M and IgG immunoblots if the first step test is positive or equivocal.[16,48,81] However, serology is insensitive in early Lyme disease, with half of patients with EM having negative serology on presentation.[47,48,79] The probability of seroreactivity has been directly linked to the duration of EM,[47,48] with all 14 of the patients presenting with EM duration of greater than or equal to 2 weeks in one study having positive ELISA and IgM immunoblot at presentation.[47] Convalescent phase testing can be used to increase the sensitivity of serologic assays.[16,48] Two-tiered testing has the disadvantages of increased cost, time, and labor, and subjectivity in the interpretation of immunoblots.[82] More recently, testing using a C6 ELISA (based on the highly conserved 25-amino-acid C6 peptide of the VlsE protein) was significantly more sensitive than 2-tier testing, with sensitivities of 66.5% (95% confidence interval [CI], 61.7–71.1) and 35.2% (95% CI, 30.6–40.1), respectively (P<.001) in sera from 403 patients with EM.[82] Specificity of the C6 ELISA assay was slightly decreased compared with 2-tier testing.[82] However, because the diagnosis of EM is usually straightforward and because all available diagnostic assays frequently yield false-negative results, the routine use of serology or any other diagnostic test (eg, PCR) cannot be recommended at present for patients with EM.[16] Diagnostic tests in patients with EM should be reserved for those in whom there is a doubt about the diagnosis (eg, difficulty in distinguishing between EM and a hypersensitivity reaction to an arthropod, or an EM-like rash in a nonendemic region), or for those in clinical trials or epidemiologic studies.

TREATMENT
Long-term Outcome of Untreated Patients with Erythema Migrans

Although EM lesions resolve spontaneously within a median of 4 weeks, most untreated patients at some point develop clinical manifestations that may cause considerable morbidity.[5,43] Of 314 patients with EM diagnosed between 1976 and 1982, 55 who did not receive antibiotics were followed prospectively (after enrollment from 1976 to 1978) for a mean duration of 6 years. Although all EM lesions resolved spontaneously, within 1 to 14 months, 9% developed recurrent EM at the site of the primary lesion, 5% had recurrence of secondary lesions, and 7% had recurrence of both, whereas 5% had recurrent evanescent lesions. Two children experienced frequent evanescent lesions for more than 3 years. Other manifestations of Lyme disease were experienced by 12 patients with recurrent skin lesions.[5] Eighty percent of all those observed without treatment developed joint symptoms ranging from arthralgias to intermittent episodes of arthritis to chronic synovitis. Of these 80%, 11% also developed neurologic abnormalities and 4% had cardiac involvement. The most typical course for Lyme arthritis, occurring in 51% of patients, was intermittent attacks of monoarticular or oligoarticular arthritis of large joints (almost invariably involving the knee), beginning months after the initial infection.[43] Although some patients experienced recurrent attacks of arthritis for many years, the number of recurrences decreased by 10% to 20% each year.[43] Severity of symptoms at onset of illness was predictive of development of late disease (arthritis).[43] However, 20% of untreated patients had no subsequent manifestations of Lyme disease over a median of 6 years (range, 3–8 years) after the resolution of their EM lesions.

Treatment Trials of Patients with Erythema Migrans

There have been several randomized prospective trials in the United States to evaluate treatment of EM. From 1980 to 1981, the first randomized trial was conducted in Connecticut in 112 patients with EM, comparing erythromycin, tetracycline, and penicillin for 10 days.[10] EM and associated symptoms resolved more rapidly in patients receiving penicillin or tetracycline compared with those receiving erythromycin. An intensification of fever, rash, or pain, noted in 15% of patients during the first 24 hours after initiation of antimicrobial therapy, was thought to represent a Jarisch-Herxheimer–like reaction. Complications such as meningitis, carditis, and arthritis were observed less frequently in patients receiving tetracycline or penicillin than in those receiving erythromycin.[10] No additional benefit was noted when the duration of treatment with tetracycline was extended from 10 to 20 days.[10] Two subsequent smaller studies evaluated amoxicillin (to which probenecid was added to increase drug levels) and doxycycline and showed efficacy of these medications with rapid resolution of rash and associated symptoms and a favorable outcome at 6 months in nearly all patients.[83,84] A similar satisfactory outcome was reported in patients receiving azithromycin in a third treatment arm in 1 of these studies.[84]

The efficacy of oral cefuroxime axetil 500 mg twice daily and doxycycline 100 mg 3 times daily were compared in a total of 364 patients (from New York, New Jersey, and Connecticut) with early Lyme disease characterized by EM in 2 subsequent randomized, multicenter, investigator-blinded, prospective, controlled studies.[85,86] A satisfactory clinical outcome (defined as resolution of EM and associated signs and symptoms by day 5 posttreatment, or improvement of these findings by day 5 and complete resolution at 1 month posttreatment) was observed in 93% and 90% of the cefuroxime axetil group and in 88% and 95% of the doxycycline group, respectively.[85,86] The two drugs seemed to be equally effective in treatment of early Lyme disease and prevention of extracutaneous disease at 1 year of follow-up.[85,86] Patients receiving cefuroxime axetil more frequently experienced diarrhea, whereas those treated with doxycycline were significantly more likely to have photosensitivity reactions; most adverse effects were mild and did not require discontinuation of treatment.[85,86]

Another prospective (but unblinded) controlled study addressed intravenous (IV) versus oral treatment of those with disseminated Lyme disease (not involving the central nervous system).[87] Of 140 patients with EM and disseminated disease, 133 had multiple EM lesions and 81 had fever. Resolution of symptoms and the prevention of complications did not differ between those patients receiving oral doxycycline 100 mg twice daily for 21 days versus ceftriaxone 2 g IV daily for 14 days.[87]

Because a significant minority of patients have allergies or are otherwise intolerant of β-lactam antimicrobials, and because tetracyclines may be associated with photosensitivity reactions during the late spring and summer months when EM is most common and also are contraindicated in pregnant women and young children, much interest has focused on the well-tolerated macrolide azithromycin for treatment of patients with EM. This drug was associated with excellent in vitro activity against B burgdorferi and was predicted to attain therapeutic levels in skin.[88] In a multicenter prospective controlled study 246 patients (from Westchester County and Long Island [NY], Connecticut, Missouri, Wisconsin, New Jersey, Minnesota, California, and Rhode Island) were randomized to receive either azithromycin 500 mg daily for 7 days or amoxicillin 500 mg 3 times daily for 20 days.[88] Azithromycin was significantly less effective than amoxicillin for the resolution of EM and associated symptoms, and in the prevention of objective relapse at 6 months[88] (in retrospect, the patients from Missouri, a nonendemic area for Lyme disease, probably had STARI rather than EM). However, in European studies, azithromycin seems to be more successful in treating early Lyme disease. Azithromycin was compared with phenoxymethylpenicillin and with doxycycline in prospective randomized trials from Germany and Slovenia, and showed comparable efficacy with possible earlier resolution of symptoms.[89–91] Another macrolide, oral clarithromycin (500 mg twice daily for 21 days), was studied in an open-labeled pilot trial in 41 patients with EM in Long Island, NewYork.[92] Symptoms resolved in 91% of the 33 evaluable patients by the end of treatment, and all 28 evaluable patients were well at 6 months.[92] However, although a semisynthetic macrolide, roxithromycin, showed good in vitro activity against B burgdorferi, a European trial comparing this drug with phenoxymethylpenicillin was interrupted because of failure in 5 of 19 enrolled patients, all of whom were receiving roxithromycin.[93]

Shorter, 10-day courses of tetracyclines have been shown to be as effective as longer courses.[10,94–97] Ten days of oral doxycycline twice daily, with or without a single 2-g IV dose of ceftriaxone, was compared with 20 days of oral doxycycline twice daily in a prospective, randomized, double-blind controlled trial.[94] All 3 treatment groups had similar rates of complete response at all assessment times over 30 months. Objective evidence of treatment failure was extremely rare regardless of the regimen.[94] It was concluded that extending the course of doxycycline from 10 to 20 days, or adding 1 dose of IV ceftriaxone at the beginning of a 10-day course of doxycycline did not enhance therapeutic efficiency in patients with EM.[94]

Doxycycline is not routinely recommended in children less than 8 years of age, which limits antibiotic options for children who are intolerant of amoxicillin. In a prospective, randomized, unblinded study in 43 children aged 6 months to 12 years, 2 different doses (20 mg/kg/d and 30 mg/kg/d) of cefuroxime axetil were compared with amoxicillin (50 mg/kg/d). All patients had good outcomes with resolution of EM and no long-term problems attributable to Lyme disease.[98] Minimal adverse effects were observed in all 3 groups.[98] Both amoxicillin and cefuroxime axetil have been recommended as the preferred regimen for pediatric patients less than 8 years old.[16]

Unlike other agents used to treat Lyme disease, doxycycline has excellent activity against A phagocytophilum, the causal agent of HGA, which may be transmitted together with B burgdorferi or separately after I scapularis tick bites.[16,58,75] Cephalexin, fluoroquinolones, metronidazole, and sulfonamides have no appreciable activity against B burgdorferi and should not be used to treat patients with Lyme disease.[16,99]

A low incidence of serious adverse effects has been observed in treatment trials for early Lyme disease. Doxycycline may cause phototoxicity, a potential concern because EM usually occurs in late spring or summer. Patients should be counseled regarding avoiding strong sunlight and using sun block. To prevent esophagitis associated with doxycycline, patients should be advised to drink a full 240 mL (8 oz) of fluid with this medication, and should avoid a recumbent position for 1 hour afterward. Doxycycline is relatively contraindicated in children less than 8 years old and in pregnant or breastfeeding women. Amoxicillin and cefuroxime axetil have been associated with rash, diarrhea, and other adverse effects. Guidelines from the Infectious Diseases Society of America (IDSA) for the treatment of EM are summarized in **Table 7**.

Long-term Outcome of Treated Patients with Erythema Migrans

Long-term outcomes are excellent for patients treated appropriately for EM.[15,18,25,85,86,94,100,101] In an observational study evaluating 118 patients (recruited in the LYMErix vaccine trial[102]), seen in 10 endemic states with culture-confirmed EM, who were mostly treated with oral doxycycline, 11% had persistent signs and symptoms for more than 30 days after treatment, decreasing to 4% at 60 days.[18] However, these symptoms were mainly subjective, including headache, fatigue, and arthralgias, or represented residual neurologic symptoms of facial numbness or weakness in the 2 patients who had experienced seventh cranial nerve palsy. At 20 months' follow-up, all but 1 of the patients had completely recovered.[18]

In another prospective study conducted in Westchester County, New York, 99 patients with EM confirmed by culture of blood or skin biopsy specimens (5 additional

Table 7
IDSA recommendations for treatment of patients with EM

Drug	Dosage for Adults	Dosage for Children
Preferred[a]		
Amoxicillin	500 mg 3 times per day	50 mg/kg per day in 3 divided doses (maximum 500 mg per dose)
Doxycycline	100 mg twice per day	Not recommended for children aged <8 y
	Relatively contraindicated in pregnant or lactating women	For children aged ≥8 y, 4 mg/kg per day, in 2 divided doses (maximum 100 mg per dose)
Cefuroxime axetil	500 mg twice per day	30 mg/kg per day in 2 divided doses (maximum 500 mg per dose)
Alternative[b]		
Azithromycin	500 mg per day for 7–10 d	10 mg/kg per day (maximum 500 mg per day)
Clarithromycin	500 mg twice per day for 14–21 d Relatively contraindicated in pregnant women	7.5 mg/kg twice per day (maximum 500 mg per dose)
Erythromycin	500 mg 4 times per day for 14–21 d	12.5 mg/kg 4 times per day (maximum 500 mg per dose)

In patients suspected of having coinfection with HGA, doxycycline is preferred if not contraindicated.

[a] Recommended duration is 14 days (10–21 days for doxycycline or 14–21 days for amoxicillin and cefuroxime axetil).

[b] Because of their lower efficacy, macrolides are reserved for patients who are unable to take, or who are intolerant of, tetracyclines, penicillins, and cephalosporins; patients treated with macrolides should be closely observe to ensure resolution of clinical symptoms.

From Wormser GP, Dattwyler RJ, Shapiro ED, et al. The clinical assessment, treatment, and prevention of Lyme disease, human granulocytic anaplasmosis, and babesiosis: clinical practice guidelines by the Infectious Diseases Society of America. Clin Infect Dis 2006;43(9):1089–134. [Erratum appears in Clin Infect Dis 2007;45(7):941].

patients who participated in a Lyme disease vaccine study[102] were excluded) were followed for a mean of 4.9 ± 2.9 years after treatment with first-line antibiotic regimens at baseline.[25] EM resolved within 3 weeks in all cases, and no patient developed extracutaneous manifestation of late Lyme disease. Within 3 months, 84% to 92% of patients were asymptomatic. Of those followed for more than 1 year, 10% were symptomatic at their last visit; symptoms were mild and intermittent. Of note, 47% of patients experienced subsequent tick bites, and 15% of patients had repeated episodes of EM (discussed later) after initial enrollment, highlighting the need for education on tick bite prevention for those persons who live, work, or have recreation in endemic areas. The number and severity of symptoms at baseline, and presentation with multiple EMs, were associated with the presence of symptoms at follow-up.[25]

A similar favorable outcome after antibiotic treatment has been observed in multiple studies from Europe. In a prospective study of French patients treated for EM, complete resolution of EM was observed with regression of associated symptoms at 6-week follow-up (except in those with preexisting rheumatologic disorders).[30] No patients developed arthritis or neurologic or cardiac manifestations of Lyme disease at 3-year follow-up.[30] Studies from other European countries showed similar excellent outcomes in patients treated for EM after 6 weeks, and at long-term follow-up (up to 27 months).[29,35,89–91,103] In one novel study, symptoms in 230 Slovenian patients with EM were compared, at baseline and at 6 and 12 months after standard antibiotic treatment of EM, with those of controls (spouse, family member, or friend within 5 years of age) without a prior history of Lyme disease.[100] Based on identical questionnaires administered to both groups, patients were less likely than controls to have subjective symptoms; none of the symptoms were severe enough to be disabling. The findings suggest that some symptoms experienced after treatment of EM may be unrelated to infection. However, this conclusion must be tempered by the fact that patients with multiple EM lesions (who may be more likely to develop symptoms after treatment) were excluded from participation.[100] The applicability to US patients of findings in European studies is uncertain because of clinical differences associated with *B burgdorferi* sensu stricto infection in the United States versus infection caused by *B afzelii* and *B garinii* in Europe.

Objective evidence of late disease almost never develops after patients with EM are treated with currently recommended regimens.[16,85–88,94,100,101] In some of the rare patients who have developed objective neurologic findings, subtle symptoms suggestive of central nervous system involvement had been present in retrospect at initiation of oral antimicrobial therapy.[84] However, approximately 10% of patients with EM experience subjective symptoms such as fatigue, myalgias, and arthralgias, and vague neurologic symptoms after treatment.[25,85,86,88,94,104] There is no evidence that ongoing infection causes these symptoms and prolonged antimicrobial treatment of these patients does not result in sustained improvement and can be harmful.[16,105–112]

Persistent fatigue was rare in patients followed prospectively for a mean of 15.4 years (range, 11–20 years) after treatment of culture-confirmed EM in Westchester County, New York.[113] Patients were evaluated using an 11-item fatigue severity scale (FSS-11) that has been used in studies of posttreatment Lyme disease syndrome[113] in which a score of greater than or equal to 4 is considered to indicate severe fatigue. Only 3 of 100 subjects (3%) were thought to have had persistent fatigue that might be attributable to Lyme disease, and the FSS-11 scores for these individuals was less than 4, averaging 2.27, with no person having functional impairment.[113] Although fibromyalgia has been postulated to be triggered by *B burgdorferi* infection, it was also exceedingly rare in this same cohort, observed in only 1 of 100 study participants.[114] The presence of chronic symptoms following treatment of EM must be interpreted in the context of similar symptoms in the general population.[115,116] Ninety percent of the general population have 1 or more somatic symptoms in a given 2-week to 4-week period and 30% report current musculoskeletal symptoms.[115] Significant fatigue is experienced by 20% of adults, and more than 75% of healthy college students report at least 1 symptom in a 3-day period.[115] Thus, outcome studies that include controls without Lyme disease may be best suited to identify sequelae that may be related to infection with B burgdorferi as opposed to coincidental.[100]

Outcome in Special Patient Groups: Pregnant and Immunocompromised Hosts

Pregnant women have been excluded from enrollment in prospective treatment studies. However, there is no reason to think that this group of patients requires different antimicrobial therapy from others, other than avoiding doxycycline in pregnancy. Epidemiologic studies of outcomes following Lyme disease during pregnancy[117–119] have been unable to corroborate an early uncontrolled report that described adverse fetal outcomes in 19 patients with EM during pregnancy.[120] Furthermore, a survey of 162 pediatric neurologists in Connecticut (the state with the second highest incidence of Lyme disease[14]) failed to identify a single child with a neurologic problem thought to be related to Lyme disease during pregnancy.[121]

Several investigations of pregnancy outcomes from Europe have been conducted.[122–124] In a retrospective study from Hungary, untreated patients with EM had worse pregnancy outcomes than women treated orally, whereas those treated with IV therapy had the best outcomes.[123] However, no consistent adverse outcome was noted and the investigators concluded that a specific congenital Lyme borreliosis syndrome was unlikely. The findings of a prospective study of 105 pregnant women with EM from Slovenia were consistent with this conclusion.[122] Excellent outcomes were achieved after antibiotic treatment in 93 (88.6%) pregnancies, and adverse outcomes (abortion, preterm birth, syndactyly, and urologic anomalies) were not clearly linked to Lyme disease.[122] Good outcomes were also reported after treatment with IV ceftriaxone in 7 pregnant women with documented spirochetemia.[124] However, in European studies of EM during pregnancy, most patients have presumably been infected with B afzelii rather than B burgdorferi sensu stricto; thus it may not be possible to generalize conclusions to the United States.

Several studies have been published in Europe regarding the response to treatment of immunocompromised patients with EM.[125–127] In a Slovenian study (again, presumably dominated by B afzelii infection), more frequent early disseminated disease and more treatment failures requiring retreatment were noted in 67 patients with a variety of causes of immunosuppression compared with the control group.[127] However, both groups had a similarly favorable outcome at 1-year follow-up.[127] A favorable outcome was also observed in a retrospective study of 33 immunosuppressed patients from Austria with EM.[126] Initial clinical presentation, response to therapy, and production of anti-Borrelia antibodies were similar in immunosuppressed patients compared with controls.[126] Excellent outcomes after treatment of EM were also noted in 6 Slovenian patients with a prior history of organ transplant.[125]

Early Borrelia burgdorferi Infection Without Erythema Migrans

Some patients from endemic areas present with nonspecific systemic symptoms without EM during tick season. Some have EM lesions that are not recognized because of an inadequate physical examination that did not include visualization of the entire body. In others, an EM rash may have come and gone. In others, EM may become noticeable some days after systemic symptoms appear. However, there is evidence that some patients with Lyme disease present with nonspecific symptoms without EM.[128] A Lyme disease vaccine trial offered a unique opportunity to study this topic because participants were followed prospectively by experts in tick-borne diseases who were familiar with the diagnosis of EM, and all patients had baseline blood samples stored that could be run in parallel after an acute illness to check for seroconversion. Of nearly 11,000 study participants in 10 states, 269 met predetermined criteria for definite, possible, or asymptomatic Lyme disease. Of these, 42 persons (16%) had systemic symptoms associated with IgM and/or IgG seroconversion but no EM. The 14 patients with only IgM seroconversions were considered to have possible Lyme disease, whereas 28 patients with IgG seroconversions on either the VlsE peptide ELISA or on sonicate Western blot were considered to be definite cases. A few patients were thought to have coinfection (ie, HGA [termed ehrlichiosis in the study] or babesiosis). Patient symptoms are summarized in **Table 8**. Symptoms resolved in a median of 3 to 7 days for almost all patients after treatment with doxycycline (34 patients) or amoxicillin (6 patients) (2 patients declined any treatment), although arthralgias or fatigue persisted for weeks to months in 7 patients. No patient developed objective manifestations (eg, arthritis or neurologic signs) of Lyme disease during the study.[128]

Reinfection

Patients may sustain a second, and occasionally more, episodes of Lyme disease after the first episode has resolved. These subsequent occurrences of Lyme disease are almost invariably associated with EM.[24] Reinfection may be defined as a new infection that occurs after successful antimicrobial treatment of a prior episode of Lyme disease.[24] In various prospective US series, the rate of reinfection ranged from 1.2% to 14.6 % over 1 to 5 years (averaging 1.2%–3.1% per year).[18,25,94] In 100

Table 8		
Characteristics of systemic symptoms in patients with early Lyme disease without EM		
	Definite Lyme Disease (n = 24) **Number (%) or Median (Range)**	**Possible Lyme Disease (n = 7)** **Number (%) or Median (Range)**
Age	53 (27–72)	48 (37–62)
Male sex	14 (58)	5 (72)
Fever	15 (63)	7 (100)
Chills	12 (50)	4 (57)
Malaise	17 (71)	7 (100)
Headache	13 (54)	6 (86)
Stiff neck	10 (42)	2 (29)
Paresthesia	7 (29)	0
Arthralgia	17 (71)	2 (29)
Myalgia	11 (46)	5 (71)
Sore throat	2 (8)	0
Dry cough	1 (4)	0
Number of symptoms per patient	4 (1–7)	5 (4–7)

Definite Lyme disease indicates seroconversion by IgG or C6 ELISA testing; possible Lyme disease indicates seroconversion only by IgM testing; patients thought to have coinfection with anaplasmosis (ehrlichiosis) or babesiosis were excluded.

Adapted from Steere AC, Dhar A, Hernandez J, et al. Systemic symptoms without erythema migrans as the presenting picture of early Lyme disease. Am J Med 2003;114(1):58–62.

patients with EM confirmed by culture and followed for 15.4 years (range, 11–20 years) after treatment, 24% reported a second episode of EM during this time, and one-third of these individuals experienced at least 2 subsequent episodes.[113] For patients with a prior history of EM, the rate of recurrent EM can exceed the incidence of Lyme disease in the general population living in the same community by a factor of 20 to 50.[24]

The most likely cause of recurrent EM is repeat tick bite. In one prospective study on the use of prophylactic doxycycline after a recognized tick bite in Westchester County, New York, 17% of 335 subjects sustained new tick bites over the 6 weeks following enrollment, despite receiving oral and written instructions on ways to reduce the risk of tick bites.[19] In addition, the human immune response is not fully protective against reinfection. Strain variability of B burgdorferi is possibly a factor; there are at least 19 OspC types causing infection in the United States.[129] Data from 17 patients with 22 paired consecutive episodes of culture-confirmed EM indicate that all second episodes were associated with an OspC type different from that of the first episode, indicating reinfection rather than a relapse.[129] Based on these findings as well as data from other patients with EM in the northeastern United States, probabilistic and simulation models suggest that strain-specific immunity develops in humans after EM and that it lasts at least 6 years.[130] Consistent with this finding is an experimental model of infection in which mice immunized with one OspC type were immune to reinfection with that strain but susceptible to infection with a different OspC type.[131] Humans with late Lyme disease (eg, arthritis) are extremely unlikely to develop reinfection as a result of an expanded immune response.[24]

Limited data are available regarding the clinical features of reinfected patients. Recurrent EM in 28 patients seen on Rhode Island was evenly divided among men and women; was unassociated with any immunodeficiency; and was almost exclusively seen in June, July, and August.[51] Preliminary experience from Westchester County, New York, indicated no differences in the occurrence of a variety of clinical signs and symptoms or in EM size in 11 men and 11 women experiencing reinfection a mean of 3.25 ± 2.65 years apart.[132] However, patients with second episodes of EM seemed less likely (3 of 11 [14%] vs 7 of 11 [32%]; $P = .15$) than those with first episodes to have multiple EM lesions (although this did not achieve statistical significance). This finding is consistent with the development of partial immunity preventing hematogenous spread during the second episode.[24] Supporting this concept is the observation in another study that patients with a prior episode of Lyme disease seemed less likely than those with first episodes to have spirochetemia (odds ratio, 2.5; 95% CI, 1.1–5.6; $P = .02$).[37]

In contrast with reinfection, relapse has not been well documented in patients receiving recommended treatment courses.[24,51] However, relapse has been well documented in patients treated with antibiotics not recommended for Lyme disease (eg, cephalexin)[99] and has been reported in patients receiving second-line agents,[16] such as macrolides.[88]

Prevention of Infection

Avoiding ticks can be difficult for people who live, work, or have recreational activities in tick-infested environments. Covering up the skin and applying acaricides or insect repellants to clothing and skin have been recommended to decrease risk.[16,133] Daily skin inspection with prompt removal of attached ticks is also recommended in order to interrupt transmission of tick-borne infection.[16,133] The chance of developing Lyme disease after a recognized bite from an I scapularis tick can be further decreased with the appropriate prophylactic use of doxycycline. In a randomized placebo-controlled trial of 503 subjects who removed attached I scapularis ticks, the risk of

EM was reduced from 3.2% to 0.4%, an 87% risk reduction, with the use of a single 200-mg dose of doxycycline, given within 3 days of a tick bite.[19] In highly endemic areas, people bitten by nymphal or adult *I scapularis* ticks that are estimated to have been attached for longer than 36 hours should be offered doxycycline prophylaxis if there are no contraindications.[16] Duration of tick attachment can be estimated when the tick is available by measuring the degree of engorgement of the tick.[16] Other preventative methods have been recommended, including application of acaricides to property and modifying the environment to exclude deer (fences) or inhibit tick movement (placing wood chip borders on property).[15,133] Vaccination was shown to be 80% effective in preventing Lyme disease but is no longer available.[15,102]

SUMMARY

In the United States, EM has only been associated with infection with *B burgdorferi* sensu stricto but, in Europe and Asia, other genospecies more commonly cause Lyme disease (often referred to in Europe as Lyme borreliosis).[26,27,29–31,33,53–55] Although distinctive in appearance, EM-like lesions should not be considered pathognomonic for Lyme disease, in part because localized arthropod bite reactions without infection may appear similar, as may STARI, which occurs in regions of the United States that are not endemic for *B burgdorferi* infection.[6,20,63,65,66]

Because appropriate treatment with oral antibiotics at this early stage of infection with *B burgdorferi* results in excellent outcomes, with objective treatment failures being exceedingly rare, it is important to recognize EM lesions.[15,16,18,83–91,94,95,98,100,113,114] Clinicians should be aware that some patients with EM may also be coinfected with the bacterium that causes HGA (which is sensitive to doxycycline, but not amoxicillin) or the parasitic causal agent of babesiosis, which may require additional specific treatment. The gold standard for the diagnosis of EM is the isolation in culture of *B burgdorferi* from a biopsy taken from a sample of the skin lesion but this is neither routinely obtainable nor necessary.[12,18,26,29,31,33,42,54,134] Serologic testing is readily available, and consists of either a 2-tier serologic testing protocol or the C6 peptide ELISA; however, although both methods are useful in the diagnosis of extracutaneous manifestations of Lyme disease, they have limited value in patients presenting with EM, in part because of poor sensitivity in this early stage of infection.[16,47,48,82] For practitioners, EM remains a clinical diagnosis.[6,16]

REFERENCES

1. Nadelman RB, Wormser GP. Lyme borreliosis. Lancet 1998;352(9127):557–65.
2. Nadelman RB, Wormser GP. Erythema migrans and early Lyme disease. Am J Med 1995;98(4A):15S–23S.
3. Steere AC, Snydman D, Murray P, et al. Historical perspectives. In: Lyme borreliosis. Proceedings of the second International symposium on Lyme disease and related disorders. Stuttgart, New York: Gustav Fischer Verlag; 1987. p. 3–6.
4. Åsbrink E, Olsson I. Clinical manifestations of erythema chronicum migrans afzelius in 161 patients. Acta Derm Venereol 1985;65(1):43–52.
5. Steere AC, Bartenhagen NH, Craft JE, et al. The early clinical manifestations of Lyme disease. Ann Intern Med 1983;99(1):76–82.
6. Nadelman RB, Wormser GP. Recognition and treatment of erythema migrans: are we off target. Ann Intern Med 2002;136(6):477–9.
7. Gerber MA, Shapiro ED, Burke GS, et al. Lyme disease in children in southeastern Connecticut. Pediatric Lyme Disease Study Group. N Engl J Med 1996;335(17):1270–4.

8. Krause PJ, Telford SR 3rd, Spielman A, et al. Concurrent Lyme disease and babesiosis. Evidence for increased severity and duration of illness. JAMA 1996;275(21):1657–60.

9. Hollström E. Successful treatment of erythema migrans Afzelius. Acta Derm Venereol 1951;31(2):235–43.

10. Steere AC, Hutchinson GJ, Rahn DW, et al. Treatment of the early manifestations of Lyme disease. Ann Intern Med 1983;99(1):22–6.

11. Berger BW. Dermatologic manifestations of Lyme disease. Rev Infect Dis 1989; 11(Suppl 6):S1475–81.

12. Nadelman RB, Nowakowski J, Forseter G, et al. The clinical spectrum of early Lyme borreliosis in patients with culture-confirmed erythema migrans. Am J Med 1996;100(5):502–8.

13. Malane MS, Grant-Kels JM, Feder HM, et al. Diagnosis of Lyme disease based on dermatologic manifestations. Ann Intern Med 1991;114(6):490–8.

14. Centers for Disease Control and Prevention (CDC). Lyme disease – United States 2003-2005. MMWR Morb Mortal Wkly Rep 2007;56:573–6.

15. Wormser GP. Early Lyme disease. N Engl J Med 2006;354:2794–801.

16. Wormser GP, Dattwyler RJ, Shapiro ED, et al. The clinical assessment, treatment, and prevention of Lyme disease, human granulocytic anaplasmosis, and babesiosis: clinical practice guidelines by the infectious diseases society of America. Clin Infect Dis 2006;43(9):1089–134 [Erratum appears in Clin Infect Dis 2007;45(7):941].

17. Feder HM, Whitaker DL. Misdiagnosis of erythema migrans. Am J Med 1995; 99(4):412–9.

18. Smith RP, Schoen RT, Rahn DW, et al. Clinical characteristics and treatment outcome of early Lyme disease in patients with microbiologically confirmed erythema migrans. Ann Intern Med 2002;136(6):421–8.

19. Nadelman RB, Nowakowski J, Fish D. Prophylaxis with single-dose doxycycline for the prevention of Lyme disease after an *Ixodes scapularis* tick bite. N Engl J Med 2001;345(2):79–84.

20. Tibbles CD, Edlow JA. Does this patient have erythema migrans? JAMA 2007; 297(23):2617–27.

21. Ribeiro JM, Mather TN, Piesman J, et al. Dissemination and salivary delivery of Lyme disease spirochetes in vector ticks. J Med Entomol 1987;24(2):201–5.

22. Habif TP. Infestations and bites. In: Clinical dermatology. 4th edition. Mosby; 2004. p. 497–546.

23. Melski JW, Reed KD, Mitchell PD, et al. Primary and secondary erythema migrans in central Wisconsin. Arch Dermatol 1993;129(6):709–16.

24. Nadelman RB, Wormser GP. Reinfection in patients with Lyme disease. Clin Infect Dis 2007;45(8):1032–8.

25. Nowakowski J, Nadelman RB, Sell R, et al. Long-term follow-up of patients with culture-confirmed Lyme disease. Am J Med 2003;115(2):91–6.

26. Strle F, Nadelman RB, Cimperman J, et al. Comparison of culture-confirmed erythema migrans caused by *Borrelia burgdorferi* sensu stricto in New York and by *Borrelia afzelii* in Slovenia. Ann Intern Med 1999;130(1):32–6.

27. Strle F, Ružić-Sabljić E, Logar M, et al. Comparison of erythema migrans caused by *Borrelia burgdorferi* and *Borrelia garinii*. Vector Borne Zoonotic Dis 2011; 11(9):1253–8.

28. Jurca T, Ruzic-Sabljic E, Lotric-Furlan S, et al. Comparison of peripheral and central biopsy sites for the isolation of *Borrelia burgdorferi* sensu lato from erythema migrans skin lesions. Clin Infect Dis 1998;27(3):636–8.

29. Kuiper H, Cairo I, Van Dam A, et al. Solitary erythema migrans: a clinical, laboratory and epidemiological study of 77 Dutch patients. Br J Dermatol 1994; 130(4):466–72.

30. Lipsker D, Antoni-Bach N, Hansmann Y, et al. Long-term prognosis of patients treated for erythema migrans in France. Br J Dermatol 2002;146(5):872–6.

31. Logar M, Ruzic-Sabljic E, Maraspin V, et al. Comparison of erythema migrans caused by Borrelia afzelii and Borrelia garinii. Infection 2004;32(1):15–9.

32. Goldberg NS, Forseter G, Nadelman RB, et al. Vesicular erythema migrans. Arch Dermatol 1992;128(11):1495–8.

33. Strle F, Nelson JA, Ruzic-Sabljic E, et al. European Lyme borreliosis: 231 culture-confirmed cases involving patients with erythema migrans. Clin Infect Dis 1996; 23(1):61–5.

34. Weber K, Preac-Mursic V, Neubert U, et al. Antibiotic therapy of early European Lyme borreliosis and acrodermatitis chronica atrophicans. Ann N Y Acad Sci 1988;539:324–45.

35. Weber K, Preac-Mursic V, Wilske B, et al. A randomized trial of ceftriaxone versus oral penicillin for the treatment of early European Lyme borreliosis. Infection 1990;18(2):91–6.

36. Strle K, Drouin EE, Shen S, et al. Borrelia burgdorferi stimulates macrophages to secrete higher levels of cytokines and chemokines than Borrelia afzelii or Borrelia garinii. J Infect Dis 2009;200(12):1936–43.

37. Wormser GP, McKenna D, Carlin J, et al. Brief communication: hematogenous dissemination in early Lyme disease. Ann Intern Med 2005;142(9):751–5.

38. Liveris D, Varde S, Iyer R, et al. Genetic diversity of Borrelia burgdorferi in Lyme disease patients as determined by culture versus direct PCR with clinical specimens. J Clin Microbiol 1999;37(3):565–9.

39. Seinost G, Dykhuizen DE, Dattwyler RJ, et al. Four clones of Borrelia burgdorferi sensu stricto cause invasive infections in humans. Infect Immun 1999;67(7): 3518–24.

40. Grimm D, Tilly K, Byram R, et al. Outer surface protein C of the Lyme disease spirochete: a protein induced in ticks for infection in mammals. Proc Natl Acad Sci U S A 2004;101(9):3142–7.

41. Margos G, Gatewood AG, Aanensen DM, et al. MLST of housekeeping genes captures geographic population structure and suggests a European origin of Borrelia burgdorferi. Proc Natl Acad Sci U S A 2008;105:8730–5.

42. Strle K, Jones KL, Drouin EE, et al. Borrelia burgdorferi RST1 (OspC type A) genotype is associated with greater inflammation and more severe Lyme disease. Am J Pathol 2011;178(6):2726–39.

43. Steere AC, Schoen RT, Taylor E, et al. The clinical evolution of Lyme arthritis. Ann Intern Med 1987;107(5):725–31.

44. Wormser GP, Kaslow R, Tang J, et al. Association between human leukocyte antigen class II alleles and genotype of Borrelia burgdorferi in patients with early Lyme disease. J Infect Dis 2005;192(11):2020–6.

45. Kuehn BM. CDC estimates 300,000 US cases of Lyme disease annually. JAMA 2013;310(11):1110.

46. Lyme disease data. Available at: http://www.cdc.gov/lyme/stats/index.html. Accessed October 13, 2014.

47. Aguero-Rosenfeld ME, Nowakowski J, McKenna D, et al. Serodiagnosis in early Lyme disease. J Clin Microbiol 1993;31(12):3090–5.

48. Aguero-Rosenfeld ME, Wang G, Schwartz I, et al. Diagnosis of Lyme borreliosis. Clin Microbiol Rev 2005;18(3):484–509.

49. Ertel SH, Nelson RS, Cartter ML. Effect of surveillance method on reported characteristics of Lyme disease, Connecticut, 1996-2007. Emerg Infect Dis 2012; 18(2):242–7.

50. Falco RC, McKenna DF, Daniels TJ, et al. Temporal relation between *Ixodes scapularis* abundance and risk for Lyme disease associated with erythema migrans. Am J Epidemiol 1999;149(8):771–6.

51. Krause PJ, Foley DT, Burke GS, et al. Reinfection and relapse in early Lyme disease. Am J Trop Med Hyg 2006;75(6):1090–4.

52. Fish D. Environmental risk and prevention of Lyme disease. Am J Med 1995; 98(4A):2S–8S.

53. Hashimoto Y, Kawagishi N, Sakai H, et al. Lyme disease in Japan. analysis of *Borrelia* species using rRNA gene restriction fragment length polymorphism. Dermatology 1995;191(3):193–8.

54. Busch U, Hizo-Teufel C, Böhmer R, et al. *Borrelia burgdorferi* sensu lato strains isolated from cutaneous Lyme borreliosis biopsies differentiated by pulsed-field gel electrophoresis. Scand J Infect Dis 1996;28(6):583–9.

55. Ornstein K, Berglund J, Nilsson I, et al. Characterization of Lyme borreliosis isolates from patients with erythema migrans and neuroborreliosis in southern Sweden. J Clin Microbiol 2001;39(4):1294–8.

56. Masuzawa T. Terrestrial distribution of the Lyme borreliosis agent *Borrelia burgdorferi* sensu lato in East Asia. Jpn J Infect Dis 2004;57(6):229–35.

57. Sharma A, Jaimungal S, Basdeo-Maharaj K, et al. Erythema migrans-like illness among Caribbean islanders. Emerg Infect Dis 2010;16(10):1615–7.

58. Nadelman RB, Horowitz HW, Hsieh TC, et al. Simultaneous human ehrlichiosis and Lyme borreliosis. N Engl J Med 1997;337(1):27–30.

59. Rubin DA, Sorbera C, Nikitin P, et al. Prospective evaluation of heart block complicating early Lyme disease. Pacing Clin Electrophysiol 1992;15(3):252–5.

60. Haddad FA, Nadelman RB. Lyme disease and the heart. Front Biosci 2003;8: s769–82.

61. Frithsen IL, Vetter RS, Stocks IC. Reports of envenomation by brown recluse spiders exceed verified specimens of *Loxosceles* spiders in South Carolina. J Am Board Fam Med 2007;20(5):483–8.

62. Vetter RS, Bush SP. Reports of presumptive brown recluse spider bites reinforce improbable diagnosis in regions of North America where the spider is not endemic. Clin Infect Dis 2002;35(4):442–5.

63. Masters E, Granter S, Duray P, et al. Physician-diagnosed erythema migrans and erythema migrans-like rashes following lone star tick bites. Arch Dermatol 1998;134(8):955–60.

64. Kirkland KB, Klimko TB, Meriwether RA, et al. Erythema migrans-like rash illness at a camp in North Carolina: a new tick-borne disease? Arch Intern Med 1997; 157(22):2635–41.

65. Wormser GP, Masters E, Nowakowski J, et al. Prospective clinical evaluation of patients from Missouri and New York with erythema migrans-like skin lesions. Clin Infect Dis 2005;41(7):958–65.

66. Wormser GP, Masters E, Liveris D, et al. Microbiologic evaluation of patients from Missouri with erythema migrans. Clin Infect Dis 2005;40(3):423–8.

67. Felz MW, Durden LA, Oliver JH Jr. Ticks parasitizing humans in Georgia and South Carolina. J Parasitol 1996;82(3):505–8.

68. Piesman J, Sinsky RJ. Ability of *Ixodes scapularis*, *Dermacentor variabilis* and *Amblyomma americanum* to acquire, maintain and transmit Lyme disease spirochetes. J Med Entomol 1988;25:336–9.

69. Barbour AG, Maupin GO, Teltow GJ, et al. Identification of an uncultivable *Borrelia* species in the hard tick *Amblyomma americanum*: possible agent of a Lyme disease-like illness. J Med Entomol 1988;25(5):336–9.
70. Steere AC, McHugh G, Suarez C, et al. Prospective study of coinfection in patients with erythema migrans. Clin Infect Dis 2003;36(8):1078–81.
71. Belongia EA, Reed KD, Mitchell PD, et al. Clinical and epidemiological features of early Lyme disease and human granulocytic ehrlichiosis in Wisconsin. Clin Infect Dis 1999;29(6):1472–7.
72. Nadelman RB, Nowakowski J, Horowitz HW, et al. Thrombocytopenia and *Borrelia burgdorferi*: an association remains unproven. Clin Infect Dis 1999;29(6):1603–5.
73. Wormser GP, Aguero-Rosenfeld ME, Cox ME, et al. Differences and similarities between culture-confirmed human granulocytic anaplasmosis and early Lyme disease. J Clin Microbiol 2013;51(3):954–8.
74. Krause PJ, Gewurz BE, Hill D, et al. Persistent and relapsing babesiosis in immunocompromised patients. Clin Infect Dis 2008;46(3):370–6.
75. Bakken JS, Dumler S. Human granulocytic anaplasmosis. Infect Dis Clin North Am 2008;22(3):433–48, viii.
76. El Khoury MY, Camargo JF, White JL, et al. Potential role of deer tick virus in Powassan encephalitis cases in Lyme disease-endemic areas of New York, U.S.A. Emerg Infect Dis 2013;19(12):1926–33.
77. Krause PJ, Narasimhan S, Wormser GP, et al, Tick Borne Diseases Group. *Borrelia miyamotoi* sensu lato seroreactivity and seroprevalence in the northeastern United States. Emerg Infect Dis 2014;20(7):1183–90.
78. Gugliotta JL, Goethert HK, Berardi VP, et al. Meningoencephalitis from *Borrelia miyamotoi* in an immunocompromised patient. N Engl J Med 2013;368(3):240–5.
79. Nowakowski J, Schwartz I, Liveris D, et al. Laboratory diagnostic techniques for patients with early Lyme disease associated with erythema migrans: a comparison of different techniques. Clin Infect Dis 2001;33(12):2023–7.
80. Liveris D, Schwartz I, McKenna D, et al. Comparison of five diagnostic modalities for direct detection of *Borrelia burgdorferi* in patients with early Lyme disease. Diagn Microbiol Infect Dis 2012;73(3):243–5.
81. Centers for Disease Control and Prevention (CDC). Recommendations for test performance and interpretation from the second national conference on serologic diagnosis of Lyme disease. MMWR Morb Mortal Wkly Rep 1995;44:590–1.
82. Wormser GP, Schriefer M, Aguero-Rosenfeld ME, et al. Single-tier testing with the C6 peptide ELISA kit compared with two-tier testing for Lyme disease. Diagn Microbiol Infect Dis 2013;75(1):9–15.
83. Dattwyler RJ, Volkman DJ, Conaty SM, et al. Amoxicillin plus probenecid versus doxycycline for treatment of erythema migrans borreliosis. Lancet 1990; 336(8728):1404–6.
84. Massarotti EM, Luger SW, Rahn DW, et al. Treatment of early Lyme disease. Am J Med 1992;92(4):396–403.
85. Nadelman RB, Luger SW, Frank E, et al. Comparison of cefuroxime axetil and doxycycline in the treatment of early Lyme disease. Ann Intern Med 1992; 117(4):273–80.
86. Luger SW, Paparone P, Wormser GP, et al. Comparison of cefuroxime axetil and doxycycline in treatment of patients with early Lyme disease associated with erythema migrans. Antimicrob Agents Chemother 1995;39(3):661–7.
87. Dattwyler RJ, Luft BJ, Kunkel MJ, et al. Ceftriaxone compared with doxycycline for the treatment of acute disseminated Lyme disease. N Engl J Med 1997; 337(5):289–94.

88. Luft BJ, Dattwyler RJ, Johnson R, et al. Azithromycin compared with amoxicillin in the treatment of erythema migrans: a double blind, randomized, controlled trial. Ann Intern Med 1996;124(9):785–91.
89. Weber K, Wilske B, Preac-Mursic V, et al. Azithromycin versus penicillin V for the treatment of early Lyme borreliosis. Infection 1993;21(6):367–72.
90. Strle F, Ruzic E, Cimperman J. Erythema migrans: comparison of treatment with azithromycin, doxycycline and phenoxymethylpenicillin. J Antimicrob Chemother 1992;30(4):543–50.
91. Strle F, Maraspin V, Lotric-Furlan S, et al. Azithromycin and doxycycline for treatment of Borrelia culture-proven erythema migrans. Infection 1996;24(1):64–8.
92. Dattwyler RJ, Grunwaldt E, Luft BJ. Clarithromycin in treatment of early Lyme disease: a pilot study. Antimicrob Agents Chemother 1996;40(2):468–9.
93. Hansen K, Hovmark A, Lebech AM, et al. Roxithromycin in Lyme borreliosis: discrepant results of an in vitro and in vivo animal susceptibility study and a clinical trial in patients with erythema migrans. Acta Derm Venereol 1992;72(4):297–300.
94. Wormser GP, Ramanathan R, Nowakowski J, et al. Duration of antibiotic therapy for early Lyme disease. Ann Intern Med 2003;138(9):697–704.
95. Stupica D, Lusa L, Ruzić-Sabljić E, et al. Treatment of erythema migrans with doxycycline for 10 days versus 15 days. Clin Infect Dis 2012;55(3):343–50.
96. Nowakowski J, Nadelman RB, Forseter G, et al. Doxycycline versus tetracycline therapy for Lyme disease associated with erythema migrans. J Am Acad Dermatol 1995;32(2 Pt 1):223–7.
97. Kowalski TJ, Tata S, Berth W, et al. Antibiotic treatment duration and long-term outcomes of patients with early Lyme disease from a Lyme disease-hyperendemic area. Clin Infect Dis 2010;50(4):512–20.
98. Eppes SC, Childs JA. Comparative study of cefuroxime axetil versus amoxicillin in children with early Lyme disease. Pediatrics 2002;109(6):1173–7.
99. Nowakowski J, McKenna D, Nadelman RB, et al. Failure of treatment with cephalexin for Lyme disease. Arch Fam Med 2000;9(6):563–7.
100. Cerar D, Cerar T, Ruzić-Sabljić E, et al. Subjective symptoms after treatment of early Lyme disease. Am J Med 2010;123(1):79–86.
101. Jares TM, Mathiason MA, Kowalski TJ. Functional outcomes in patients with Borrelia burgdorferi reinfection. Ticks Tick Borne Dis 2014;5(1):58–62.
102. Steere AC, Sikand VK, Meurice F, et al. Vaccination against Lyme disease with recombinant Borrelia burgdorferi outer-surface lipoprotein A with adjuvant. Lyme disease vaccine study group. N Engl J Med 1998;339(4):209–15.
103. Hulshof MM, Vandenbroucke JP, Nohlmans LM, et al. Long-term prognosis in patients treated for erythema chronicum migrans and acrodermatitis chronica atrophicans. Arch Dermatol 1997;133(1):33–7.
104. Feder HM Jr, Johnson BJ, O'Connell S, et al. A critical appraisal of "chronic Lyme disease." N Engl J Med 2007;357(14):1422–30.
105. Nadelman RB, Arlin Z, Wormser GP. Life-threatening complications of empiric ceftriaxone therapy for 'seronegative Lyme disease.' South Med J 1991;84(10):1263–5.
106. Fallon BA, Keilp JG, Corbera KM, et al. A randomized, placebo-controlled trial of repeated IV antibiotic therapy for Lyme encephalopathy. Neurology 2008;70:992–1003.
107. Klempner MS, Hu LT, Evans J, et al. Two controlled trials of antibiotic treatment in patients with persistent symptoms and a history of Lyme disease. N Engl J Med 2001;345(2):85–92.

108. Krupp LB, Hyman LG, Grimson R, et al. Study and treatment of post Lyme disease (STOP-LD): a randomized double masked clinical trial. Neurology 2003; 60(12):1923–30.
109. Ettestad PJ, Campbell GL, Welbel SF, et al. Biliary complications in the treatment of unsubstantiated Lyme disease. J Infect Dis 1995;171(2):356–61.
110. Patel R, Grogg KL, Edwards WD, et al. Death from inappropriate therapy for Lyme disease. Clin Infect Dis 2000;31(4):1107–9.
111. Halperin JJ. Prolonged Lyme disease treatment: enough is enough. Neurology 2008;70(13):986–7.
112. Holzbauer SM, Kemperman MM, Lynfield R. Death due to community-associated *Clostridium difficile* in a woman receiving prolonged antibiotic therapy for suspected Lyme disease. Clin Infect Dis 2010;51(3):369–70.
113. Wormser GP, Weitzner E, McKenna D, et al. Long-term assessment of fatigue in patients with culture-confirmed Lyme disease. Am J Med 2015;128:181–4.
114. Wormser GP, Weitzner E, McKenna D, et al. Long-term assessment of fibromyalgia in patients with culture-confirmed Lyme disease. Arthritis Rheumatol 2014. [Epub ahead of print].
115. Barsky AJ, Borus JF. Functional somatic syndromes. Ann Intern Med 1999; 130(11):910–21.
116. Seltzer EG, Gerber MA, Cartter ML, et al. Long-term outcomes of persons with Lyme disease. JAMA 2000;283(5):609–16.
117. Williams CL, Strobino B, Weinstein A, et al. Maternal Lyme disease and congenital malformation: a cord blood serosurvey in endemic and control areas. Paediatr Perinat Epidemiol 1995;9(3):320–30.
118. Strobino B, Abid S, Gewitz M. Maternal Lyme disease and congenital heart disease: a case-control study in an endemic area. Am J Obstet Gynecol 1999;180(3 Pt 1):711–6.
119. Strobino BA, Williams CL, Abid S, et al. Lyme disease and pregnancy outcome: a prospective study of two thousand prenatal patients. Am J Obstet Gynecol 1993;169(2 Pt 1):367–74.
120. Markowitz LE, Steere AC, Benach JL, et al. Lyme disease during pregnancy. JAMA 1986;255(24):3394–6.
121. Gerber MA, Zalneraitis EL. Childhood neurologic disorders and Lyme disease during pregnancy. Pediatr Neurol 1994;11(1):41–3.
122. Maraspin V, Cimperman J, Lotric-Furlan S, et al. Erythema migrans in pregnancy. Wien Klin Wochenschr 1999;111(22–23):933–40.
123. Lakos A, Solymosi N. Maternal Lyme borreliosis and pregnancy outcome. Int J Infect Dis 2010;14(6):e494–8.
124. Maraspin V, Ružić-Sabljić E, Pleterski-Rigler D, et al. Pregnant women with erythema migrans and isolation of borreliae from blood: course and outcome after treatment with ceftriaxone. Diagn Microbiol Infect Dis 2011;71(4):446–8.
125. Maraspin V, Cimperman J, Lotric-Furlan S, et al. Erythema migrans in solid organ transplant recipients. Clin Infect Dis 2006;42(12):1751–4.
126. Fürst B, Glatz M, Kerl H, et al. The impact of immunosuppression on erythema migrans. A retrospective study of clinical presentation, response to treatment and production of Borrelia antibodies in 33 patients. Clin Exp Dermatol 2006; 31(4):509–14 [Erratum appears in Clin Exp Dermatol 2006;31(5):751].
127. Maraspin V, Lotric-Furlan S, Cimperman J, et al. Erythema migrans in the immunocompromised host. Wien Klin Wochenschr 1990;111(22–23):923–32.
128. Steere AC, Dhar A, Hernandez J, et al. Systemic symptoms without erythema migrans as the presenting picture of early Lyme disease. Am J Med 2003; 114(1):58–62.

129. Nadelman RB, Hanincová K, Mukherjee P, et al. Differentiation of reinfection from relapse in recurrent Lyme disease. N Engl J Med 2012;367(20):1883–90.
130. Khatchikian CE, Nadelman RB, Nowakowski J, et al. Evidence for strain-specific immunity in patients treated for early Lyme disease. Infect Immun 2014;82(4): 1408–13.
131. Probert WS, Crawford M, Cadiz RB, et al. Immunization with outer surface protein (Osp) A but not OspC provides cross-protection of mice challenged with North American isolates of *Borrelia burgdorferi*. J Infect Dis 1997;175(2):400–5.
132. Nadelman RB, Gaidici AT, McKenna D, et al. Comparison of clinical manifestations of 1st and 2nd episodes of erythema migrans (EM). In: Program and abstracts of the 9th International conference on Lyme borreliosis and other tick-borne diseases. New York, August 18-22, 2002. abstract P-51.
133. Hayes EB, Piesman J. How can we prevent Lyme disease? N Engl J Med 2003; 348(24):2424–30.
134. Berger BW, Johnson RC, Kodner C, et al. Cultivation of *Borrelia burgdorferi* from erythema migrans lesions and perilesional skin. J Clin Microbiol 1992;30(2): 359–61.

Nervous System Lyme Disease

John J. Halperin, MD[a,b],*

KEYWORDS

- Lyme disease • *Borrelia burgdorferi* • Neuroborreliosis
- Garin-Bujadoux Bannwarth syndrome • Nervous system
- Peripheral nervous system • Central nervous system • Intrathecal antibody

KEY POINTS

- The nervous system is involved in 10% to 15% of patients with untreated *Borrelia burgdorferi* infection. This proportion is similar in Eurasian and North American patients.
- Nervous system infection causes either meningitis or multifocal inflammatory changes in the peripheral nervous system (frequent) or central nervous system (CNS; rare), as shown by objective changes on neurologic examination or other objective tests.
- As in many other systemic infectious and inflammatory states, patients may experience cognitive and memory difficulty; these symptoms do not indicate CNS infection and alone are not diagnostic of Lyme disease.
- Treatment with standard courses of oral antimicrobials cures approximately 95% of patients with neuroborreliosis. Parenteral treatment may be needed in those rare patients with parenchymal CNS involvement but some evidence supports the use of oral therapy in these individuals as well.

INTRODUCTION

"It was the best of times, it was the worst of times, it was the age of wisdom, it was the age of foolishness, it was the epoch of belief, it was the epoch of incredulity..." These famous opening words of Dickens' *A Tale of Two Cities* aptly describe a great deal of what is currently said about Lyme disease and its effects on the nervous system. Numerous factors contribute to this[1,2]; probably the single most important is that patients, the public in general, and even many physicians struggle with the concept

Disclosures: The author has been an expert witness defending physicians in medical malpractice cases in which they have been accused of failure to diagnose or treat Lyme disease; the author has equity in several pharmaceutical companies, none of which is relevant to this topic. The author receives royalties from Up-to-date and *Lyme Disease: an Evidence-based Approach*, published by CABI in 2011.
[a] Department of Neurosciences, Overlook Medical Center, 99 Beauvoir Avenue, Summit, NJ 07902, USA; [b] Department of Neurology and Medicine, Icahn School of Medicine at Mount Sinai, New York, NY 10029, USA
* Department of Neurosciences, Overlook Medical Center, 99 Beauvoir Avenue, Summit, NJ 07902.
E-mail address: john.halperin@atlantichealth.org

Infect Dis Clin N Am 29 (2015) 241–253
http://dx.doi.org/10.1016/j.idc.2015.02.002
0891-5520/15/$ – see front matter © 2015 Elsevier Inc. All rights reserved.

id.theclinics.com

of what does and does not constitute nervous system disease. Although nervous system function is essential for all behavior, many things affect behavior in the absence of damage to the nervous system, which is the defining requirement of neurologic disorders. Conditions as diverse as sleep deprivation, sepsis, depression, uremia, psychosis, and learned behaviors can profoundly alter how people function, but none of these necessarily implies the presence of neurologic disease. Because the possibility of neurologic diseases (eg, stroke, Alzheimer, Parkinson) is terrifying to most people, it could be argued that these misconceptions about nervous system Lyme disease, or neuroborreliosis, contribute substantially to the widespread fear of this tick-borne infection, and some patients' and physicians' willingness to use highly unconventional therapies to try to eradicate what is, in reality, a straightforward infection.

HISTORICAL BACKGROUND

Although the term Lyme disease was coined in the 1970s, with the initial reports of nervous system involvement appearing shortly thereafter,[3,4] the first description of neuroborreliosis was published in 1922 in a case report[5] that both was brilliant in its insights and foreshadowed how misunderstandings about the specifics of neurologic diagnosis can result in confusion.

Three weeks following the bite of an *Ixodes* tick on his left buttock, a French sheep farmer developed severe pain at the site of the bite and an erythroderm that expanded to cover the entire buttock, much of the thigh, and the lower abdomen. The distribution of the pain expanded; he developed bilateral sciatica and severe and intractable pain in the trunk and right arm. When evaluated, his examination was normal except for marked right deltoid atrophy and weakness. He had a neutrophilic cerebrospinal fluid (CSF) pleocytosis with increased protein and normal glucose levels. In light of a slightly positive Wasserman test the investigators concluded this was a spirochetosis, but went to great pains to explain why this could not possibly have been syphilis, and treated him with neoarsphenamine (state-of-the-art syphilis treatment in 1922) with rapid resolution of his pain.

Although this case succinctly captured most of the key elements of neuroborreliosis, the investigators' discussion also revealed several logical flaws. In attributing the infection to a spirochetosis, they considered spirochetes to be a type of virus, reflecting the limitations of medical knowledge at that time. They went on to equate this patient's problem with tick bite paralysis; a disorder that occurs while a tick is still attached, not weeks later; is associated with *Dermacentor* ticks, not *Ixodes*; and is not associated with a rash, pain, or a CSF pleocytosis. Such inappropriate linking of superficially similar disorders continues to this day.

As European clinical experience with this illness grew, these misunderstandings were increasingly unimportant. The disorder became known as Garin-Bujadoux (and subsequently Bannwarth) syndrome and by the 1950s was routinely recognized by European neurologists, and treated with penicillin.[6] In the 1970s and 1980s, the essentially identical neurologic syndrome was described in US patients in association with Lyme disease, and similarly found to be responsive to penicillin.[3]

It would be reasonable to assume that there could be little controversy surrounding an illness that has been well characterized for nearly a century and is caused by a known, antibiotic-sensitive microorganism. The more than 10,000 book citations on the subject of Lyme disease at Amazon.com (a number similar to the total published scientific articles listed in Medline in a search on the same day [August 17, 2014]) suggests otherwise.

In summarizing what is known about neuroborreliosis, the goal of this article is to address 4 key fallacies (**Box 1**): (1) that nervous system infection with *Borrelia*

Box 1
Neuroborreliosis fallacies (ie, all are incorrect)

- Nervous system Lyme disease:
  - Can cause every imaginable neurobehavioral abnormality
  - Is incurable and causes progressive brain deterioration
- Symptoms of fatigue, memory or cognitive disorders, or other neurobehavioral changes
  - In patients with Lyme disease are evidence of nervous system infection
  - Are sufficiently specific for Lyme disease that they support the diagnosis absent any other laboratory or clinical support

---

burgdorferi can cause every imaginable neurologic presentation, without any pattern or specificity; (2) that nervous system Lyme disease, like some neurologic disorders, is inexorably progressive and difficult, if not impossible, to cure; (3) that, in a patient with Lyme disease, nonspecific cognitive symptoms indicate nervous system disease; and (4) that such nonspecific symptoms are sufficiently indicative of Lyme disease that treatment is appropriate even in the absence of other evidence supporting the diagnosis. Addressing these fallacies requires 1 key understanding -that for patients to be diagnosed with nervous system Lyme disease they must have (**Box 2**) both nervous system disease and Lyme disease and there must be a rational basis for believing the two are causally linked.

Requirement #1: Nervous System Disease

An underlying premise of neurology is that neurologic disease is caused by structural damage to the nervous system at either a macroscopic or microscopic level. The clinical signs and symptoms of nervous system disorders can vary widely, reflecting the specific structures involved and the severity of the damage. One patient with a stroke on MRI imaging may have no demonstrable symptoms, but another may be incapacitated with a hemiparesis and aphasia. The range of clinical presentations does not reflect a biological mystery but rather that, for any given pathophysiologic process, the size, site, and severity of damage may vary widely. However, if considered within a logical framework, specific patterns are usually evident and can be helpful in inferring an appropriate differential diagnosis, pathophysiology, and therapy.

This framework typically begins with categorization based on either structural or functional neuroanatomy. At its most basic, neuroanatomic localization begins with separating central nervous system (CNS) from peripheral nervous system (PNS)

Box 2
Prerequisites to diagnose nervous system Lyme disease

Objective evidence of:

- Lyme disease (erythema migrans, diagnostic testing)
- Nervous system disease
- Causal relation between the two
  - Syndrome within the clinical/pathophysiologic spectrum linked to Lyme disease

    And/or
  - In central nervous system (CNS) disorders, evidence of CNS inflammation and intrathecal antibody production

disorders. Primary nervous system disorders usually affect the CNS or the PNS, only rarely both, frequently with localizing patterns within the affected system. A single localized site of a CNS lesion suggests, in the appropriate context, a stroke, tumor, or other structural abnormality. Localization of a single PNS lesion suggests a nerve entrapment, nerve root irritation, or other focal abnormality. Recognition that a disorder involves the meninges suggests an infectious, hemorrhagic, or rarely neoplastic cause. Involvement of function-related populations of neurons can point to specific neurodegenerative processes, such as amyotrophic lateral sclerosis (upper and lower motor neurons) and Parkinson disease (substantia nigra).

In contrast with these localizable primary disorders of the nervous system, systemic illnesses often affect the nervous system in a more widespread fashion. Despite being well protected mechanically by the skull and vertebral column and physiologically by the blood-brain and blood-nerve barriers, the CNS and PNS are occasionally involved in systemic inflammatory or infectious processes. Some infectious agents have developed highly specific mechanisms to invade the nervous system. In some circumstances, circulating immune molecules and cells, although normally excluded from the nervous system, enter the CNS and PNS and contribute to damage. Consequently the absence of a well-defined anatomic pattern usually suggests a disseminated process, such as the immune dysregulation of Guillain-Barré syndrome, or the widespread involvement of CNS and PNS in vasculitis or diabetic vasculopathy.

In contrast, many systemic illnesses can affect behavior without causing CNS damage. From psychiatric disease to altered mental status in hypoglycemia, there is a broad range of biochemical, medical, environmental, and physiologic alterations that affect behavior but are not neurologic. One of the most frequently seen in medicine is the encephalopathy that accompanies a systemic inflammatory state. Patients with pneumonia, particularly if older, can easily develop delirium, which does not indicate CNS infection but is the effect of fever and circulating cytokines on the nervous system.

Requirement #2: Lyme Disease Involving the Nervous System

The diagnosis of Lyme disease is well addressed elsewhere in this issue; the diagnosis of nervous system Lyme disease requires compelling evidence that the patient has Lyme disease, and also has causally related nervous system involvement. European and US neurologists have adopted slightly different diagnostic criteria for neuroborreliosis (**Boxes 3** and **4**)[7,8] but differences relate more to emphasis than substance.

Neuroborreliosis occurs with any of the 3 most common strains of *B burgdorferi* (*B burgdorferi* sensu stricto, *Borrelia garinii*, and *Borrelia afzelii*). In Europe, neuroborreliosis seems to be more common with *B garinii* than *B afzelii*.[9] *B burgdorferi* sensu stricto rarely causes neuroborreliosis in Europe, but it is an infrequent human

---

Box 3
European Federation of Neurological Societies (EFNS) criteria for the diagnosis of neuroborreliosis

1. Neurologic disorder within the spectrum of those known to be caused by neuroborreliosis without other apparent cause

2. CSF pleocytosis

3. Intrathecal antibody production

Definite neuroborreliosis if 3 out of 3; possible if 2 out of 3.
   Data from Mygland A, Ljostad U, Fingerle V, et al. EFNS guidelines on the diagnosis and management of European Lyme neuroborreliosis. Eur J Neurol 2010;17:8–16, e1–4.

> **Box 4**
> **American Academy of Neurology criteria for the diagnosis of neuroborreliosis (update in progress)**
>
> 1. Possible exposure to *Ixodes* ticks in Lyme-endemic area
> 2. One or more of the following:
>   a. Erythema migrans
>   b. Histopathologic, microbiologic, or polymerase chain reaction proof of *B burgdorferi* infection
>   c. Immunologic evidence of exposure to *B burgdorferi*
> 3. Occurrence of a clinical disorder within the realm of those associated with Lyme disease, without other apparent cause
>
> *Data from* Halperin J, Logigian E, Finkel M, et al. Practice parameter for the diagnosis of patients with nervous system Lyme borreliosis (Lyme disease). Neurology 1996;46:619–27.

pathogen there. In the United States, where Lyme disease is caused solely by *B burgdorferi* sensu stricto, neuroborreliosis occurs in about 12% of untreated infected patients,[10] which is essentially the same proportion as described in Europe. Although much is made of the differences between European and US *B burgdorferi* infection symptoms, from a neurologic perspective they are remarkably similar. US patients probably more often have multifocal erythema migrans and arthritis, but the range and frequency of neurologic manifestations seem to be similar.

Once the diagnosis of Lyme disease is established, it is helpful to recognize the common neurologic presentations of this infection. Nervous system involvement most commonly occurs early in infection and is acute in nature; as a result, most patients present in warm weather months when ticks are most likely to feed.[10] Because neurologic symptoms, by definition, require disseminated infection, which takes time to develop, peripheral blood serologic testing is much more likely to be positive than in erythema migrans. Serologies are often markedly positive often with a prominent immunoglobulin (Ig) M component. Very rarely, neurologic symptoms precede development of a measurable antibody response,[11] so convalescent serologies may be necessary.

Although the neurologic manifestations of neuroborreliosis are often described as protean, this is no more meaningful than it is in any systemic disorder affecting the nervous system. Although Lyme disease can affect any nervous system structure, there are meaningful patterns, presumably reflecting the ability of *B burgdorferi*, and the host response to it, to affect specific parts of the nervous system preferentially. Recognition of these patterns is useful in diagnosis.

Involvement can conveniently be considered (**Box 5**, **Tables 1** and **2**) to affect 1 or more of 3 separate compartments: the meninges and subarachnoid space, the PNS,

> **Box 5**
> **Alterations of nervous system function in Lyme disease**
>
> • Focal/multifocal PNS inflammation/infection (common)
> • Diffuse meningeal inflammation (common)
> • Focal/multifocal CNS inflammation/infection (rare)
> • Chronic low-grade encephalopathy in the absence of nervous system infection or inflammation

Table 1
PNS disorders associated with Lyme disease

Pathophysiology	Clinical Presentation
Mononeuropathy multiplex	Cranial neuropathy (particularly VII)
	Radiculoneuropathy (painful mono- or oligoradiculopathy)
	Brachial plexopathy
	Mononeuropathy
	Mononeuropathy multiplex
	Confluent mononeuropathy multiplex (mimicking diffuse axonal polyneuropathy)
	Possibly acute inflammatory demyelinating polyneuropathy (rare if ever)

and the parenchymal CNS. The classic triad of neuroborreliosis (meningitis, cranial neuritis, and radiculoneuritis) involves the meninges and the PNS; parenchymal CNS involvement is rare.

Subarachnoid space

Just as in Garin and Bujadoux's[5] patient, a CSF pleocytosis (the defining characteristic of meningitis) is common, being found in 5% to 10% of infected, untreated patients. The pleocytosis is typically lymphocyte predominant with modest numbers of white cells per cubic millimeter (50–200), normal CSF glucose level, and modest protein concentration increase. Symptoms vary widely. Some patients with bland CSF have severe headaches, photophobia, and meningismus; others, such as the one described by Garin and Bujadoux,[5] have a significant pleocytosis but no symptoms typical of meningitis. Because neuroborreliosis typically occurs in warm weather months, the most common concern in endemic areas is whether a given patient's aseptic meningitis is caused by Lyme disease or an enteroviral infection. Although clinical algorithms[12–14] have been proposed to differentiate between these two, the most useful element of these is the presence of other components of the triad; particularly a cranial neuropathy or radiculoneuropathy. In endemic areas the occurrence of either of these in a patient with clinically symptomatic meningitis should lead to a preliminary diagnosis of neuroborreliosis.

More specific diagnosis of Lyme meningitis usually depends on indirect diagnostic evidence, in particular measurement of the intrathecal antibody response (discussed later). Although *B burgdorferi* sensu lato can be cultured, culture of these slowly reproducing organisms is rarely clinically helpful. Even when technically feasible, CSF cultures are only positive in about 10% of definite cases of Lyme meningitis. Using polymerase chain reaction (PCR)–based testing improves sensitivity minimally. Given

Table 2
CNS disorders associated with Lyme disease

Pathophysiology	Clinical Presentation
Inflammation in subarachnoid space	Meningitis
	Pseudotumor cerebri–like (children)
Parenchymal CNS inflammation and presumably infection	Short segmental spinal cord inflammation in Garin-Bujadoux Bannwarth syndrome (primarily in European patients)
	Encephalomyelitis (active brain inflammation with focally abnormal neurologic examination and MRI imaging with inflammatory CSF; extremely rare)

the technical sensitivity of PCR, the number of organisms in CSF is presumably so small that they are not present in the obtained samples.

The other CSF-space disorder linked to neuroborreliosis, primarily in children, is pseudotumor cerebri. The clinical presentation is typical, with headaches, papilledema, increased intracranial pressure, and visual obscurations. Visual loss can occur, so accurate, timely diagnosis and treatment are critically important.[15] Virtually all reported children have had a significant CSF pleocytosis at the time of presentation, suggesting that it would be more accurate to think of these patients as having Lyme meningitis with secondarily increased intracranial pressure (ICP), rather than true pseudotumor. This distinction is probably prognostically important, because the increased ICP of meningitis may be more self-limited than pseudotumor. Regardless, immediate management needs to address both the causative infection and the increased pressure.

Peripheral nervous system

Peripheral and cranial nerves are both frequently involved. Facial nerve (seventh cranial nerve, controlling facial muscle function) paresis is the most commonly recognized, probably accounting for three-quarters of patients with cranial nerve involvement, and can be bilateral in up to a quarter of affected individuals.

Facial nerve palsy consists of marked paresis or paralysis of 1 side of the face, including lip movement, eye closure, and forehead wrinkling. Patients occasionally receive this diagnosis based on a subtle, often subjective, sense of facial asymmetry, or even facial paresthesias. Neither of these warrants a diagnosis of seventh nerve palsy. Most patients with facial nerve palsies (of any cause) describe pain behind the ear ipsilateral to the palsy, often preceding weakness by a day or two. Hyperacusis on the symptomatic side is common, as is a perceived (but often difficult for the patient to characterize) alteration in the sense of taste.

Idiopathic facial nerve palsy is uncommon in young children; bilateral facial palsies are uncommon at any age, occurring primarily in Lyme disease, sarcoid, human immunodeficiency virus infection, other less common basal meningitides, and Guillain-Barré syndrome. In Lyme-endemic areas in warm weather months, it is reasonable to entertain a preliminary diagnosis of Lyme disease, and even to begin antibiotic treatment pending serologic test results, in adults with otherwise unexplained bilateral facial palsies or young children with either unilateral or bilateral facial palsies.

Other cranial neuropathies occur much less frequently and are insufficiently predictive of a diagnosis of Lyme disease to warrant even a preliminary diagnosis. The nerves to the extraocular muscles (III, IV, and VI) can be involved, causing diplopia. Occasionally the trigeminal nerve (V) can be involved, causing unilateral facial paresthesias, pain, and/or hypoesthesia. The acoustovestibular (VIII) nerve is involved occasionally as well, affecting hearing and balance. Involvement of the lower cranial nerves (IX–XII) is highly uncommon. The optic nerve (II; technically a CNS tract and not a peripheral nerve) is involved so rarely that it is questionable whether the anecdotal reports are anything but coincidental.[16,17]

The radiculoneuropathy of Lyme disease is probably the most commonly misdiagnosed form of nervous system involvement. As described by Garin and Bujadoux,[5] patients present with severe, often intractable, neuropathic pain, typically in a radicular distribution, often involving 1 but occasionally several contiguous dermatomes. The European literature suggests that this most often affects the limb that was the site of the tick bite; there are insufficient data in the United States to know whether that is the case with *B burgdorferi* sensu stricto infection.

Pain is identical in character to that of mechanical radiculopathies: superficial, burning, or shocklike, and often with hyperpathia. Typically there are sensory, motor (eg, the deltoid weakness and atrophy in Garin and Bujadoux's[5] patient), and reflex changes appropriate to the involved dermatome. Symptoms can involve the trunk; as in diabetic truncal neuropathies, this often leads to a focus on possible visceral causes of the pain, resulting in prolonged pursuit of other irrelevant diagnoses. As in patients with Lyme disease–associated cranial neuropathies there is often, but not invariably, an accompanying CSF pleocytosis, which may help in guiding the diagnosis.[18] When a patient in an endemic area in warm weather months develops otherwise unexplained radicular symptoms or symptoms with no relevant changes on spine imaging, the diagnosis of Lyme radiculoneuropathy should be seriously considered.

In approximately the same time frame as the acute radicular symptoms, patients may develop other acute focal PNS symptoms. Brachial and lumbosacral plexopathies occur, as do acute mononeuropathies. Occasionally patients have clinical evidence of multiple mononeuropathies, a picture usually associated with a vasculitic process, and rarely (in developed countries) in infectious neuropathies such as leprosy. Detailed neurophysiologic studies in large numbers of patients with PNS neuroborreliosis indicate that all these presentations (cranial neuropathies, radiculopathies, plexopathies, and mononeuropathies) represent varying presentations of a mononeuropathy multiplex.[19] Rare patients have been described with an acute presentation resembling the Guillain-Barré syndrome.[20] Only 1 small series[20] from a Lyme-endemic area suggested this was an acute demyelinating polyneuropathy. Because other studies of PNS neuroborreliosis do not suggest demyelination, the implication of these isolated observations remains unclear.

Early in the development of the understanding of Lyme disease, patients who had been undiagnosed and untreated for several years presented with more indolent neuropathic symptoms, typically stocking-glove numbness, paresthesias, and occasionally weakness and reflex changes.[21] Neurophysiologic testing in such individuals showed a confluent mononeuropathy multiplex (the same pathophysiologic process found in acute Lyme radiculoneuropathy) and changes improved following antimicrobial treatment.[19,22] Because it is now uncommon to see patients who have had long-standing untreated Lyme disease, this entity is now seen rarely, if ever. Patients presenting with nothing but acral paresthesias, who lack any objective evidence of PNS dysfunction, should not be diagnosed with PNS neuroborreliosis, or a neuropathy of any kind.

Parenchymal central nervous system involvement

Patients with European neuroborreliosis-associated radicular symptoms may have findings that indicate spinal cord involvement at the same spinal level as the symptomatic nerve root, suggesting contiguous spread of the inflammatory process. This condition has been observed anecdotally in the United States but systematic data are unavailable. Other than this, parenchymal CNS involvement is very unusual. Reports in the 1980s and 1990s primarily involved patients with long-standing untreated infection,[23] which occurs rarely today. Occasional patients with acute to subacute focal encephalitis have been described. Affected individuals have all had focally abnormal brain MRI scans; abnormalities more commonly, but not exclusively, affecting white matter than gray. Clinical neurologic examinations are significantly abnormal, with findings congruous with the MRI abnormalities. Brain PET and single-photon emission computed tomography scans have found hypermetabolism in the affected areas.[24] CSF is invariably inflammatory, typically with increased IgG synthesis and oligoclonal bands, which are findings seen in other chronic CNS infections such as neurosyphilis and subacute sclerosing panencephalitis. The increased production of antibodies within the CNS in these patients typically specifically targets the causative organism (ie, there is increased intrathecal synthesis of organism-specific antibody).

Behavioral change without central nervous system infection: Lyme encephalopathy
Patients with serious infections not directly affecting the CNS, such as pneumonia or sepsis; inflammatory states such as lupus or active rheumatoid arthritis; or even individuals receiving immunomodulatory therapy such as interferons commonly describe marked fatigue and cognitive difficulty. In most instances this relates to physiologic effects on the CNS and not anything that would be considered nervous system involvement or a neurologic process. The state is generally reversible with elimination (or suppression) of the causative process and has no long-term neurologic implications.

In the 1980s and 1990s, when diagnosis and treatment of Lyme disease were still inconsistent, it was common to see patients with several years of relapsing, primarily rheumatologic symptoms who were then diagnosed with Lyme disease, were treated, and improved. Before treatment, many experienced fatigue and cognitive slowing that interfered with their daily functioning.[21,25,26] Detailed investigations found:

1. Their perceived difficulties were quantifiable and verifiable with formal neuropsychological testing
2. In most instances neurologic examinations, brain MRI and CSF examinations were normal
3. The state was reversible with antibiotic therapy

Nothing about the state was considered unique or diagnostic of Lyme disease; this was viewed as an opportunity to better understand this commonplace phenomenon in patients in whom the symptoms were both persistent and not particularly time varying (and therefore measurable), and also reversible with treatment. Exhaustive studies found evidence of CNS infection (past or present) in a few but nothing to suggest this in most. The entity was labeled Lyme encephalopathy to distinguish it from Lyme encephalitis; the latter term being reserved for individuals with brain infection.[27]

Some clinicians took this ubiquitous symptom complex to be diagnostic of Lyme disease and began treating such patients, in the absence of anything else to suggest this infection, with ever more aggressive courses of antibiotics. The epidemiology of Lyme disease and of this symptom complex makes the futility of this approach obvious. The annual incidence of cases of Lyme disease confirmed by the US Centers for Disease Control and Prevention is approximately 0.01% (although some recent estimates suggest 10 times that number of patients may be treated for the diagnosis[28]). Population studies suggest that, at any given time, 2% of the population experiences these symptoms to a disabling extent.[29] This finding suggests that no more than 1 in 200 (or possibly 1 in 20) patients with these symptoms might have Lyme disease, indicating that the symptoms have no predictive value for the diagnosis of Lyme disease. Despite this, the notion that patients with this symptom complex have Lyme disease and require prolonged antibiotic (and other) treatment is one of the major drivers of the Lyme controversy.

Requirement #3: Causal Relationship Between Lyme Disease and the Neurologic Process

The third element in diagnosing a patient with nervous system Lyme disease is the plausibility of their nervous system disease and their Lyme disease being causally related. Laboratory support can be challenging. Serologies, particularly using 2-tier testing, have high sensitivity and specificity beyond the first few weeks of infection, but, like any antibody-based measure, can remain elevated long after microbiologic cure.

CSF studies can be more helpful but have distinct limitations as well. The approach that is most helpful is measurement of intrathecal antibody production (production of specific antibody within the CNS). There are technically several different ways of quantifying this; all rely on finding proportionately more specific anti–B burgdorferi antibody in CSF than in serum. All require measuring both specific and total antibody in serum and CSF and determining whether there is proportional excess in CSF. It is essential to recognize that simply measuring CSF antibody by itself is uninformative if either the peripheral blood specific antibody level is increased, or if there is increased blood-brain barrier permeability. Either of these circumstances results in artifactually increased CSF antibody measures that are not necessarily evidence of intrathecal antibody production.

There are several important limitations of this approach. Most importantly if there is no CNS infection, there should be no expectation that CSF will be informative. Specifically, if the patient's Lyme disease does not affect the nervous system, or if their neuroborreliosis is limited to the PNS, or if their only neurologic symptom is fatigue and cognitive slowing with an otherwise normal neurologic evaluation, CSF will predictably be normal. The technique is useful in patients with demonstrable inflammatory CNS disease; however, in the absence of another gold standard diagnostic test for CNS infection, estimates of the sensitivity of this measure in true CNS neuroborreliosis vary from 50% to nearly 100%.

Two observations related to the time course of the intrathecal antibody response are particularly problematic. As with peripheral blood serologies, patients have been found to have increased intrathecal antibody production for a decade or more following clearly successful treatment.[30] At the other extreme, European series describe patients with very early infection in whom CSF antibodies are increased before peripheral blood antibody is detectable. This finding has been observed very rarely in the United States but, if a patient has a clinically compatible acute (symptoms of <3–6 weeks' duration) disorder in which the CNS is likely involved, a CSF examination with measurement of the CSF/serum Lyme antibody index might be informative.

These issues notwithstanding, there are several ways this measurement is clearly useful. In a patient with an active CNS inflammatory process (eg, a picture that resembles multiple sclerosis), whose CSF is clearly inflammatory with increased total antibody production, if the process is caused by this infection, it can be reliably assumed that the antibodies present should be specific for B burgdorferi. Similarly, and by analogy to neurosyphilis, if the antibodies are being produced in response to an infection, the more general evidence of the immune response to the infection (CSF pleocytosis and increased protein levels) should slowly normalize following successful treatment, regardless of whether or not clones of B cells and plasma cells continue to produce specific antibody, providing a means of determining whether the intrathecal antibody production is evidence of current versus prior infection.

Beyond this laboratory support for CNS infection, inferring causality must rely on a logical approach. If the patient's neurologic symptoms are within the range of those described in Lyme disease, and epidemiologic, serologic, and other clinical data support the diagnosis, then prudence dictates treatment. If the disorder is outside the realm of disorders known to be causally related, but other data support the diagnosis, then careful case-by-case deliberation, including considering biological plausibility, are in order.

Treatment

Although treatment is dealt with in detail elsewhere, treatment of nervous system infection requires special comment (**Box 6**). The initial use of high-dose parenteral

---

Box 6
Treatment of nervous system Lyme disease in adults

Acute neuroborreliosis (meningitis, radiculitis, cranial neuritis)

Ceftriaxone,[a] 2 g/d intravenously for 2 to 4 weeks, or

Cefotaxime, 2 g intravenously every 8 hours for 2 to 4 weeks, or

Penicillin, 20 million to 24 million units/d intravenously for 2 to 4 weeks

Or

Probably doxycycline[b] 100 mg orally twice to 4 times a day for 3 to 4 weeks

Possible alternatives:

    Amoxicillin, 500 mg orally 3 times a day for 21 days, or

    Cefuroxime axetil, 500 mg orally twice a day for 21 days

Encephalomyelitis or treatment failure

Intravenous ceftriaxone[a] or cefotaxime or intravenous penicillin (as listed earlier)

  [a] Ceftriaxone should not be used late in pregnancy.
  [b] Doxycycline should not be used in pregnant women, or children with Lyme disease before the age of 8 years.

---

penicillin, then ceftriaxone, was based on the presumption that in some patients the presence of CNS infection required treatment with regimens known to achieve high levels in the CSF. Numerous European studies have now convincingly shown that oral doxycycline is as effective as parenteral regimens in patients with Lyme meningitis, cranial neuritis, and radiculoneuritis.[31,32] Although there are no studies of amoxicillin or cefuroxime axetil, innumerable patients with Lyme disease have been treated with these regimens and none has progressed to develop neuroborreliosis, which suggests that these are effective as well.

There are no high-level studies addressing the use of oral regimens in the rare individuals who have parenchymal CNS infection. However, there is at least 1 longitudinal study supporting the role of oral doxycycline in treatment of these patients as well.[33] As more data are accrued in coming years it may be that oral treatment will be considered appropriate first-line treatment in all but the most severely affected patients with neuroborreliosis.

SUMMARY

The CNS or PNS may be involved in up to 15% of patients with untreated infection with *B burgdorferi*. The efficacy of antimicrobial therapy (which is curative in almost all patients) in reversing the resulting disorders supports the hypothesis that these are caused by direct infection of the nervous system and not by immune or other indirect mechanisms. Neurologic involvement often includes meningitis (inflammation of the meninges) and/or multifocal inflammatory changes in peripheral nerves or, rarely, in the brain or spinal cord. PNS involvement most often presents as a cranial neuropathy, particularly the facial nerve, or other peripheral mononeuropathies. Other peripheral mononeuropathies frequently present as painful dysfunction of one or several spinal nerve roots, mimicking a mechanical radiculopathy. All but the most severely affected patients with neuroborreliosis respond well to oral antimicrobial therapy.

REFERENCES

1. Halperin JJ, Baker P, Wormser GP. Common misconceptions about Lyme disease. Am J Med 2013;126:264.e1–7.
2. Halperin JJ. Lyme disease – neurology, neurobiology and behavior. Clin Infect Dis 2014;58:1267–72.
3. Steere AC, Pachner AR, Malawista SE. Neurologic abnormalities of Lyme disease: successful treatment with high-dose intravenous penicillin. Ann Intern Med 1983;99:767–72.
4. Reik L, Steere AC, Bartenhagen NH, et al. Neurologic abnormalities of Lyme disease. Medicine 1979;58:281–94.
5. Garin C, Bujadoux A. Paralysie par les tiques. J Med Lyon 1922;71:765–7.
6. Hollstrom E. Successful treatment of erythema migrans Afzelius. Acta Derm Venereol 1951;31:235–43.
7. Halperin J, Logigian E, Finkel M, et al. Practice parameter for the diagnosis of patients with nervous system Lyme borreliosis (Lyme disease). Neurology 1996;46:619–27.
8. Mygland A, Ljostad U, Fingerle V, et al. EFNS guidelines on the diagnosis and management of European Lyme neuroborreliosis. Eur J Neurol 2010;17: 8–16 e1–4.
9. Ogrinc K, Lotric-Furlan S, Maraspin V, et al. Suspected early Lyme neuroborreliosis in patients with erythema migrans. Clin Infect Dis 2013;57:501–9.
10. Bacon RM, Kugeler KJ, Mead PS. Surveillance for Lyme Disease – United States, 1992–2006. MMWR Morb Mortal Wkly Rep 2008;57:1–9.
11. Halperin JJ, Golightly M. Lyme borreliosis in Bell's palsy. Long Island Neuroborreliosis Collaborative Study Group. Neurology 1992;42:1268–70.
12. Tuerlinckx D, Bodart E, Garrino MG, et al. Clinical data and cerebrospinal fluid findings in Lyme meningitis versus aseptic meningitis. Eur J Pediatr 2003;162: 150–3.
13. Shah SS, Zaoutis TE, Turnquist J, et al. Early differentiation of Lyme from enteroviral meningitis. Pediatr Infect Dis J 2005;24:542–5.
14. Garro AC, Rutman M, Simonsen K, et al. Prospective validation of a clinical prediction model for Lyme meningitis in children. Pediatrics 2009;123:e829–34.
15. Kan L, Sood SK, Maytal J. Pseudotumor cerebri in Lyme disease: a case report and literature review. Pediatr Neurol 1998;18:439–41.
16. Sibony P, Halperin J, Coyle P, et al. Reactive Lyme serology in patients with optic neuritis and papilledema. J Neuroophthalmol 2005;25:71–82.
17. Blanc F, Ballonzoli L, Marcel C, et al. Lyme optic neuritis. J Neurol Sci 2010;295: 117–9.
18. Halperin JJ. Facial nerve palsy associated with Lyme disease. Muscle Nerve 2003;28:516–7.
19. Halperin JJ, Luft BJ, Volkman DJ, et al. Lyme neuroborreliosis - peripheral nervous system manifestations. Brain 1990;113:1207–21.
20. Muley SA, Parry GJ. Antibiotic responsive demyelinating neuropathy related to Lyme disease. Neurology 2009;72:1786–7.
21. Logigian EL, Kaplan RF, Steere AC. Chronic neurologic manifestations of Lyme disease. N Engl J Med 1990;323:1438–44.
22. Halperin JJ, Little BW, Coyle PK, et al. Lyme disease - a treatable cause of peripheral neuropathy. Neurology 1987;37:1700–6.
23. Ackermann R, Rehse KB, Gollmer E, et al. Chronic neurologic manifestations of erythema migrans borreliosis. Ann N Y Acad Sci 1988;539:16–23.

24. Kalina P, Decker A, Kornel E, et al. Lyme disease of the brainstem. Neuroradiology 2005;47:903–7.
25. Halperin JJ, Luft BJ, Anand AK, et al. Lyme neuroborreliosis: central nervous system manifestations. Neurology 1989;39:753–9.
26. Kaplan RF, Jones-Woodward L. Lyme encephalopathy: a neuropsychological perspective. Semin Neurol 1997;17:31–7.
27. Halperin JJ, Krupp LB, Golightly MG, et al. Lyme borreliosis-associated encephalopathy. Neurology 1990;40:1340–3.
28. Hinckley AF, Connally NP, Meek JI, et al. Lyme disease testing by large commercial laboratories in the United States. Clin Infect Dis 2014;59:676–81.
29. Luo N, Johnson J, Shaw J, et al. Self-reported health status of the general adult U.S. population as assessed by the EQ-5D and Health Utilities Index. Med Care 2005;43:1078–86.
30. Hammers Berggren S, Hansen K, Lebech AM, et al. *Borrelia burgdorferi*-specific intrathecal antibody production in neuroborreliosis: a follow-up study. Neurology 1993;43:169–75.
31. Halperin JJ, Shapiro ED, Logigian EL, et al. Practice parameter: treatment of nervous system Lyme disease. Neurology 2007;69:91–102.
32. Ljostad U, Skogvoll E, Eikeland R, et al. Oral doxycycline versus intravenous ceftriaxone for European Lyme neuroborreliosis: a multicentre, non-inferiority, double-blind, randomised trial. Lancet Neurol 2008;7:690–5.
33. Bremell D, Dotevall L. Oral doxycycline for Lyme neuroborreliosis with symptoms of encephalitis, myelitis, vasculitis or intracranial hypertension. Eur J Neurol 2014; 21:1162–7.

Lyme Carditis

Matthew L. Robinson, MD[a], Takaaki Kobayashi, MD[b],
Yvonne Higgins, PA, MAS, MS/ITS[b], Hugh Calkins, MD, FHRS[c], Michael T. Melia, MD[a],*

KEYWORDS

- Lyme carditis • Lyme disease • Heart block • AV block • Pericarditis

KEY POINTS

- Lyme carditis most commonly manifests as atrioventricular (AV) block.
- Lyme carditis is readily treatable with antibiotic therapy and supportive care measures.
- Although temporary pacemaker placement may be needed for patients with Lyme carditis manifesting as high-grade second- or third-degree AV block with debilitating symptoms and/or hemodynamic instability, permanent pacemaker placement is not recommended.

EPIDEMIOLOGY

Although Lyme disease is common in North America and Europe, affecting as many as 1 in 1000 people in certain American states and 1 in 300 people in parts of Southern Europe annually, its cardiac manifestations that predominantly include conduction disturbances affect only a small minority of patients.[1,2] Such conduction disturbances were first described in 1977, and in 1980 the term, Lyme carditis, was coined to describe the variety of cardiac abnormalities found in patients with Lyme disease.[3,4] Reported rates of cardiac involvement in incident Lyme disease have declined since the initial descriptions of Borrelia burgdorferi infection. In the mid-1980s, 10% of Lyme disease cases reported to the Centers for Disease Control and Prevention (CDC) included cardiac symptoms, but most of these cases consisted of palpitations alone.[5] Although standardized surveillance and reporting for Lyme disease cases began in 1991, reporting of clinical manifestations, including only second- or third-degree AV block among the cardiac manifestations, has since been optional.[6,7] Using this more narrow definition, 1.1% of Lyme disease cases reported to the CDC between 2001 and 2010 included cardiac manifestations.[8] The reported frequency of cardiac involvement in Europe has ranged from 1% to 2%.[9,10]

Disclosure Statement: None of the authors have anything to disclose.
[a] Division of Infectious Diseases, Department of Medicine, Johns Hopkins University, 1830 East Monument Street, Room 448, Baltimore, MD 21287, USA; [b] The Sherrilyn and Ken Fisher Center for Environmental Infectious Diseases, Division of Infectious Diseases, Department of Medicine, Johns Hopkins University, 725 North Wolfe Street, PTCB - Room 231, Baltimore, MD 21287, USA; [c] Division of Cardiology, Department of Medicine, Johns Hopkins University, 600 North Wolfe Street, Sheikh Zayed Tower, Room 7125R, Baltimore, MD 21287, USA
* Corresponding author. 1830 East Monument Street, #448, Baltimore, MD 21287.
E-mail address: mmelia4@jhmi.edu

Infect Dis Clin N Am 29 (2015) 255–268
http://dx.doi.org/10.1016/j.idc.2015.02.003
0891-5520/15/$ – see front matter © 2015 Elsevier Inc. All rights reserved.

id.theclinics.com

Although numbers of all Lyme disease cases are split almost evenly between the genders, Lyme carditis is more common among men, who constitute 65% of patients with cardiac manifestations reported to the CDC between 2001 and 2010.[8,11] A systematic review of Lyme-related third-degree heart block cases found that 84% of reported cases were male.[12] Although children as well as adults may develop Lyme carditis, pediatric cases are less common than adult cases.[8] Children under 14 years of age are least likely to come to attention with cardiac manifestations of Lyme disease.[8] The clinical manifestations, however, seem similar.[13]

PATHOGENESIS

Understanding of the pathogenesis of Lyme carditis has been obtained primarily from study of mouse models. After mice are inoculated with B burgdorferi, sacrificed murine hearts demonstrate peak inflammatory changes at 2 to 3 weeks. During the first month postinoculation, inflammatory infiltrates have been demonstrated within the connective tissue of the heart base, aortic root, atrial and ventricular epicardium, endocardium, myocardium, and perivascular spaces, with notable foci at the AV junction.[14,15] Unlike the neutrophil-predominant inflammation of Lyme arthritis, macrophages predominate in murine cardiac inflammation, and chemokines may play an important role recruiting macrophages to the heart.[14,16] Few lymphocytes and neutrophils have been observed in the heart; the presence of inflammatory cardiac infiltrates among class II major histocompatibility complex–deficient mice indicates that antigen presentation to CD4+ T lymphocytes is not essential to the pathogenesis of murine Lyme carditis.[14]

Demonstration of B burgdorferi spirochetes by indirect immunofluorescence in these mouse models has suggested the presence of active cardiac infection, and there is mounting evidence of B burgdorferi persisting in the extracellular matrix.[14,17] Using immunofluorescence, spirochetes have been identified in murine cardiac connective tissues, particularly at the AV junction, and in the epicardium and occasionally myocardium.[14,18]

In mouse models, B burgdorferi spirochetes undergo phagocytosis by macrophages. Recognition of B burgdorferi by the membrane-spanning Toll-like receptor 2 and the intracellular receptor Nod2 has been implicated in activating the innate inflammatory response by activating nuclear factor (NF)-κB, leading to cytokine release.[19,20] Unlike mouse models of Lyme arthritis wherein miR-146a helps to control inflammation through negative regulation of NF-κB signaling, NF-κB modulation by miR-146a was not shown to affect murine cardiac disease manifestations, further highlighting the complex, differential patterns of B burgdorferi–induced inflammation in different organ systems.[21]

Although lymphocytes comprise a small proportion of the cells within inflammatory infiltrates of Lyme carditis, invariant natural killer T (iNKT) cells also modify the inflammatory response to B burgdorferi infection of the heart. Transgenic mice without iNKT cells, for example, showed higher numbers of spirochetes invading cardiac tissue than those with iNKT cells. These iNKT cells have also been shown to localize to the heart after B burgdorferi infection and become activated by CD1d-expressing macrophages. Such activation of iNKT cells is believed to produce interferon gamma, which in turn leads to enhanced immunologic control of the infection and modulation of the inflammatory response by increasing both the phagocytic activity of macrophages and surface expression of CD1d.[22]

Although inflammation and spirochete infiltration is seen in murine Lyme carditis models, few studies have evaluated for functional effects of these phenomena on the cardiac conduction system. In a study of 76 mice infected with *B burgdorferi* and negative controls, infected mice were found to have wider QRS complexes than control mice, but no conduction abnormalities at the level of the AV node were seen despite the widespread epicardial and subepicardial inflammation at the base of the heart, in the atria, in the basal interventricular septum, and in the perivascular regions.[23]

DEMONSTRATION OF MYOCARDIAL INVOLVEMENT IN HUMANS

Pathologic features of Lyme carditis in humans have been described in small numbers of patients who have undergone myocardial biopsy or autopsy. In the few patients whose deaths were attributed to Lyme carditis, autopsies showed infiltration of the endocardium, myocardium, and pericardium with lymphocytes, plasma cells, and macrophages. Perivascular inflammation has been prominent in most cases reported within the United States, and interstitial infiltration and inflammation have been observed in 1 patient from Austria and in another with an extensive travel history.[24–27] One case of a patient from the United Kingdom was notable for fibrinous pericarditis, endocardial fibrosis, and endodermal heterotopia of the AV node.[28]

As part of the evaluation of unexplained cardiogenic shock, 3 children who were ultimately diagnosed with Lyme carditis underwent diagnostic endomyocardial biopsies that demonstrated extensive, predominantly lymphocytic infiltrates with myocyte damage and necrosis. There was a small predominance of B lymphocytes over T lymphocytes, and plasma cells were present.[13] Adults with complete heart block who have undergone biopsies have also been shown to have lymphoplasmacytic infiltration of the endocardium and perivascular myocardium, with varying degrees of myocyte injury.[29–31] Evidence of cardiac inflammation has also been demonstrated by indium 111–monoclonal antimyosin antibody scanning, MRI, and gallium scanning.[27,29–33] In pathologic examinations of cardiac tissue, the presence of *B burgdorferi* has been variably proved by polymerase chain reaction (PCR) and direct visualization of spirochetes.[13,25,27,34,35]

CLINICAL MANIFESTATIONS

Although there is pathologic evidence of diffuse carditis in mouse models and case reports of myocardial injury on human biopsy specimens, a vast majority of Lyme carditis that come to clinical attention involve a fairly narrow spectrum of manifestations; these predominantly include derangements of cardiac conduction, including varying degrees of heart block (**Box 1**).[36,37] This array of clinical manifestations arises within a prescribed timeline after initial infection.

Usually, Lyme disease first manifests in an early, localized stage with the characteristic erythema migrans (EM) rash a median of 12 days (range 5–48 days) after acquisition of infection owing to a tick bite.[10] A flulike illness with fever often accompanies this rash. These signs and symptoms of early, localized disease, including the EM rash, typically resolve after 3 to 4 weeks even without antibiotic therapy.[34] Several weeks to months after infection acquisition, involvement of organ systems, such as the cardiac or neurologic systems, may come to attention among untreated patients as part of early disseminated disease.[38]

These cardiac disease manifestations typically arise 2 to 5 weeks after the EM rash appears, but cardiac pathology may come to attention as few as 2 days or as many as 7 months after initial infection.[4,12,39] Patients who develop Lyme disease–related complete heart block may first manifest some degree of AV block a median of 14 days (range 2–24 days) after the onset of any Lyme disease symptom.[12] Only

---

Box 1
Manifestations of Lyme carditis

Most common

Conduction system disturbances

- Heart block (any degree)—most common
- Atrial fibrillation
- Bundle branch block
- Intraventricular conduction delay
- Prolonged QTc interval
- Supraventricular tachycardia
- Ventricular tachycardia

Infrequent

Myocarditis

Myopericarditis

Pericarditis

Rare

Acute heart failure (cardiogenic shock)

Possible (further confirmation needed)

Chronic DCM

Infective endocarditis

Recurrent pericardial effusions

---

one-third of patients, however, who developed Lyme carditis remembers having a tick bite.[35]

Because the time course for resolution of the EM rash overlaps with the timeline for cardiac disease manifestations, some but not all patients who present with Lyme carditis may have a concurrent EM rash. Additional signs and symptoms may be present as well. For example, in the initial description of Lyme carditis before antibiotics were routinely prescribed, at the onset of cardiac symptoms, 79% of patients still had skin lesions, 68% had joint involvement, 53% were febrile, and 37% had neurologic symptoms.[4] In 2 case series of Lyme carditis, 44% to 85% of reported cases were associated with an EM rash concurrent with the carditis or at some point during the illness.[12,39]

In carditis cases reported to CDC, 69% had palpitations.[5] The frequency of cardiopulmonary symptoms described in a systematic review of 45 patients with complete heart block included such anticipated problems as syncope (40%), lightheadedness (33%), dyspnea (33%), palpitations (22%), and chest pain (20%).[12] Other associated symptoms included arthralgia (6%), headache (18%), and fever (36%).[12]

Disease manifestations and symptoms among children are similar to those experienced by adults. In a series of 207 children admitted to the hospital with early disseminated Lyme disease, carditis defined by ECG changes, myocardial dysfunction, or pericarditis was found in 33 (16%), second- or third-degree heart block meeting the CDC criteria for cardiac involvement was found in 7%, and 2% had complete heart block.[13] Of these 33 children ages greater than 10 years with Lyme carditis, 18%

had palpitations, 6% dyspnea, 15% chest pain, 12% syncope, 6% near syncope, and 42% any cardiopulmonary symptom.[13] In this series, arthralgia and any cardiopulmonary symptom were associated with the presence of carditis.[13]

RISK OF DEVELOPING CARDITIS

Carditis is a rare occurrence after a diagnosis of Lyme disease has been made. In the era before antibiotic treatment of Lyme disease, 2 of 55 (4%) prospectively followed patients with EM manifested cardiac involvement during a mean duration of 6 years of follow-up. One patient developed Wenckebach rhythm and the other complete heart block. Both were symptomatic.[3,40]

Although no study has ever proved that antibiotic therapy for Lyme disease prevents cardiac manifestations, in a study of 61 patients with EM, 1 had AV block on presentation (before initiation of antibiotics). Of 54 patients who underwent repeat ECG after a 20-day course of antibiotics, none developed new ECG abnormalities.[41] In another study of 118 patients who received antibiotics for EM, microbiologically confirmed as B burgdorferi infection, none developed cardiac symptoms.[42] Carditis is thus unlikely to occur as a complication of Lyme disease if antibiotics are given.

CONDUCTION SYSTEM DISEASE

In a compilation of 875 Lyme disease cases reported to the CDC from 1983 to 1986 wherein information about cardiac manifestations was provided, 84 cases of cardiac involvement were reported, including 16 (19%) with conduction defects.[5] Since that early case series, reporting guidelines have changed, such that currently only Lyme disease cases with associated second- or third-degree heart block are reported as having cardiovascular involvement for surveillance purposes.[7]

Because Lyme carditis is uncommon, most knowledge about the frequency with which patients experience cardiac conduction disturbances has been derived from case reports and series. In 1 early series of 52 cases of Lyme carditis, 45 (87%) patients had some degree of AV block, of whom 28 (62%) had high-grade or complete block.[39] In another series of 105 patients with Lyme carditis, 49% had third-degree heart block, 16% second-degree, and 12% first-degree.[35] The degree of AV block can fluctuate rapidly over minutes to hours and days.[34,39,43,44]

In the few electrophysiology studies of patients with Lyme carditis reported in the literature, AV block has usually been above the bundle of His in the AV node, but block frequently occurs simultaneously in multiple locations and may occur in the sinoatrial node, within the atrium, and in the bundle of His, bundle branches, and fascicles.[29,31,39,44,45] Bundle branch block and intraventricular conduction delay have also been reported; in 2 series, they occurred in 13% of Lyme carditis cases.[3,35,39,46]

For patients with high-grade or complete heart block, escape rhythms may be slow, with heart rates less than 40 beats per minute in 7 of 28 (25%) cases and wide complex QRS morphologies on ECG in 9 of 28 (32%) cases in 1 series.[39] Failure to generate an escape rhythm can result in prolonged periods of asystole.[29,39,45,47] Fortunately, AV block is a transient phenomenon. It typically resolves within 1 to 6 weeks in a stepwise progression from complete heart block, to Wenckebach AV block, to first-degree heart block, and on to decreasing PR interval back to normal.[39] Although patients with Lyme carditis are now treated with antibiotic therapy, resolution of the heart block without antibiotics has been described.[39] Examples of AV block in Lyme carditis patients are shown in Fig. 1.

Other arrhythmias have infrequently been attributed to Lyme disease (Fig. 2). Atrial fibrillation has rarely been reported.[46] Ventricular tachycardia has been reported in a

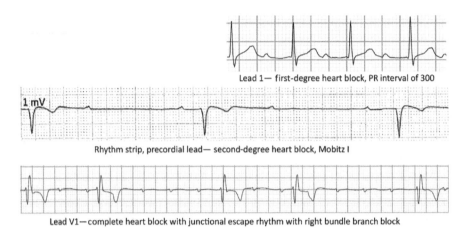

Lead 1— first-degree heart block, PR interval of 300

Rhythm strip, precordial lead— second-degree heart block, Mobitz I

Lead V1—complete heart block with junctional escape rhythm with right bundle branch block

Fig. 1. ECGs demonstrating AV block in patients with Lyme carditis. The first and third ECGs are from the same patient at different times. (*Courtesy of* Matthew Robinson, MD.)

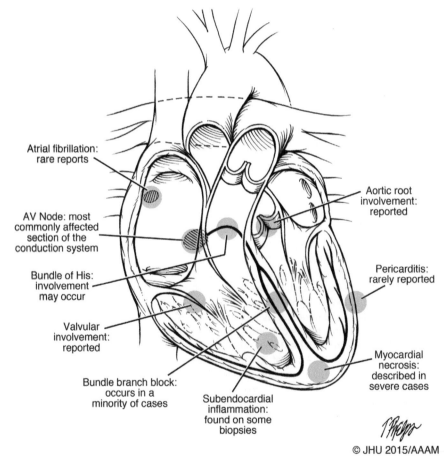

Atrial fibrillation: rare reports

AV Node: most commonly affected section of the conduction system

Bundle of His: involvement may occur

Valvular involvement: reported

Bundle branch block: occurs in a minority of cases

Subendocardial inflammation: found on some biopsies

Aortic root involvement: reported

Pericarditis: rarely reported

Myocardial necrosis: described in severe cases

© JHU 2015/AAAM

Fig. 2. Potential effects of *B burgdorferi* on cardiac tissue. (*Artwork copyright* Johns Hopkins University, 2015, created by Tim Phelps, MS, FAMI, Associate Professor and Medical Illustrator, Department of Art as Applied to Medicine.)

few cases, including 1 case that promptly followed antibiotic therapy and was attributed to a Jarisch-Herxheimer reaction.[47,48]

MYOPERICARDITIS AND VALVULAR DISEASE

Although myocardial inflammation is commonly seen on histopathologic analysis of cardiac tissue obtained via biopsy from patients with Lyme carditis, clinically apparent acute myocarditis is uncommon. Myocarditis was reported in only 8 of 84 (10%) cases reported to the CDC in a series from the mid-1980s.[5] Some patients thought to have symptoms attributable to conduction disease have also been found to have transiently and reversibly decreased left ventricular cardiac function; symptomatic myocarditis in such cases cannot be excluded.[39]

Signs and symptoms of Lyme myopericarditis have rarely been found to mimic acute coronary syndrome, with ECG ST segment elevations and elevated peripheral blood cardiac biomarkers; in such cases, echocardiography has shown diffuse ventricular hypokinesis rather than the focal wall motion abnormalities expected with an acute coronary syndrome.[33,49] Lyme disease is not thought to be a cause of severe congestive heart failure, although cases of acute heart failure have been reported.[48,50] Among children, cases of fulminant myocarditis leading to cardiogenic shock requiring extracorporeal membrane oxygenation have been published.[13,47] In the few cases of death attributable to Lyme carditis, extensive myocardial inflammation has been found at autopsy.[24–26]

Pericarditis seems even less common than myocarditis; it was reported in 2 of 84 (2%) reported cases of Lyme carditis.[5] Small pericardial effusions have been reported in some patients with Lyme carditis.[4] One case of pericarditis complicated by cardiac tamponade has been attributed to Lyme disease; the patient had positive serologic testing, and spirochetes were seen in pericardial fluid and synovium.[51]

Although Lyme disease is generally not thought of as a cause of valvular heart disease, reports of European-acquired B afzelli and B bissettii DNA have been found by PCR in explanted heart valves.[52,53] In another patient who was Lyme seropositive and underwent mitral valve replacement, lymphocytic infiltration of the explanted mitral leaflet and pericardium were found, although no spirochetes were seen.[54]

CHRONIC DILATED CARDIOMYOPATHY

Whether Lyme disease can cause chronic dilated cardiomyopathy (DCM) is controversial. In 1990, an Austrian group suggested a link between Lyme disease and idiopathic DCM after culturing B burgdorferi from a myocardial biopsy of a patient with idiopathic DCM and a positive Lyme serology.[55] Spirochetes were also identified by silver staining of endomyocardial biopsies obtained by the same group from DCM patients with B burgdorferi seropositivity.[56–58] This group also found that 19 of 72 (26%) consecutive patients with chronic heart failure due to DCM were seropositive for B burgdorferi by ELISA compared with 7 (13%) with coronary disease and 5 (8%) without heart disease.[56]

In a separate Austrian report of 42 patients with DCM, 9 (21%) were seropositive for B burgdorferi by ELISA, of whom 7 (17%) had a history of ECM. These 9 patients were treated with ceftriaxone for 2 weeks. Six patients recovered completely and showed a normal EF after 6 months, 2 had some improvement in left ventricular function, and 1 did not improve.[59]

Two separate Czech studies demonstrated evidence of B burgdorferi by PCR or electron microscopy on 21% to 24% of endomyocardial biopsy specimens taken from patients with recent-onset, unexplained DCM in an area in which Lyme disease is endemic.[60,61] No native hearts explanted from 15 patients undergoing cardiac transplantation for coronary artery disease were positive for *B burgdorferi* by PCR.[61]

Further investigations conducted in both Europe and America, however, have not reproduced these early studies. Among 175 patients in Minnesota, 125 (71%) of whom were from Lyme-endemic regions, 77 idiopathic cardiomyopathy patients did not have greater rates of seropositivity for Lyme disease than 73 patients with ischemic cardiomyopathy (8% vs 10%, respectively). Of 6 seropositive patients (including 2 with ischemic disease) treated with antibiotics, only 1 demonstrated a modest improvement in left ventricular ejection fraction, from 6% to 13%.[62] Another American study comparing current cardiac symptoms and ECG findings among 176 seropositive patients previously treated for Lyme disease and 160 seronegative controls found no differences between the 2 groups.[63] In another study conducted in Europe, 64 German patients with suspected inflammatory cardiomyopathy and IgM immunoblot positivity for *B burgdorferi* underwent endomyocardial biopsies, and none showed evidence of *B burgdorferi* DNA by PCR.[64]

Although isolation of *B burgdorferi* from a myocardial biopsy specimen taken from a patient with idiopathic DCM was a provocative finding, it has not been reproduced in the 25 years since these early reports. The serologic studies of Lyme disease (discussed previously) are also fraught with lack of specificity without immunoblot confirmation. Further clouding this picture, a recent nonhuman primate investigation demonstrated evidence of Lyme disease persistence by presence of *B burgdorferi* DNA, RNA transcripts, immunofluorescence assay, and hematoxylin-eosin staining 1 to 2 years after inoculation among several primates; in some cases, persistence was seen after antibiotic treatment.[65] Given these discrepant data and the geographic variability in incidence and causative *Borrelia* species, whether borrelia infection can cause chronic DCM remains uncertain; it is not inconceivable that a true clinical entity observed in 1 region may not be found in another.

DIAGNOSIS

Establishing a diagnosis of Lyme carditis can be difficult, because serologic testing for Lyme disease is incompletely reliable for the diagnosis of early disease in the first few weeks after acquiring infection. Furthermore, evidence supporting a diagnosis of cardiac involvement may be nonspecific. As with all manifestations of Lyme disease, epidemiologic risk for acquisition of *B burgdorferi* infection is essential. If the person has not been to a Lyme disease–endemic area within the past 6 months, a diagnosis of Lyme carditis can almost unequivocally be excluded.[1] If acquisition of infection is epidemiologically plausible and if the clinical manifestations are compatible with the diagnosis, serologic testing for Lyme disease should be performed. This is a first-tier screen, such as ELISA, which, if sufficiently elevated, is followed by *B burgdorferi*–specific immunoblots for IgM and IgG. Although this 2-tier diagnostic algorithm is standard of care, IgG immunoblot testing is poorly sensitive within the first 2 to 3 weeks after acquisition of infection and poorly specific in diagnosing cardiac disease, especially in high-prevalence areas where background seropositivity rates may be 4%.[1] In early illness, the presence or recent history of an EM rash may be used to diagnose Lyme disease. A majority of Lyme carditis patients in 1 series, however, did not have an EM rash.[12] The presence of other associated early Lyme disease symptoms, such as fever and arthralgia, may also suggest an infectious process, such as Lyme disease. Additional symptoms may help clinicians hone in on a diagnosis of Lyme carditis: lightheadedness, dizziness, syncope, and dyspnea were each present among greater than or equal to 33% of patients with complete heart block caused by *B burgdorferi* infection.[12] As such, Lyme disease complicated by carditis should be considered alongside infective endocarditis (with or without an aortic valve ring abscess causing heart block), acute myocarditis, and acute pericarditis in the infectious differential diagnosis for any patient with some combination of these signs and symptoms.

Although typically advanced heart block and positive Lyme serology bring most patients to proper diagnosis, other ECG changes may be witnessed, including a wide spectrum of AV block (described previously). In 1 of the early reports of Lyme carditis, 10% of cases included ECG ST segment depressions, and 50% showed T-wave inversions.[4] ST segment elevations may be present in cases of myopericarditis; other ST changes have also been seen but are nonspecific.[27,34] Echocardiographic findings are variable, with some cases showing minimal left ventricular or right ventricular dilatation, although most patients have normal-sized ventricles.[4,29,66] LV function is typically normal and without wall motion abnormalities, although patients with myopericarditis may show diffuse hypokinesis, and other patients with depressed left ventricular systolic function have been described.[4,5,29,32,49,66] Cardiac MRI may show areas of increased signal intensity and focal late gadolinium enhancement with subendocardial sparing in some cases.[27,32,33]

TREATMENT

On diagnosing Lyme carditis, a decision must be made regarding a need for inpatient hospitalization. Current guidelines recommend that any patient with cardiac symptoms, such as syncope, dyspnea, or chest pain; patients with first-degree heart block and a PR interval greater than or equal to 300 milliseconds; and patients with second- or third-degree heart block be admitted for continuous telemetry monitoring.[50] The rationale for admitting such a broad range of patients, including some with seemingly minor symptoms and ECG findings, is the highly variable course observed in some patients, including the possibility of rapid fluctuations in the severity of heart block.

The indication for placement of a temporary pacemaker in Lyme disease is the combination of high-grade second- or third-degree AV block with debilitating symptoms and/or hemodynamic instability. This indication is similar to that for other causes of heart block.[45] A recent review showed that transvenous pacing was required in 40% of patients with complete heart block.[12] Because of the transient nature of complete heart block in Lyme carditis, placement of a permanent pacemaker should not be performed, save for the most exceptional circumstances (eg, the advanced heart block does not resolve within 6 weeks). The 2008 American College of Cardiology/American Heart Association/Heart Rhythm Society Guidelines for Device-Based Therapy of Cardiac Rhythm Abnormalities specifically cite Lyme disease as a condition for which permanent pacemaker placement is not indicated because heart block is transient and resolves without expectation for recurrence over time.[67] For this reason it is listed as a class 3 indication (placement of a permanent pacemaker should not be performed).

Options for achieving temporary pacing include placement of a standard percutaneous temporary pacemaker lead attached to an external pacemaker or modified temporary transvenous pacing.[12,39,50,68] Modified temporary transvenous pacing refers to the placement of an active fixation permanent pacemaker lead into a patient and attaching it to a resterilized permanent pacemaker, which is used as a temporary external pacemaker and taped to the skin.[67] This modified approach allows patients to be hospitalized on a monitored floor without the need for bed rest, as is typically required for a conventional temporary pacemaker system. Permanent pacemaker implantation was undertaken in a handful of cases reported in the 1980s and early 1990s, with subsequent spontaneous resolution of complete heart block in all but 2 cases.[31,35,39,69]

All patients with Lyme carditis should receive at least a 14-day course of antibiotics; the treatment course may be extended up to 21 days. Although hospitalized patients should be treated with intravenous ceftriaxone, this recommendation is based on expert opinion alone; there are no data comparing oral versus intravenous antibiotic therapy in Lyme carditis. On resolution of concerning heart block and hospital discharge, usually the remainder of the treatment course may be completed with standard oral dosing of doxycycline, amoxicillin, or cefuroxime.[50] Although corticosteroids have previously been used, they are no longer a recommended treatment of Lyme carditis.[12,35,45,50]

PROGNOSIS

Lyme carditis has an excellent prognosis. In patients with third-degree heart block, the median time to improvement to first-degree heart block or normal sinus rhythm is 6 days (range 1–42 days).[12] Persistent heart block has been described after 7 weeks and 1 year of follow-up but is exceedingly rare.[31,69] Acute, but transient, worsening after initiation of antibiotics has rarely been reported and is attributed to a Jarisch-Herxheimer–like reaction.[48,66]

Although the prognosis of Lyme carditis is excellent, there have been some reports of attributed deaths.[8,24–26] All but 1 of these patients had antecedent symptoms suggesting acute borreliosis; the 1 patient for whom there was no available information regarding preceding symptoms had a history of underlying cardiac disease (hypertension and Wolff-Parkinson-White syndrome). Although these deaths highlight the importance of including early Lyme disease as a diagnostic consideration for patients with appropriate epidemiologic risk and a flulike illness and/or symptoms of acute myocarditis, sudden cardiac death without premonitory symptoms has not been described, and mortality related to Lyme carditis seems exceedingly rare. A review of US death certificates over a 4-year period found only 1 death likely due to Lyme disease.[70] After the 2013 report of 3 deaths from Lyme carditis, only 2 cases (0.001%) of suspected Lyme carditis–associated mortality were identified from 1696 cases of Lyme carditis reported to the CDC from 7 high-incidence states between 1995 and 2013.[8,26]

SUMMARY

Lyme disease is a common disease that uncommonly affects the heart. Because of the rarity of this diagnosis, and given the frequent absence of other concurrent clinical manifestations of early Lyme disease, consideration of Lyme carditis demands a high level of suspicion when patients in endemic areas come to attention with cardiovascular symptoms and evidence of higher-order heart block. When present, a majority of cases manifest as AV block ranging from asymptomatic first-degree heart block to complete heart block, with asystole requiring temporary pacemaker placement. Placement of a permanent pacemaker is not recommended. The degree of AV block in individual patients may fluctuate rapidly and unpredictably, necessitating inpatient telemetry monitoring for some patients. A minority of Lyme carditis cases have also been associated with myopericarditis. Although cases of genuine Lyme carditis–associated mortality have been described, exceedingly few deaths are attributable to this diagnosis. Like other manifestations of Lyme disease, carditis can readily be managed with antibiotic therapy and supportive care measures, such that affected patients almost always completely recover.

REFERENCES

1. Stanek G, Wormser GP, Gray J, et al. Lyme borreliosis. Lancet 2012;379(9814): 461–73.
2. Centers for Disease Control and Prevention (CDC). Reported cases of lyme disease by state or locality, 2004–2013. Available at: http://www.cdc.gov/lyme/stats/chartstables/reportedcases_statelocality.html. Accessed January 3, 2015.
3. Steere AC, Malawista SE, Hardin JA, et al. Erythema chronicum migrans and lyme arthritis. The enlarging clinical spectrum. Ann Intern Med 1977;86(6): 685–98.
4. Steere AC, Batsford WP, Weinberg M, et al. Lyme carditis: cardiac abnormalities of lyme disease. Ann Intern Med 1980;93(1):8–16.
5. Ciesielski CA, Markowitz LE, Horsley R, et al. Lyme disease surveillance in the united states, 1983–1986. Rev Infect Dis 1989;11(Suppl 6):S1435–41.
6. Wharton M, Chorba TL, Vogt RL, et al. Case definitions for public health surveillance. MMWR Recomm Rep 1990;39(RR-13):1–43.
7. Council of State and Territorial Epidemiologists. Public health reporting and national notification for lyme disease. Available at: http://c.ymcdn.com/sites/www.cste.org/resource/resmgr/PS/10-ID-06.pdf. Accessed January 3, 2015.
8. Forrester JD, Meiman J, Mullins J, et al. Notes from the field: update on lyme carditis, groups at high risk, and frequency of associated sudden cardiac death–united states. MMWR Morb Mortal Wkly Rep 2014;63(43):982–3.
9. Cimmino MA. Relative frequency of lyme borreliosis and of its clinical manifestations in Europe. European community concerted action on risk assessment in lyme borreliosis. Infection 1998;26(5):298–300.
10. Oschmann P, Dorndorf W, Hornig C, et al. Stages and syndromes of neuroborreliosis. J Neurol 1998;245(5):262–72.
11. Bacon RM, Kugeler KJ, Mead PS, Centers for Disease Control and Prevention (CDC). Surveillance for lyme disease–united states, 1992–2006. MMWR Surveill Summ 2008;57(10):1–9.
12. Forrester JD, Mead P. Third-degree heart block associated with lyme carditis: review of published cases. Clin Infect Dis 2014;59(7):996–1000.
13. Costello JM, Alexander ME, Greco KM, et al. Lyme carditis in children: presentation, predictive factors, and clinical course. Pediatrics 2009;123(5):e835–41.
14. Ruderman EM, Kerr JS, Telford SR 3rd, et al. Early murine lyme carditis has a macrophage predominance and is independent of major histocompatibility complex class II-CD4+ T cell interactions. J Infect Dis 1995;171(2):362–70.
15. Barthold SW, de Souza MS, Janotka JL, et al. Chronic lyme borreliosis in the laboratory mouse. Am J Pathol 1993;143(3):959–71.
16. Montgomery RR, Booth CJ, Wang X, et al. Recruitment of macrophages and polymorphonuclear leukocytes in L:yme carditis. Infect Immun 2007;75(2):613–20.
17. Cabello FC, Godfrey HP, Newman SA. Hidden in plain sight: Borrelia burgdorferi and the extracellular matrix. Trends Microbiol 2007;15(8):350–4.
18. Imai DM, Feng S, Hodzic E, et al. Dynamics of connective-tissue localization during chronic borrelia burgdorferi infection. Lab Invest 2013;93(8):900–10.
19. Petnicki-Ocwieja T, DeFrancesco AS, Chung E, et al. Nod2 suppresses borrelia burgdorferi mediated murine lyme arthritis and carditis through the induction of tolerance. PLoS One 2011;6(2):e17414.
20. Oosting M, Berende A, Sturm P, et al. Recognition of borrelia burgdorferi by NOD2 is central for the induction of an inflammatory reaction. J Infect Dis 2010;201(12):1849–58.

21. Lochhead RB, Ma Y, Zachary JF, et al. MicroRNA-146a provides feedback regulation of lyme arthritis but not carditis during infection with borrelia burgdorferi. PLoS Pathog 2014;10(6):e1004212.
22. Olson CM Jr, Bates TC, Izadi H, et al. Local production of IFN-gamma by invariant NKT cells modulates acute lyme carditis. J Immunol 2009;182(6):3728–34.
23. Saba S, VanderBrink BA, Perides G, et al. Cardiac conduction abnormalities in a mouse model of lyme borreliosis. J Interv Card Electrophysiol 2001;5(2): 137–43.
24. Marcus LC, Steere AC, Duray PH, et al. Fatal pancarditis in a patient with coexistent lyme disease and babesiosis. Demonstration of spirochetes in the myocardium. Ann Intern Med 1985;103(3):374–6.
25. Tavora F, Burke A, Li L, et al. Postmortem confirmation of lyme carditis with polymerase chain reaction. Cardiovasc Pathol 2008;17(2):103–7.
26. Centers for Disease Control and Prevention (CDC). Three sudden cardiac deaths associated with lyme carditis - united states, november 2012-july 2013. MMWR Morb Mortal Wkly Rep 2013;62(49):993–6.
27. Bergler-Klein J, Sochor H, Stanek G, et al. Indium 111-monoclonal antimyosin antibody and magnetic resonance imaging in the diagnosis of acute lyme myopericarditis. Arch Intern Med 1993;153(23):2696–700.
28. Cary NR, Fox B, Wright DJ, et al. Fatal lyme carditis and endodermal heterotopia of the atrioventricular node. Postgrad Med J 1990;66(772):134–6.
29. Reznick JW, Braunstein DB, Walsh RL, et al. Lyme carditis. Electrophysiologic and histopathologic study. Am J Med 1986;81(5):923–7.
30. de Koning J, Hoogkamp-Korstanje JA, van der Linde MR, et al. Demonstration of spirochetes in cardiac biopsies of patients with lyme disease. J Infect Dis 1989; 160(1):150–3.
31. van der Linde MR, Crijns HJ, de Koning J, et al. Range of atrioventricular conduction disturbances in lyme borreliosis: a report of four cases and review of other published reports. Br Heart J 1990;63(3):162–8.
32. Mener DJ, Mener AS, Daubert JP, et al. Tick tock. Am J Med 2011;124(4):306–8.
33. Maher B, Murday D, Harden SP. Cardiac MRI of lyme disease myocarditis. Heart 2012;98(3):264.
34. Cox J, Krajden M. Cardiovascular manifestations of lyme disease. Am Heart J 1991;122(5):1449–55.
35. van der Linde MR. Lyme carditis: clinical characteristics of 105 cases. Scand J Infect Dis Suppl 1991;77:81–4.
36. Harburger JM, Halperin JL. Chapter 11: cardiac involvement. In: Halperin JJ, editor. Lyme disease: an evidence-based approach. Cambridge (MA): CAB International; 2011. p. 179.
37. Fish AE, Pride YB, Pinto DS. Lyme carditis. Infect Dis Clin North Am 2008;22(2): 275–88, vi.
38. Steere AC. Lyme disease. N Engl J Med 2001;345(2):115–25.
39. McAlister HF, Klementowicz PT, Andrews C, et al. Lyme carditis: an important cause of reversible heart block. Ann Intern Med 1989;110(5):339–45.
40. Steere AC, Schoen RT, Taylor E. The clinical evolution of lyme arthritis. Ann Intern Med 1987;107(5):725–31.
41. Rubin DA, Sorbera C, Nikitin P, et al. Prospective evaluation of heart block complicating early lyme disease. Pacing Clin Electrophysiol 1992;15(3):252–5.
42. Smith RP, Schoen RT, Rahn DW, et al. Clinical characteristics and treatment outcome of early lyme disease in patients with microbiologically confirmed erythema migrans. Ann Intern Med 2002;136(6):421–8.

43. Manzoor K, Aftab W, Choksi S, et al. Lyme carditis: sequential electrocardiographic changes in response to antibiotic therapy. Int J Cardiol 2009;137(2): 167–71.
44. van der Linde MR, Crijns HJ, Lie KI. Transient complete AV block in lyme disease. Electrophysiologic observations. Chest 1989;96(1):219–21.
45. Sigal LH. Early disseminated lyme disease: cardiac manifestations. Am J Med 1995;98(4A):25S–8S [discussion: 28S–9S].
46. Wenger N, Pellaton C, Bruchez P, et al. Atrial fibrillation, complete atrioventricular block and escape rhythm with bundle-branch block morphologies: an exceptional presentation of lyme carditis. Int J Cardiol 2012;160(1):e12–4.
47. Wolf GK, Frakes MA, Gallagher M, et al. Management of suspected myocarditis during critical-care transport. Pediatr Emerg Care 2010;26(7):512–7.
48. Koene R, Boulware DR, Kemperman M, et al. Acute heart failure from lyme carditis. Circ Heart Fail 2012;5(2):e24–6.
49. Horowitz HW, Belkin RN. Acute myopericarditis resulting from lyme disease. Am Heart J 1995;130(1):176–8.
50. Wormser GP, Dattwyler RJ, Shapiro ED, et al. The clinical assessment, treatment, and prevention of lyme disease, human granulocytic anaplasmosis, and babesiosis: clinical practice guidelines by the Infectious Diseases Society of America. Clin Infect Dis 2006;43(9):1089–134.
51. Bruyn GA, De Koning J, Reijsoo FJ, et al. Lyme pericarditis leading to tamponade. Br J Rheumatol 1994;33(9):862–6.
52. Maczka I, Chmielewski T, Walczak E, et al. Tick-borne infections as a cause of heart transplantation. Pol J Microbiol 2011;60(4):341–3.
53. Rudenko N, Golovchenko M, Mokracek A, et al. Detection of Borrelia bissettii in cardiac valve tissue of a patient with endocarditis and aortic valve stenosis in the czech republic. J Clin Microbiol 2008;46(10):3540–3.
54. Canver CC, Chanda J, DeBellis DM, et al. Possible relationship between degenerative cardiac valvular pathology and lyme disease. Ann Thorac Surg 2000; 70(1):283–5.
55. Stanek G, Klein J, Bittner R, et al. Isolation of Borrelia burgdorferi from the myocardium of a patient with longstanding cardiomyopathy. N Engl J Med 1990;322(4):249–52.
56. Stanek G, Klein J, Bittner R, et al. Borrelia burgdorferi as an etiologic agent in chronic heart failure? Scand J Infect Dis Suppl 1991;77:85–7.
57. Bergler-Klein J, Glogar D, Stanek G. Clinical outcome of Borrelia burgdorferi related dilated cardiomyopathy after antibiotic treatment. Lancet 1992; 340(8814):317–8.
58. Klein J, Stanek G, Bittner R, et al. Lyme borreliosis as a cause of myocarditis and heart muscle disease. Eur Heart J 1991;12(Suppl D):73–5.
59. Gasser R, Dusleag J, Reisinger E, et al. Reversal by ceftriaxone of dilated cardiomyopathy borrelia burgdorferi infection. Lancet 1992;339(8802):1174–5.
60. Palecek T, Kuchynka P, Hulinska D, et al. Presence of borrelia burgdorferi in endomyocardial biopsies in patients with new-onset unexplained dilated cardiomyopathy. Med Microbiol Immunol 2010;199(2):139–43.
61. Kubanek M, Sramko M, Berenova D, et al. Detection of Borrelia burgdorferi sensu lato in endomyocardial biopsy specimens in individuals with recent-onset dilated cardiomyopathy. Eur J Heart Fail 2012;14(6):588–96.
62. Sonnesyn SW, Diehl SC, Johnson RC, et al. A prospective study of the seroprevalence of borrelia burgdorferi infection in patients with severe heart failure. Am J Cardiol 1995;76(1):97–100.

63. Sangha O, Phillips CB, Fleischmann KE, et al. Lack of cardiac manifestations among patients with previously treated lyme disease. Ann Intern Med 1998; 128(5):346–53.

64. Karatolios K, Maisch B, Pankuweit S. Suspected inflammatory cardiomyopathy: prevalence of borrelia burgdorferi in endomyocardial biopsies with positive serological evidence. Herz 2014. [Epub ahead of print].

65. Embers ME, Barthold SW, Borda JT, et al. Persistence of borrelia burgdorferi in rhesus macaques following antibiotic treatment of disseminated infection. PLoS One 2012;7(1):e29914.

66. Hajjar RJ, Kradin RL. Case records of the massachusetts general hospital. Weekly clinicopathological exercises. Case 17-2002. A 55-year-old man with second-degree atrioventricular block and chest pain. N Engl J Med 2002; 346(22):1732–8.

67. Epstein AE, DiMarco JP, Ellenbogen KA, et al. ACC/AHA/HRS 2008 guidelines for device-based therapy of cardiac rhythm abnormalities: a report of the american college of Cardiology/American Heart Association task force on practice guidelines (writing committee to revise the ACC/AHA/NASPE 2002 guideline update for implantation of cardiac pacemakers and antiarrhythmia devices): developed in collaboration with the American Association for Thoracic Surgery and Society of Thoracic Surgeons. Circulation 2008;117(21):e350–408.

68. Rosenfeld LE. Temporary permanent or permanent temporary pacing? Pacing Clin Electrophysiol 2011;34(6):670–1.

69. Artigao R, Torres G, Guerrero A, et al. Irreversible complete heart block in lyme disease. Am J Med 1991;90(4):531–3.

70. Kugeler KJ, Griffith KS, Gould LH, et al. A review of death certificates listing lyme disease as a cause of death in the united states. Clin Infect Dis 2011;52(3):364–7.

Diagnosis and Treatment of Lyme Arthritis

Sheila L. Arvikar, MD, Allen C. Steere, MD*

KEYWORDS

- Lyme disease • *Borrelia burgdorferi* • Lyme arthritis • Antibiotic-refractory arthritis
- Inflammatory arthritis

KEY POINTS

- Lyme arthritis is a late disease manifestation, usually beginning months after the tick bite. Patients may not report an antecedent tick bite or erythema migrans.
- Patients have intermittent or persistent attacks of joint swelling and pain, primarily in 1 or a few large joints, especially the knee, without prominent systemic manifestations.
- The diagnosis is supported by 2-tier serologic testing for *Borrelia burgdorferi* by enzyme-linked immunosorbent assay and immunoglobulin G Western blotting.
- Initial treatment is a 30-day course of oral doxycycline or amoxicillin. For patients with an insufficient response to oral treatment, intravenous therapy with ceftriaxone is recommended.
- A minority of patients may have persistent synovitis for months or several years after oral and intravenous antibiotic therapy, which is treated with antiinflammatory agents, disease-modifying antirheumatic drugs, or synovectomy.

INTRODUCTION/NATURE OF THE PROBLEM
Epidemiology

Lyme arthritis was recognized originally because of an outbreak of monoarticular and oligoarticular arthritis in children in Lyme, Connecticut, in the 1970s.[1] It then became apparent that Lyme disease was a complex, multisystem illness affecting primarily skin, nervous system, heart, or joints.[2] Before the use of antibiotic therapy for treatment of the disease, about 60% of untreated patients developed Lyme arthritis, a late disease manifestation.[3] In recent years, more than 30,000 cases of Lyme disease have been reported annually to the Centers for Disease Control and Prevention (CDC), and in one-third of reported cases, arthritis was a manifestation of the disease.[4] However, recent CDC estimates suggest the actual number of infections with the Lyme disease spirochete may be 10-fold higher.[5]

Center for Immunology and Inflammatory Diseases, Division of Rheumatology, Allergy, and Immunology, Massachusetts General Hospital, Harvard Medical School, 55 Fruit Street, Boston, MA 02114, USA
* Corresponding author.
E-mail address: asteere@mgh.harvard.edu

Infect Dis Clin N Am 29 (2015) 269–280
http://dx.doi.org/10.1016/j.idc.2015.02.004
0891-5520/15/$ – see front matter © 2015 Elsevier Inc. All rights reserved.

id.theclinics.com

The infection is transmitted primarily by nymphal *Ixodes scapularis* ticks, which quest in the late spring and early summer.[6] However, Lyme arthritis can present at any time of the year. The majority of cases occur in the northeastern United States, from Maine to Virginia.[5] Other affected areas in the United States include the northern mid-Western states of Minnesota, Wisconsin, and Michigan, and the West coast in northern California.

In the United States, *Borrelia burgdorferi* is the sole cause of the disease, but subtypes of *B burgdorferi* differ in pathogenicity.[7,8] OspC type A (RST1) strains, which account for 30% to 50% of the infections in the northeastern United States,[7,8] but only 3% in mid-Western states,[9] are particularly virulent and arthritogenic. These strains are thought to have played an important role in the emergence of the Lyme disease epidemic in the northeastern United States in the late 20th century.[10]

Pathogenesis

In the northeastern United States, *B burgdorferi* strains often disseminate to joints, tendons, or bursae early in the infection.[3,6] Although this event is frequently asymptomatic, transient or migratory arthralgias may occur at that time. Lyme arthritis, a late disease manifestation, usually occurs months later accompanied by intense innate and adaptive immune responses.[11] The adaptive immune response leads to the production of specific antibodies that opsonize the organism, facilitating phagocytosis and effective spirochetal killing.

With appropriate oral and, if necessary, intravenous (IV) antibiotic therapy, spirochetes are eradicated, and joint inflammation resolves in the great majority of patients. However, in a small percentage of patients, particularly in those who were infected with highly inflammatory *B burgdorferi* RST1 strains, synovial inflammation persists for months or several years despite receiving oral and IV antibiotic therapy for 2 or 3 months, called antibiotic-refractory arthritis.[12] A refractory outcome is likely to require multiple factors, and may include some combination of pathogen-associated, genetic, and immunologic factors (**Box 1**).

Although antibiotic-refractory arthritis is associated with highly inflammatory strains of *B burgdorferi*, persistent infection in the postantibiotic period does not seem to play role in this outcome. Polymerase chain reaction (PCR) testing of synovial fluid for *B burgdorferi* DNA, which is often positive before treatment, is usually negative after antibiotic treatment, and both culture and PCR testing of synovial tissue have been

---

Box 1
Factors associated with antibiotic-refractory Lyme arthritis

Pathogen

- *Borrelia burgdorferi*, particularly OspC type A (RST-1) type strain[8]
- Possible retained spirochetal antigens[18,19]

Genetic

- Certain HLA-DR alleles that bind *B burgdorferi* outer surface protein A (OspA)[14]
- Toll-like receptor 1-1805 GG polymorphism[17]

Immunologic

- Endothelial cell growth factor autoantibodies[20]
- Decreased ratio of T-regulatory/T-effector cells among synovial fluid mononuclear cells[16,17]

uniformly negative from synovectomy specimens obtained months to years after anti-biotic therapy.[13]

Rather, excessive inflammation during the infection, infection-induced autoimmunity, and failure to downregulate inflammatory responses appropriately after spirochetal killing seem to be critical factors. Specifically, antibiotic-refractory arthritis is associated with specific HLA-DR alleles that bind an epitope of *B burgdorferi* outer surface protein A (OspA), leading to particularly strong T helper type 1 cell responses.[14] Additionally, this outcome occurs more often in patients with a Toll-like receptor 1 polymorphism (1805 GG) that is found in one-half of the European Caucasian population and leads to exceptionally high levels of cytokines and chemokines in affected joints.[15] As evidence of immune dysregulation, patients with antibiotic-refractory arthritis have low frequencies of FoxP3$^+$ regulatory T cells in synovial fluid; the lower the frequency, the longer the posttreatment duration of arthritis.[16,17] In MyD88$^{-/-}$ mice, spirochetal antigens are retained on cartilage surfaces,[18,19] but it is not yet clear whether retained spirochetal antigens play a role in the postantibiotic period in human Lyme arthritis. Finally, a novel human autoantigen, endothelial cell growth factor, was recently identified as a target of T-cell and B-cell responses in a subset of patients with Lyme disease, which provides the first direct evidence for autoimmune T-cell and B-cell responses in this illness.[20] Additionally, synovial tissue in Lyme arthritis often shows obliterative microvascular lesions, and this finding correlates directly with the magnitude of endothelial cell growth factor antibody responses.[21]

Despite heightened immune reactivity, antibiotic-refractory arthritis eventually resolves. Thus, it seems that spirochetal killing, either by the immune system or with the assistance of antibiotic therapy, removes the innate immune "danger" signals. Without these signals, the adaptive immune response to autoantigens eventually regains homeostasis, and the arthritis resolves. This process may be facilitated by therapy with disease-modifying antirheumatic drugs (DMARDs).

PATIENT HISTORY

During the 1970s, before the cause of the disease was known, the natural history of Lyme arthritis was elucidated in a study of 55 non–antibiotic-treated patients who were followed prospectively from onset of erythema migrans (EM), the initial skin lesion, through the period of arthritis.[3] Clinical features of the infection in these patients included the following:

- Arthritis began from 4 days to 2 years (mean, 6 months) after the EM skin lesion.
- Patients had intermittent or persistent attacks of joint swelling and pain, primarily in 1 or a few large joints, especially the knee, over a period of several years.[3] However, particularly in earlier episodes, other large or small joints, the temporomandibular joint, or periarticular sites (bursa, tendons) were sometimes affected.
- Generally, fewer than 5 joints were affected at 1 time.
- Knee joints were often very swollen, but not particularly painful, and ruptured Baker's cysts were common.
- By the time arthritis was present, systemic manifestations (fever or other constitutional symptoms) were uncommon.

Differential Diagnosis

In addition to serologic testing, clinical features may distinguish Lyme arthritis from other arthritides. A common concern is mechanical injury in an active individual;

therefore, orthopedists are often the first specialist to see a patient with Lyme arthritis. However, the clinical picture of Lyme arthritis is most like reactive arthritis in adults or pauciarticular juvenile idiopathic arthritis in children, and serologic testing is essential to distinguish Lyme arthritis from these entities. Children may have a more acute presentation, with higher synovial white blood cell counts, which may suggest a diagnosis of acute septic arthritis.[22–24] However, Lyme arthritis typically causes only minimal pain with passive range of motion, and involvement of more than 1 joint (currently or by history) may help to distinguish Lyme arthritis from septic bacterial arthritis.[22–24] Lyme arthritis rarely, if ever, causes chronic, symmetric polyarthritis, which helps to distinguish Lyme arthritis from rheumatoid arthritis. Fibromyalgia is sometimes misdiagnosed as Lyme disease, but patients with fibromyalgia generally have diffuse pain, and they lack objective evidence of joint inflammation.

Other inflammatory arthritides, such as rheumatoid arthritis, reactive arthritis, or psoriatic arthritis may develop within months after Lyme disease, seemingly triggered by the spirochetal infection. Thus, these entities should be considered in the differential diagnosis. In endemic areas, concomitant positive serologic results for Lyme disease in patients with other inflammatory arthritides can present a diagnostic challenge, because antibody responses to *B burgdorferi* after antibiotic-treated Lyme arthritis typically persist for many years.[25]

PHYSICAL EXAMINATION

Patients with Lyme arthritis typically have the following features on physical examination.

- Monoarthritis or oligoarthritis most commonly affecting the knees, but other large or small joints may be affected, such as an ankle, shoulder, elbow, or wrist.
- Affected knees may have very large effusions with warmth, but in contrast with typical bacterial (eg, staphylococcal) septic arthritis, they are not particularly painful with range of motion or weight bearing. Baker's cysts may be present in the knees given the large size of effusions.
- Fever is usually not present.

Typical knee swelling in Lyme arthritis is shown in **Fig. 1**.

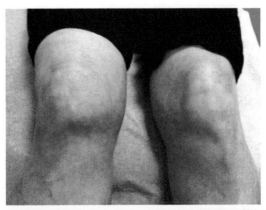

Fig. 1. Lyme arthritis. Swollen knee of a patient with Lyme arthritis. Patients have intermittent or persistent attacks of joint swelling and pain, primarily in 1 or a few large joints, especially the knee, during a period of several years, with few systemic manifestations.

IMAGING AND ADDITIONAL TESTING
Serologic Testing for Lyme Disease

The mainstay in diagnosing Lyme arthritis is serologic testing. In the United States, the CDC currently recommends a 2-test approach in which samples are first tested for antibodies to *B burgdorferi* by enzyme-linked immunosorbent assay and those with equivocal or positive results are subsequently tested by Western blotting, with findings interpreted according to the CDC criteria.[26] In contrast with early infection, when some patients may be seronegative, all patients with Lyme arthritis, a late disease manifestation, have positive serologic results for immunoglobulin (Ig)G antibodies to *B burgdorferi*, with expansion of the response to many spirochetal proteins.[27] When serum samples were tested with microarrays of more than 1200 spirochetal proteins, 120 proteins, primarily outer membrane lipoproteins, were found to be immunogenic, and patients with Lyme arthritis had IgG reactivity to as many as 89 proteins.[28] Serologic testing should be performed only in serum, because serologic tests in synovial fluid are not accurate.[29]

In addition to IgG antibody responses to *B burgdorferi*, patients with Lyme arthritis may also have low-titer IgM reactivity with the spirochete. On the other hand, a positive IgM response alone in a patient with arthritis is likely to be a false-positive response or one indicative of previous, antibiotic-treated early Lyme disease in a patient who now has another type of arthritis. Therefore, positive IgM antibody responses alone should not be used to support the diagnosis of Lyme arthritis. After spirochetal killing with antibiotics, antispirochetal antibody titers decline gradually, but both the IgG and IgM responses in patients with past Lyme arthritis may remain positive for years,[29] which seems to be an indicator of immune memory rather than active infection. We have not observed reinfection in patients with the expanded immune response generated in patients with Lyme arthritis. Therefore, a persistent, expanded IgG antibody response seems to be protective against reinfection, whereas the limited response seen in patients with EM is not.

Synovial Fluid Polymerase Chain Reaction for Borrelia burgdorferi

Although reported in a few patients,[30] it is exceedingly difficult to culture *B burgdorferi* from synovial fluid in patients with Lyme arthritis. This is presumably because joint fluid, with its many inflammatory mediators, is an extremely hostile environment. In spiked cultures, adding small amounts of joint fluid results in rapid killing of spirochetes.[13] In contrast, PCR testing of synovial fluid for *B burgdorferi* DNA often yields positive results before antibiotic therapy (range, 40%–96%),[13,31] and usually becomes negative after antibiotic treatment.[12,13] However, spirochetal DNA may persist after spirochetal killing, which limits its use as a test for active infection. Moreover, PCR testing has not been standardized for routine clinical use. Therefore, in most cases, the appropriate clinical picture and a positive serologic result are sufficient for diagnosis of Lyme arthritis, and PCR testing serves as an optional test to further support the diagnosis.

Synovial Fluid Analysis, Imaging, and Other Tests

On presentation, joint aspiration is usually done for diagnostic purposes to rule out the presence of other arthritides, such as crystalline arthropathy or staphylococcal septic arthritis. Joint fluid white cell counts are usually inflammatory in the range of 10,000 to 25,000 cells/mm^3, but cell counts as low as 500 or as high as 100,000 cells/mm^3 have been reported.[3] Although tests for rheumatoid factor or antinuclear antibodies typically yield negative results, antinuclear antibodies in low titer may be detected.

Peripheral white blood cell counts are usually within the normal range, but inflammatory markers, such as an erythrocyte sedimentation rate and C-reactive protein, may be increased. Imaging studies are not required for diagnosis or are not performed typically. The major reason for imaging studies in Lyme arthritis is when there are concerns for alternative diagnoses.

In patients with Lyme arthritis, plain films, MRI, or ultrasonography typically show nonspecific joint effusions, whereas MRI studies with contrast dye may display synovial thickening or enhancement. In adult patients, imaging studies may show coincidental degenerative changes or chronic mechanical injuries, but these abnormalities would not be expected to cause significant synovitis or inflammation. Lyme arthritis is not rapidly erosive, but with longer arthritis durations, joint damage can be seen on radiographic studies.[32] Finally, MRI may be useful in the planning of synovectomies by determining the extent of synovitis within the joint.

TREATMENT

Treatment of Lyme arthritis is based on several small, double-blind or randomized studies and observational studies (summarized in **Table 1**). The efficacy of antibiotics was first demonstrated in a double-blind, placebo-controlled trial of intramuscular benzathine penicillin, 2.4 million units weekly for 3 weeks versus placebo. In that study, 7 of 20 antibiotic-treated patients (35%) had complete resolution of arthritis, whereas all 20 placebo treatment patients continued to have arthritis.[33] Subsequently, 11 of 20 patients (55%) treated with IV penicillin, 20 million U daily in 6 divided doses for 10 days, had resolution of arthritis.[33] It was then reported that IV ceftriaxone, 2 g daily, was effective in 90% of patients who were given 2 to 4 weeks of therapy.[34] In a later randomized trial, treatment with 30 days of doxycycline, 100 mg twice daily, or amoxicillin, 500 mg 4 times daily, also led to resolution of arthritis in 90% of patients.[35]

According to current recommendations from the Infectious Diseases Society of America,[36] patients with Lyme arthritis should be treated initially with a 30-day course of oral doxycycline, 100 mg twice daily, or amoxicillin, 500 mg 3 times daily. In patients who are unable to take either of these oral agents, cefuroxime axetil, 500 mg twice daily, may be an acceptable alternative. This medication was shown to be equivalent to treatment with doxycycline or amoxicillin in patients with EM,[37] but has not been studied systematically in patients with Lyme arthritis. Unless there are concomitant neurologic abnormalities, oral regimens are the initial treatment of choice because such therapy is safer and more cost effective.

In our experience, some patients do require longer courses of antibiotic therapy for effective treatment of Lyme arthritis.[12] Thus, if there is mild residual joint swelling after a 30-day course of oral antibiotics, we repeat the oral antibiotic regimen for another 30 days. However, for patients who continue to have moderate to severe joint swelling after a 30-day course of oral antibiotics, we treat with IV ceftriaxone, 2 g/d. Although there is trend toward greater efficacy with 4 weeks compared with 2 weeks of antibiotics, there is also a greater frequency of adverse events.[38] Thus, our practice is to prescribe a 4-week course of IV therapy, but to monitor the patient closely and to stop the antibiotic if complications occur.

Even in patients who had minimal or no improvement with oral doxycycline, we observe typically moderate improvement or even complete resolution of arthritis with IV therapy. Moreover, even in those with persistent joint inflammation, the synovitis tends to change after IV therapy with decreased size of effusions but continued synovial tissue hypertrophy and inflammation. Courses of longer than 30 days of IV antibiotics

Table 1
Prospective studies of antibiotic therapy in Lyme arthritis

Author, Year	Trial Type/Treatment	Patients	Outcomes
Steere et al,[33] 1985	Double-blind, placebo-controlled trial of intramuscular benzathine PCN for 3 wk vs placebo Additional 20 patients received IV PCN 20 million U/d for 10 d	40 with Lyme arthritis 20 with Lyme arthritis	7/20 (35%) PCN-treated patients had complete response vs 0/20 in placebo arm ($P = .02$) 11/20 (55%) had complete resolution
Dattwyler et al,[34] 1988	Randomized to IV treatment with PCN (10 d) or CTX (14 d) Additional nonrandomized cohort treated with CTX 2 or 4 g	23 patients with late Lyme (16 with arthritis) 31 patients (23 with arthritis)	5/10 responded to PCN vs 12/13 responded to CTX 27/31 patients responded to CTX Overall >90% response to CTX
Steere et al,[35] 1994	Randomized trial of doxycycline or amoxicillin plus probenecid for 30 d, or 2 wk of IV CTX for patients with persistent arthritis 3 mo after oral antibiotics or PCN	50 with Lyme arthritis	18/20 patients receiving doxycycline and 16/18 receiving amoxicillin had complete response by 3 mo; 5 patients later developed neuroborreliosis 0/16 patients treated with IV CTX had resolution with 3 mo
Dattwyler et al,[38] 2005	Randomized trial of CTX, 14- vs 28-d regimen	143 patients with late Lyme disease	5 failures out of 80 patients in 14-d group, but 0 failures out of 63 patients in 28-d group ($P = .07$) Increased adverse events in 28-d group ($P = .02$)
Oksi et al,[40] 2007	Double-blind, randomized, placebo-controlled trial of adjunct oral antibiotic therapy (amoxicillin) vs placebo for 100 d after 3 wk of IV CTX	107 patients with definite disseminated Lyme disease, including 45 with arthritis	Excellent/good response in 49/53 in amoxicillin group and 47/54 in placebo treated groups (NS) 37/45 Lyme arthritis patients had excellent or good responses

Abbreviations: CTX, ceftriaxone; IV, intravenous; NS, not significant; PCN, penicillin.

seem not to be beneficial and may be associated with a still greater frequency of adverse effects.[39] Additionally, a recent double-blind, randomized, placebo-controlled study of patients in Europe did not find a benefit of additional oral amoxicillin therapy after treatment with IV ceftriaxone.[40] A number of newer oral antibiotics in a drug library approved by the US Food and Drug Administration, including daptomycin, carbomycin, and cefoperazone, have been shown to have marked efficacy against persisting spirochetes in culture,[41] but it is not yet known whether such antibiotics would be effective in patients with Lyme arthritis that is more difficult to treat.

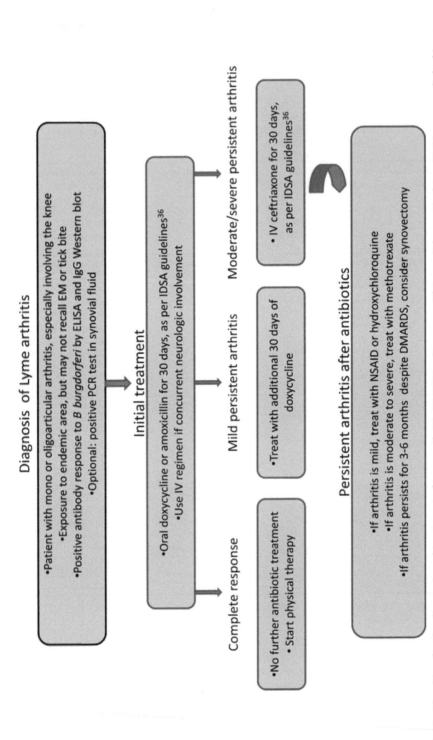

Fig. 2. Algorithm for the diagnosis and treatment of Lyme arthritis. DMARDs, disease modifying antirheumatic drugs; ELISA, enzyme-linked immuno-sorbent assay; EM, erythema migrans; IDSA, Infectious Disease Society of America; IV, intravenous; NSAID, nonsteroidal antiinflammatory drug; PCR, polymerase chain reaction.

Adjunctive Therapy

During treatment, nonsteroidal antiinflammatory drugs, such as ibuprofen or naproxen, may be used for pain. We rarely give oral or intraarticular corticosteroids, and not until antibiotic treatment is completed, because these drugs permit greater growth of spirochetes,[42] and because of the association of intraarticular steroid injections with a longer duration of arthritis in some studies.[12,43] When joints are inflamed, reduction of activity is important. If patients are limping, we advise crutch walking. Children may be more likely to regain normal function within 4 weeks after the initiation of antibiotic treatment,[23] but especially in adults, inflamed joints typically lead to quadriceps atrophy. Therefore, after the completion of antibiotic treatment and resolution of joint inflammation, formal physical therapy, including bicycle riding, is often needed.

Therapy for Antibiotic-Refractory Arthritis

The algorithm that we use for the diagnosis and treatment of antibiotic-refractory arthritis is shown in **Fig. 2**.[12] If synovitis persists after 2 or more months of oral antibiotics and 1 month of IV antibiotics, we use a similar approach to that used in the treatment of other forms of chronic inflammatory arthritis, including rheumatoid arthritis and reactive arthritis. The agents used include nonsteroidal antiinflammatory drugs, such as ibuprofen or naproxen, and DMARDs, such as hydroxychloroquine or methotrexate (MTX), depending on the severity of arthritis. Although there have been no formal trials with these agents, in practice they reduce the severity of inflammation and have not resulted in breakthrough cases of active infection. We generally do not give oral or intraarticular injections of corticosteroids, even in the postantibiotic period, although others have reported clinical utility, particularly in the pediatric popultion.[44,45]

In more recent years, with greater experience using more potent DMARD agents, we have developed an enhanced treatment strategy, now more commonly choosing low-dose MTX, typically 15 to 20 mg per week, over hydroxychloroquine as the initial DMARD, and reserving hydroxychloroquine, typically 400 mg daily, for cases with milder synovitis. Moreover, in a few patients who had incomplete responses to MTX or in those with contraindications to MTX, we have used tumor necrosis factor inhibitors, generally injectable forms such as entanercept or adalimumab.[12] The onset of action of MTX and other DMARDs can be slow, but we expect to see a significant response in 1 to 3 months. Because antibiotic-refractory arthritis has resolved after a median duration of 9 to 14 months (range, 4 months to 4 years) after the start of antibiotic therapy,[12] long courses of DMARD therapy are generally not needed. We typically prescribe these medications for only 6 to 12 months rather than indefinitely, as in the treatment of patients with rheumatoid arthritis. If the response to a DMARD agent is incomplete and if the arthritis is limited to 1 joint, primarily the knee, arthroscopic synovectomy is an option.[46] By removing most of the inflamed synovial tissue in both the anterior and posterior compartments of the knee, the arthritis does not usually recur when synovial tissue grows back.

SUMMARY

Arthritis is a late manifestation of Lyme disease, usually beginning months after the tick bite. However, a history of EM or tick bite may be lacking. Patients have intermittent or persistent attacks of joint swelling and pain, primarily in 1 or a few large joints, often the knee, over a period of months to several years, with few systemic manifestations. The diagnosis is established by 2-tier serologic testing for *B burgdorferi* by enzyme-linked immunosorbent assay and IgG Western blotting, which typically shows strong responses to many spirochetal proteins with many bands present. PCR testing of synovial fluid for *B burgdorferi* DNA is often positive before antibiotic therapy, but the test is not a reliable indicator of spirochetal eradication after antibiotic treatment, because spirochetal DNA may persist after spirochetal killing. Initial recommended therapies include a 30-day course of oral doxycycline or amoxicillin. However, for patients with persistent joint swelling despite oral therapy, IV ceftriaxone for 2 to 4 weeks may be needed for successful treatment. A small percentage of patients may have persistent arthritis for months or several years after both oral and IV antibiotic therapy, which may be treated successfully with antiinflammatory agents, DMARDs, or synovectomy. The antibody response to *B burgdorferi* declines slowly after treatment, but the test typically remains positive for years after therapy.

REFERENCES

1. Steere AC, Malawista SE, Snydman DR, et al. Lyme arthritis: an epidemic of oligoarticular arthritis in children and adults in three Connecticut communities. Arthritis Rheum 1977;20(1):7–17.
2. Steere AC, Malawista SE, Hardin JA, et al. Erythema chronicum migrans and Lyme arthritis. The enlarging clinical spectrum. Ann Intern Med 1977;86(6):685–98.
3. Steere AC, Schoen RT, Taylor E. The clinical evolution of Lyme arthritis. Ann Intern Med 1987;107(5):725–31 [Key article].
4. Bacon RM, Kugeler KJ, Mead PS, Centers for Disease Control and Prevention (CDC). Surveillance for Lyme disease–United States, 1992–2006. MMWR Surveill Summ 2008;57(10):1–9.
5. CDC estimates of Americans diagnosed with Lyme disease each year. Press release from the Centers for Disease Control and Prevention, August 13, 2013. Available at: http://www.cdc.gov/media/releases/2013/p0819-lyme-disease.html.
6. Steere AC. Lyme disease. N Engl J Med 1989;321(9):586–96 [Key article].
7. Wormser GP, Brisson D, Liveris D, et al. *Borrelia burgdorferi* genotype predicts the capacity for hematogenous dissemination during early Lyme disease. J Infect Dis 2008;198(9):1358–64.
8. Jones KL, McHugh GA, Glickstein LJ, et al. Analysis of *Borrelia burgdorferi* genotypes in patients with Lyme arthritis: high frequency of ribosomal RNA intergenic spacer type 1 strains in antibiotic-refractory arthritis. Arthritis Rheum 2009;60(7):2174–82.
9. Hanincova K, Mukherjee P, Ogden NH, et al. Multilocus sequence typing of *Borrelia burgdorferi* suggests existence of lineages with differential pathogenic properties in humans. PLoS One 2013;8(9):e73066.
10. Hoen AG, Margos G, Bent SJ, et al. Phylogeography of *Borrelia burgdorferi* in the eastern United States reflects multiple independent Lyme disease emergence events. Proc Natl Acad Sci U S A 2009;106(35):15013–8.
11. Steere AC, Coburn J, Glickstein L. The emergence of Lyme disease. J Clin Invest 2004;113(8):1093–101.
12. Steere AC, Angelis SM. Therapy for Lyme arthritis: strategies for the treatment of antibiotic-refractory arthritis. Arthritis Rheum 2006;54(10):3079–86 [Key article].
13. Li X, McHugh G, Damle N, et al. Burden and viability of *Borrelia burgdorferi* in skin or joints of patients with erythema migrans or Lyme arthritis. Arthritis Rheum 2011;63(8):2238–47.
14. Steere AC, Drouin EE, Glickstein LJ. Relationship between immunity to *Borrelia burgdorferi* outer-surface protein A (OspA) and Lyme arthritis. Clin Infect Dis 2011;52(Suppl 3):S259–65.

15. Strle K, Shin JJ, Glickstein LJ, et al. Association of a toll-like receptor 1 polymorphism with heightened Th1 inflammatory responses and antibiotic-refractory Lyme arthritis. Arthritis Rheum 2012;64(5):1497–507.

16. Shen S, Shin JJ, Strle K, et al. Treg cell numbers and function in patients with antibiotic-refractory or antibiotic-responsive Lyme arthritis. Arthritis Rheum 2010;62(7):2127–37.

17. Vudattu NK, Strle K, Steere AC, et al. Dysregulation of CD4+CD25(high) T cells in the synovial fluid of patients with antibiotic-refractory Lyme arthritis. Arthritis Rheum 2013;65(6):1643–53.

18. Bockenstedt LK, Gonzalez DG, Haberman AM, et al. Spirochete antigens persist near cartilage after murine Lyme borreliosis therapy. J Clin Invest 2012;122(7): 2652–60.

19. Wormser GP, Nadelman RB, Schwartz I. The amber theory of Lyme arthritis: initial description and clinical implications. Clin Rheumatol 2012;31(6):989–94.

20. Drouin EE, Seward RJ, Strle K, et al. A novel human autoantigen, endothelial cell growth factor, is a target of T and B cell responses in patients with Lyme disease. Arthritis Rheum 2013;65(1):186–96.

21. Londoño D, Cadavid D, Drouin EE, et al. Antibodies to endothelial cell growth factor and obliterative microvascular lesions in the synovium of patients with antibiotic-refractory Lyme arthritis. Arthritis Rheumatol 2014;66(8):2124–33.

22. Aiyer A, Hennrikus W, Walrath J, et al. Lyme arthritis of the pediatric lower extremity in the setting of polyarticular disease. J Child Orthop 2014;8:359–65.

23. Daikh BE, Emerson FE, Smith RP, et al. Lyme arthritis: a comparison of presentation, synovial fluid analysis, and treatment course in children and adults. Arthritis Care Res 2013;65(12):1986–90.

24. Deanehan JK, Kimia AA, Tan Tanny SP, et al. Distinguishing Lyme from septic knee monoarthritis in Lyme disease-endemic areas. Arthritis Rheumatol 2014; 66(8):2124–33.

25. Kalish RA, McHugh G, Granquist J, et al. Persistence of immunoglobulin M or immunoglobulin G antibody responses to *Borrelia burgdorferi* 10–20 years after active Lyme disease. Clin Infect Dis 2001;33(6):780–5.

26. Centers for Disease Control and Prevention. Recommendations for test performance and interpretation from the Second International Conference on Serologic Diagnosis of Lyme Disease. MMWR Morb Mortal Wkly Rep 1995;44(31):590–1.

27. Steere AC, McHugh G, Damle N, et al. Prospective study of serologic tests for Lyme disease. Clin Infect Dis 2008;47(2):188–95.

28. Barbour AG, Jasinskas A, Kayala MK, et al. A genome-wide proteome array reveals a limited set of immunogens in natural infections of humans and white-footed mice with *Borrelia burgdorferi*. Infect Immun 2008;76(8):3374–89.

29. Barclay SS, Melia MT, Auwaerter PG. Misdiagnosis of late-onset Lyme arthritis by inappropriate use of *Borrelia burgdorferi* immunoblot testing with synovial fluid. Clin Vaccine Immunol 2012;19(11):1806–9.

30. Snydman DR, Schenkein DP, Berardi VP, et al. *Borrelia burgdorferi* in joint fluid in chronic Lyme arthritis. Ann Intern Med 1986;104(6):798.

31. Nocton JJ, Dressler F, Rutledge BJ, et al. Detection of *Borrelia burgdorferi* DNA by polymerase chain reaction in synovial fluid in Lyme arthritis. N Engl J Med 1994;330(4):229–34.

32. Lawson JP, Steere AC. Lyme arthritis: radiologic findings. Radiology 1985; 154(1):37–43.

33. Steere AC, Green J, Schoen RT, et al. Successful parenteral penicillin therapy of established Lyme arthritis. N Engl J Med 1985;312(14):869.

34. Dattwyler RJ, Halperin JJ, Volkman DJ, et al. Treatment of late Lyme borreliosis–randomised comparison of ceftriaxone and penicillin. Lancet 1988;1(1896): 1191–4.
35. Steere AC, Levin RE, Molloy PJ, et al. Treatment of Lyme arthritis. Arthritis Rheum 1994;37(6):878–88.
36. Wormser GP, Dattwyler RJ, Shapiro ED, et al. The clinical assessment, treatment, and prevention of Lyme disease, human granulocytic anaplasmosis, and babesiosis: clinical practice guidelines by the Infectious Diseases Society of America. Clin Infect Dis 2006;43(9):1089–134 [Key article].
37. Nadelman RB, Luger SW, Frank E, et al. Comparison of cefuroxime axetil and doxycycline in the treatment of early Lyme disease. Ann Intern Med 1992; 117(4):273–80.
38. Dattwyler RJ, Wormser GP, Rush TJ, et al. A comparison of two treatment regimens of ceftriaxone in late Lyme disease. Wien Klin Wochenschr 2005; 117(11–12):393–7.
39. Fallon BA, Keilp JG, Corbera KM, et al. A randomized, placebo-controlled trial of repeated IV antibiotic therapy for Lyme encephalopathy. Neurology 2008;70(13): 992–1003.
40. Oksi J, Nikoskelainen J, Hiekkanen H, et al. Duration of antibiotic treatment in disseminated Lyme borreliosis: a double-blind, randomized, placebo-controlled, multicenter clinical study. Eur J Clin Microbiol Infect Dis 2007;26(8): 571–81.
41. Feng J, Wang T, Shi W, et al. Identification of novel activity against *Borrelia burgdorferi* persisters using an FDA approved drug library. Emerg Microb Infect 2014; 3:e49.
42. Pachner AR, Delaney E, O'Neill T. Neuroborreliosis in the nonhuman primate: *Borrelia burgdorferi* persists in the central nervous system. Ann Neurol 1995; 38(4):667–9.
43. Bentas W, Karch H, Huppertz HI. Lyme arthritis in children and adolescents: outcome 12 months after initiation of antibiotic therapy. J Rheumatol 2000; 27(8):2025–30.
44. Nimmrich S, Becker I, Horneff G. Intraarticular corticosteroids in refractory childhood Lyme arthritis. Rheumatol Int 2014;34(7):987–94.
45. Tory HO, Zurakowski D, Sundel RP. Outcomes of children treated for Lyme arthritis: results of a large pediatric cohort. J Rheumatol 2011;37(5):1049–55.
46. Schoen RT, Aversa JM, Rahn DW, et al. Treatment of refractory chronic Lyme arthritis with arthroscopic synovectomy. Arthritis Rheum 1991;34(8):1056–60.

Lyme Disease in Children

Sunil K. Sood, MBBS, DCH, MD[a,b,c,*]

KEYWORDS

- Children • Tick bite prevention • Tick bite management
- Increased intracranial pressure • Optic nerve • Lyme meningitis

KEY POINTS

- The diagnosis and management of Lyme disease in children in general is similar to that in adults, but it should be noted that doxycycline is not an initial empiric choice for children 8 years and younger.
- The prognosis of Lyme disease is excellent in almost all children, including for those who present with the late disseminated manifestation of Lyme arthritis.
- Increased intracranial pressure is observed frequently in children as a complication of acute disseminated Lyme disease, usually in acute neurologic disease, and entails a risk of visual loss.
- Serologic tests are often ordered inappropriately, and should be done only if a child's signs and symptoms are consistent with Lyme disease.
- Children frequently get tick bites, so pediatricians and family practitioners should be familiar with the prevention and management of tick bites.

Lyme disease or Lyme borreliosis owes its name to the investigation of an unusual cluster of children with unexplained arthritis occurring in Lyme, Connecticut and surrounding communities.[1] Some of the first cases of erythema migrans (EM; the characteristic rash of localized Lyme disease) in the United States also were observed in children, in Connecticut and Massachusetts in 1975.[2,3] Lyme arthritis was subsequently recognized to be part of this multisystem disease. The age-specific incidence of Lyme disease is higher in children than in adults (**Fig. 1**), presumably because of their increased exposure to ticks. About a quarter of all reported cases in the United States occur in children who are younger than 14 years of age.[4]

CLINICAL MANIFESTATIONS

As in adults, children have signs and symptoms of either early localized, early disseminated, or late Lyme disease. Early disseminated disease manifests in the skin, nervous system, heart, or with musculoskeletal symptoms, in those who develop

[a] Hofstra North Shore-LIJ School of Medicine, Hempstead, NY 11549, USA; [b] Department of Pediatrics, Southside Hospital, 301 East Main Street, Bay Shore, NY 11706, USA; [c] Pediatric Infectious Diseases, Cohen Children's Medical Center, New Hyde Park, NY 11040, USA
* Department of Pediatrics, Southside Hospital, 301 East Main Street, Bay Shore, NY 11706.
E-mail address: SSood@nshs.edu

Infect Dis Clin N Am 29 (2015) 281–294
http://dx.doi.org/10.1016/j.idc.2015.02.011
0891-5520/15/$ – see front matter © 2015 Elsevier Inc. All rights reserved.

id.theclinics.com

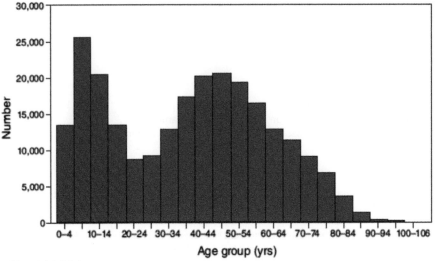

N = 241,931.

Fig. 1. Number of Lyme disease cases reported, by age group, 1992–2006. (*From* Bacon RM, Kugeler KJ, Mead PS, Centers for Disease Control and Prevention (CDC). Surveillance for Lyme disease—United States, 1992–2006. MMWR Surveill Summ 2008;57(10):1–9.)

spirochetemia after the tick bite. Some children present with more than one manifestation. A prospective study of children in five pediatric practices in hyperendemic towns of Southern Connecticut provided valuable information on the spectrum of clinical presentation of Lyme disease in children.[5] Most (89%) presented with either single or multiple EM and more than a third presented with a sign of dissemination as the presenting manifestation (multiple EM, arthritis, facial palsy, meningitis, or carditis). Children with multiple EM had a higher incidence of systemic symptoms than those with a solitary lesion. There are a few differences in the spectrum for Lyme disease acquired in Europe, where neurologic manifestations are notably more common in children (17%–38% of cases) than in adults, and Bannwarth polyradiculoneuritis also is a manifestation of Lyme disease in children.[6,7] Borrelial lymphocytoma, a localized tumor-like growth most commonly found on the nipple or earlobe, is common in children and only occurs on the Eurasian continent.[8]

Erythema Migrans

EM is a roughly circular or oval lesion that appears at the site of the tick bite after an incubation of about 1 to 31 days (mean, 10 days). At least two-thirds of solitary EM lesions are initially erythematous plaques with or without an enhanced central erythema, rather than a "bull's eye" or ring shape.[9] Because small ring-shaped lesions from insect bites are more common than Lyme disease in children, pediatricians should not rush to treat a lesion as EM. The differential diagnosis includes insect and tick-bite skin reactions. Unlike these reactions, EM enlarges gradually, and close follow-up establishes the diagnosis if the lesion attains a diameter of at least 5 cm, the minimum diameter required to meet the Centers for Disease Control and Prevention case definition of EM. Rarely, the lesion may have a somewhat atypical presentation with a central vesicular or necrotic area.[10] There can be mild pruritus or a stinging sensation. EM can occur anywhere on the body, but about half of tick bites in children are sustained on the head or neck, so an EM lesion on the scalp could be obscured

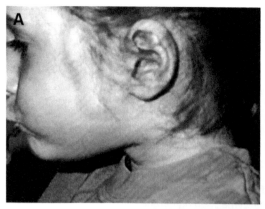
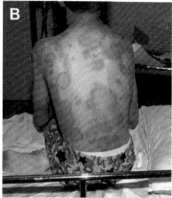
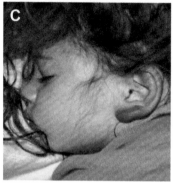

Fig. 2. (*A*) Erythema migrans: scalp lesion only partially visible on the face (*B*) Multiple erythema migrans (*C*) Borrelial lymphocytoma. (*Courtesy of* [*A*] Vijay Sikand, MD, Connecticut; [*B*] Lorry Rubin, MD, New York; and [*C*] Mark Salzman, MD, California. *From* [*A, B*] Sikand V, Mullegger R. Early Lyme borreliosis. In: Sood SK, editor. Lyme borreliosis in Europe and North America. Hoboken (NJ): John Wiley & Sons, Inc; 2011. p. 53–79; and [*C*] Salzman MB, Mullegger RR. Borrelial lymphocytoma and acrodermatitis chronica atrophicans. In: Sood SK, editor. Lyme borreliosis in Europe and North America. Hoboken (NJ): John Wiley & Sons, Inc; 2011. p. 135–48, with permission.)

(**Fig. 2**A). Lesions that resemble EM were observed in nonendemic southern states and in a child on Long Island, New York following bites of Lone Star ticks.[11] This entity was provisionally named southern tick-associated rash illness, but the causative organism is unknown.

Multiple Erythema Migrans

A multiple EM rash is the most common form of early disseminated Lyme disease in children (see **Fig. 2**B). Although the lesions can resemble erythema multiforme, they are distinct because each lesion is ring-like, although varying in size and shape. A single secondary lesion can replace a primary lesion that has since disappeared. The child may experience mild to moderate constitutional symptoms. In a prospective study of 553 children in Slovenia, 333 had solitary and 220 had multiple EM, a proportion similar to solitary and disseminated EM observed in Connecticut.[12] This was the case even though the predominant genospecies in Slovenia was *Borrelia afzelii* (40/44 blood isolates), whereas the genospecies in North America is *Borrelia burgdorferi* sensu stricto. In a related study from the same group, cerebrospinal fluid (CSF) pleocytosis was detected in a quarter of children with multiple EM, indicating possible subclinical central nervous system dissemination, which could have implications for treatment.[13] Systemic symptoms were present in fewer than 50%, and meningeal signs in only 11%.

Neuroborreliosis

Nervous system infection in Lyme disease is also known as neuroborreliosis. Acute neuroborreliosis most commonly manifests as unilateral seventh cranial nerve palsy that resembles Bell palsy, bilateral seventh nerve palsy, lymphocytic meningitis, or any combination thereof.[14] In endemic areas, Lyme facial palsy should be strongly considered in children who present with facial palsy, especially if they present during peak Lyme disease season or with a headache.[15] Children with facial palsy should be assessed clinically for presence of neck stiffness or severe headache to decide the need for lumbar puncture. Because Lyme meningitis and enteroviral meningitis are common in Lyme disease–endemic areas, it is important to appreciate their distinguishing clinical and laboratory features in the absence of EM. The course of Lyme meningitis is more indolent than that of viral meningitis.[16] Children with Lyme meningitis could experience headache, neck pain, or listlessness for several days before coming to medical attention. Signs of meningismus, such as Kernig and Brudzinski signs, are less common. The CSF pleocytosis consists predominantly of mononuclear cells (mostly lymphocytes), compared with the relative prominence of neutrophils often found early in the course of viral meningitis. In one study, the negative predictive value for Lyme meningitis was 99% when neutrophils comprised more than 10% of the cells in the CSF.[16] Clinical prediction algorithms based on these features have been developed to help in the diagnosis of Lyme meningitis in the emergency department setting.[17,18] One of these is termed the "rule of 7s."[18] In a child with meningitis if greater than or equal to 7 days of headache, greater than or equal to 70% mononuclear cells, and seventh (or other) cranial nerve palsy are all present there is a 77% likelihood of Lyme meningitis, whereas absence of these predictors is highly sensitive (96%) for identifying a low risk of Lyme meningitis.

Another important difference between Lyme meningitis and viral meningitis is the increased risk of increased intracranial pressure and papilledema in Lyme meningitis. Most published reports of raised intracranial pressure in Lyme disease have been in children, and the complication has been observed in the absence of meningitis.[7,19] The pathogenesis is unknown but deposition of immune complexes in the arachnoid villi has been speculated to be an underlying mechanism. Headache is prominent in these children. A rare but ominous complication of increased intracranial pressure is transient or permanent impairment of vision.[20] A child in whom increased intracranial pressure persisted despite treatment with ceftriaxone and steroids became permanently blind. In rare cases, objective evidence of optic nerve inflammation has been documented in a few children, occurring in either early or late disease. These observations make it vital to examine the optic discs and to monitor visual acuity in every child with acute disseminated Lyme disease, whether or not they have meningitis. Measurement of the opening CSF pressure should be part of the lumbar puncture, and if elevated, treatment to lower intracranial pressure should be immediately initiated. Close follow-up with a neurologist and an ophthalmologist is crucial.

Bannwarth syndrome, a common neurologic manifestation of Lyme disease in Europe, results from inflammation of peripheral nerves.[21] It should be considered in children who have recently traveled to Europe and present with neuralgia, paresthesias, and motor or sensory impairment, mostly affecting cervical and thoracic dermatomes. Low-grade encephalopathy and peripheral neuropathy occasionally are reported as late sequelae of Lyme disease in adults. In contrast, the neurologic and neuropsychological outcomes of children after recovery from acute neurologic disease are excellent.[22] Cognitive disorders, processing deficits on a battery of neuropsychological tests, or persistent fatigue in children should not be routinely attributed to Lyme disease. Moreover, there is minimal evidence that incidentally detected nonspecific white matter changes on MRI of the brain are caused by Lyme disease.

The association of Lyme disease with Guillain-Barré–like syndrome, acute meningo-encephalitis, transverse myelitis, and multiple cranial nerve palsies is described in published reports, but it is uncertain that this is causal or commonplace. A child with cerebellitis (manifested as cerebellar signs, multiple enhancing lesions on MRI, monocytic pleocytosis, and intrathecal production of B burgdorferi–specific antibodies) has been described.[23]

Lyme Carditis

Lyme carditis is the least commonly encountered manifestation of early disseminated Lyme disease. Cardiac involvement is usually first-, second-, or third-degree atrioventricular conduction block or bundle branch block.[24] Rare presentations are myocarditis, myopericarditis, left ventricular dysfunction, or cardiomegaly. Carditis occurs either in association with EM or acute nervous system involvement, or as the sole manifestation with symptoms of syncope or malaise attributable to symptomatic heart block. Because cardiac conduction abnormalities can be subclinical, obtaining an electrocardiogram should be considered in any child with acute disseminated Lyme disease.

Acute Constitutional Illness

An acute constitutional illness without EM or other focal manifestations, previously termed a flulike illness, is well documented in children as a form of early Lyme disease. Twenty-four untreated children 4 years and older in Connecticut were enrolled in a study if they had at least one of the following symptoms: myalgias, arthralgias, neck pain, headache, or fatigue.[25] Five children who developed self-limited fever and fatigue that lasted 5 to 21 days were confirmed by immunoblot (paired acute and convalescent sera) to have evidence of acute B burgdorferi infection. It is likely that fewer than 10% of children with B burgdorferi infection present with this form of the infection. In tick-endemic areas, babesiosis, human granulocytic anaplasmosis, or ehrlichiosis should also be considered in a child with exposure who presents with an acute constitutional illness.[26]

Lyme Arthritis

Arthritis can be the presenting symptom of Lyme disease. The mean incubation period after the tick bite is about 4 months, but the range is much wider.[27] The clinical onset of Lyme arthritis can be with sudden appearance of joint swelling, or with intermittent and migratory arthralgias or mild periarticular inflammation in the weeks leading up to frank arthritis. It is a monoarthritis in two-thirds of cases, and an oligoarthritis (fewer than four joints) in the remainder.[28] The knee is the presenting joint in 90% of the cases. In contrast to septic arthritis or rheumatic fever, there is joint swelling, effusion, and stiffness that is disproportionate to the relatively mild degree of pain. The child typically continues to ambulate and may be initially evaluated by an orthopedic surgeon for suspected traumatic injury, rather than be brought to emergency care. Basic laboratory analyses of synovial fluid are not very helpful in distinguishing

Lyme arthritis from septic or rheumatic arthritis.[29] Elevated markers and neutrophil-predominant exudates are common to all these conditions.

Lyme arthritis in children was first described as part of the investigation of an outbreak of recurrent monoarticular or oligoarticular arthritis in 39 children and 12 adults in Connecticut, where it was ultimately distinguished from juvenile rheumatoid arthritis.[1] Juvenile rheumatoid arthritis is associated with a polyclonal antibody activation that can cause a positive antibody screen for *B burgdorferi* infection, but immunoblot testing distinguishes this response from Lyme disease.[30] In addition, clinical diagnostic criteria were proposed for diagnosis of Lyme arthritis in children.[31] However, serologic confirmation should remain the gold standard, because almost 100% are seropositive by IgG immunoblot testing.[32]

The pathophysiology and clinical course of Lyme arthritis is consistent with a reactive arthritis.[33] Effusion typically reaccumulates if arthrocentesis is performed, and some degree of inflammation often persists for several weeks after appropriate treatment. Recurrent episodes can involve the same joint or a different joint, which is consistent with reactive arthritis. The severity and duration of arthritis is increased in adolescents, but the antibiotic-refractory arthritis known to occur in up to 10% of adults is not characteristic in pediatric Lyme arthritis.[34,35]

Borrelial Lymphocytoma

Borrelial lymphocytoma, which was historically known as lymphadenosis benigna cutis, is an uncommon manifestation of Lyme borreliosis and occurs more commonly in children than in adults. It is seen solely in Eurasia, because of the prevalence of causative genospecies there (*B afzelii* and *Borrelia garinii*). Borrelial lymphocytoma presents as a painless solitary bluish red plaque or nodule from 1 to 5 cm in diameter, which develops 1 to 6 months after the tick bite and mimics a benign tumor of the skin (see **Fig. 2**C). It occurs almost exclusively on the ear lobes or breast areolae but lesions on scrotum, nose, arm, and scalp have been described.[36] There are generally no constitutional symptoms, but some children may have other manifestations of dissemination. Although generally considered a form of disseminated infection, the lesion has been noted at the site of a tick bite, or at the site of a previous EM lesion.

Acrodermatitis Chronica Atrophicans

Acrodermatitis chronica atrophicans is a late manifestation of Lyme borreliosis that develops months to years after a tick bite. This skin condition is the result of chronic, active infection with *B afzelii* that results in thinning and fibrosis of skin that can become translucent with coloration acquired from underlying muscle and vascular structures. Most patients are older than 40 years but cases in children have been described.[37,38]

Asymptomatic Seroconversion

The finding of seropositivity to *B burgdorferi* is common in persons who live in endemic areas, and can be termed asymptomatic seroconversion if the patient had no symptoms attributable to Lyme disease. It is indicative of past subclinical infection, and is often discovered incidentally when serology for Lyme disease is ordered as part of evaluation for an illness of uncertain cause. The ratio of symptomatic infection to asymptomatic Lyme disease was about 9:1 in a prospective study in an endemic area.[39] Because the asymptomatic state indicates there has been successful clearance of the spirochete, there is no evidence that such children should be treated with antibiotics, which could place them at risk for adverse effects.

Lyme Disease in Pregnancy

Maternal to fetal transmission of B burgdorferi has never been definitively documented, and it may not occur at all, even after untreated Lyme disease during pregnancy.[40,41] Moreover, comprehensive epidemiologic investigations failed to show an association between maternal infection during pregnancy and fetal death, prematurity, congenital malformations, or infant neurologic disorders.[42,43] There is no evidence that transmission of B burgdorferi occurs via breastfeeding.

DIAGNOSIS

There are no separate diagnostic tests or criteria for Lyme disease in children. Children with single or multiple EM in Slovenia are often bacteremic, but blood culture for B burgdorferi is not recommended for diagnosis of EM.[44] For borrelial lymphocytoma, a biopsy may be indicated if the location is atypical, or if a tumor is in the differential diagnosis. Histologically the lesion consists of a dense polyclonal predominantly B-lymphocytic infiltration of the cutis and subcutis, usually with germinal centers.[36]

It is important for pediatricians to use serologic testing appropriately, and for them to be comfortable with interpretation of results in common clinical scenarios. Serologic testing should be ordered only if the current signs and symptoms are consistent with Lyme disease. For those without findings of EM, the results of confirmatory immuno-blot (Western blot) testing should be awaited before treatment is initiated, with the exception of the child who presents early in the course of neurologic dissemination or advanced heart block.[45] Serologic confirmation is unnecessary if the child presents with EM. Lyme disease may not be the cause of a child's current symptoms even if a test is positive, because antibodies can persist after past treatment or subclinical B burgdorferi infection, and because false-positive results on screening enzyme-linked immunosorbent assay tests are common. A common scenario is a child who has positive (immunoblot confirmed) serology for B burgdorferi infection, because the tests were ordered as part of a work-up for constitutional symptoms or atypical rash, but has no objective symptoms attributable to Lyme disease. Many clinicians treat such children even as they consider other conditions, for fear of the emergence of late manifestations, but there is scant evidence for this practice. The common practice of ordering antibody tests for Lyme disease for nonspecific or febrile illnesses is strongly discouraged, especially if the opportunity for tick exposure has not even been evaluated. The consequences of such indiscriminate testing can be harmful to the child's health. Besides being subjected to unnecessary antibiotic treatment, a child with a false-positive test could be labeled as having Lyme disease, which in the mind of many parents and practitioners, erroneously connotes a chronic illness.

TREATMENT AND PROGNOSIS

Treatment for children who have Lyme disease should follow the evidence-based guideline of the Infectious Diseases Society of America. **Table 1** is based upon this guideline.[46] Treatment of Lyme disease is effective at all stages of the infection, and treatment failures are very uncommon. B burgdorferi is highly susceptible to β-lactam antibiotics and to tetracyclines.

Doxycycline and amoxicillin are equivalent choices for treatment of early Lyme disease, and most experts prefer doxycycline for children 8 years or older. Doxycycline has the advantages of being effective for treatment of anaplasmosis that may simultaneously occur with Lyme disease, and superior central nervous system penetration. Although intravenous ceftriaxone is the initial treatment of choice for early

Table 1
Treatment of Lyme borreliosis

Manifestation	First-Line Drugs	Equivalent Alternate Drugs	Second-Line Drugs
Early localized EM*	Amoxicillin PO 10–21 d or doxycycline PO 10–21 d	Cefuroxime axetil PO[a] 10–21 d	Azithromycin PO 7–10 d, clarithromycin PO 14–21 d, or erythromycin PO 14–21 d
Early disseminated			
Multiple EM	Amoxicillin PO 21–28 d or doxycycline PO 21–28 d	Cefuroxime axetil PO[a] 21–28 d or ceftriaxone IV 14 d or cefotaxime IV 14 d	Azithromycin PO 7–10 d, clarithromycin PO 14–21 d, or erythromycin PO 14–21 d
Facial palsy	Amoxicillin PO 21–28 d or doxycycline PO 21–28 d	Ceftriaxone IV 14–28 d or cefotaxime IV 14–28 d	Azithromycin PO 7–10 d, clarithromycin PO 14–21 d, or erythromycin PO 14–21 d
Meningitis/facial palsy with meningitis/ polyneuropathy	Ceftriaxone IV 14–28 d or cefotaxime IV 14–28 d	Doxycycline PO 28 d	Penicillin IV 14–28 d
Cardiac[b]	Amoxicillin PO 21 d or doxycycline PO 21 d or ceftriaxone IV 14 d or cefotaxime IV 14 d		Azithromycin PO 7–10 d, clarithromycin PO 14–21 d, or erythromycin PO 14–21 d
Late			
Arthritis	Amoxicillin PO 28 d or doxycycline PO 28 d	Ceftriaxone[c] IV 14–28 d or cefotaxime[c] IV 14–28 d	Penicillin IV 14–28 d
Neurologic	Ceftriaxone IV 14–28 d or cefotaxime IV 14–28 d	Doxycycline PO 28 d	Penicillin IV 14–28 d
Other			
Asymptomatic seroconversion or acute constitutional illness	Amoxicillin PO 21–28 d or doxycycline PO 21–28 d	Cefuroxime axetil PO[a] 21–28 d	Azithromycin PO 7–10 d, clarithromycin PO 14–21 d, or erythromycin PO 14–21 d

Doses: Doxycycline 2–4 mg/kg/day divided into two doses, up to adult dose of 200 mg a day; amoxicillin 40–50 mg/kg/day divided into three doses, up to adult dose of 2 g a day; cefuroxime axetil 30 mg/kg/day divided into two doses, up to adult dose of 1 g a day; azithromycin 10 mg/kg once daily (maximum of 500 mg per day); erythromycin 30–40 mg/kg/day divided into four doses, up to adult dose of 1 g a day; clarithromycin 15 mg/kg/day divided into two doses, up to adult dose of 1 g a day; ceftriaxone 100 mg/kg/day once daily, up to adult dose of 2 g a day; cefotaxime 180 mg/kg/day, up to adult dose of 6 g a day; penicillin 200,000–400,000 units/kg/day, divided into four doses, up to adult dose of 24 million units a day.

Abbreviations: EM, erythema migrans; IV, intravenous; PO, by mouth.

* Use same treatment regimens as EM for borrelial lymphocytoma.

[a] Cefuroxime axetil was tested in children 12 and older.

[b] First-degree block with PR interval less than 0.3 seconds, PO therapy; PR greater than 0.3 seconds or higher grade, IV initially, then PO if responds rapidly.

[c] For oral therapy failures only.

disseminated Lyme disease with meningitis, doxycycline can be a latter part of therapy, such as when parenteral therapy becomes unfeasible. If a child who presents with Lyme facial palsy has concomitant meningitis by the presence of CSF pleocytosis, treatment with parenteral ceftriaxone is preferred. Children with Lyme carditis manifesting as second- or third-degree atrioventricular block, or with first-degree heart block when the PR interval is prolonged to ≥ 30 milliseconds, should be continuously monitored in the hospital and treated with intravenous ceftriaxone until resolution of symptomatic block. In some patients, temporary pacing may be indicated.

Most children with Lyme arthritis are effectively treated with oral therapy (doxycycline or amoxicillin). Persistent or recurrent joint swelling after antibiotic therapy is usually an indication of posttreatment reactive arthritis or patellofemoral inflammation, but if retreatment is considered, the options are a repeat 4-week course of oral antibiotics or a 2- to 4-week course of ceftriaxone. Nonsteroidal anti-inflammatory agents, intra-articular corticosteroids, disease-modifying antirheumatic drugs, such as hydroxychloroquine, and arthroscopic synovectomy are adjunct treatments considered for children with significant pain or limitation of movement.[47]

Published treatment trials and cumulative clinical experience have demonstrated that children who receive appropriate antibiotic treatment of Lyme disease have an excellent prognosis. This is also true for Lyme arthritis, a late disseminated stage of the infection. Chronic arthritis, joint deformities, or recurrences of infection were not observed even among children who experienced antibiotic-refractory arthritis.[47] In an earlier telephone follow-up study of Lyme arthritis, only 4 of 90 children reported ongoing musculoskeletal complaints, and none had evidence of arthritis, 2 to 12 years following treatment.[28] Older age and female gender were associated with persistent arthritis in a series of 55 children in Germany.[48] No cardiac, neurologic, or arthritic sequelae were identified among 63 children 11 months to 22 years old treated for physician-documented EM in a practice in southeastern Connecticut.[49] In children in Sweden with confirmed neuroborreliosis, mild persistent motor or sensory deficits were detected in about a quarter of children at 5-year follow up. Half of these were persistent facial nerve palsy, and the deficits did not affect daily activities or school performance more often in patients than in controls. Nonspecific subjective symptoms such as headache, fatigue, or memory or concentration problems were not more common in patients than in controls.[50] There is no evidence that persistence of fatigue, musculoskeletal pain, or difficulties with concentration or short-term memory after treatment of Lyme disease are caused by persistence of B burgdorferi.[51] The pathogenesis of these symptoms is likely similar to other postinfectious conditions in which persistent immune-mediated inflammation occurs after resolution of an infection.[52] Reinfection has been noted in fewer children than in adults, occurring in about 3%.[5]

PREVENTION AND MANAGEMENT OF IXODES TICK BITES

Avoidance of exposure to tick-infested vegetation is the ideal prevention, but children in endemic areas have many opportunities for tick bites in recreational and residential spaces.[53] The key to prevention is the use of repellents in conjunction with daily tick checks and prompt removal of attached ticks. Diethyltoluamide (DEET) is the most effective repellent, but has been underused because of exaggerated concerns about potential toxicity. Only very small amounts are absorbed after topical application and the compound is rapidly eliminated. A 25% to 35% formulation, which provides about 6 hours of protection, should be used with care to avoid application near mucosal surfaces in young children (**Box 1**, **Table 2**). Because some DEET-sunscreen combinations and topical retinoids can enhance the absorption of DEET, the use of

---

Box 1
Use of repellents and insecticides to prevent *Ixodes* tick bites in children

DEET

- Use any formulation of DEET with concentration between 25% and 35%
  - American Academy of Pediatrics recommends 10%–30% DEET for children 2 months of age and older[59]
  - Health Canada recommends using a product containing no more than 10% DEET for children ≤12 years of age; note that DEET concentration of ≤10% does not provide protection for more than 1–2 h (see **Table 2**)[60]
- When using on babies, avoid face and mucosal surfaces
- Do not use on open wounds, inflamed or sunburned skin, and do not leave on overnight
- Do not use preparations that are premixed with sunscreens or other active ingredients; apply sunscreen before applying DEET

Permethrin (a repellent and insecticide)

- Apply liberally on clothes, shoes, surfaces of equipment, and patio surfaces

Other products registered for use as tick repellents by the US Environmental Protection Agency are picaridin (KBR 3023), the plant-based oil of eucalyptus, and IR3535 (3-[N-butyl-N-acetyl]-aminopropionic acid, ethyl ester); data on their efficacy against ticks are limited.

---

combination DEET-sunscreen preparations is not recommended.[54,55] Permethrin applied to or impregnated in clothing is a highly effective adjunct. Tick checks should be performed under bright lighting and ticks removed with an ordinary pair of thin-tipped tweezers. Bathing with a washcloth with special attention to armpit, groin, back, and scalp areas is effective to dislodge unattached ticks. Early removal of an *Ixodes* tick minimized the risk of acquiring *B burgdorferi* infection.[56,57]

Despite the very low incidence of *B burgdorferi* infection following an *Ixodes* tick bite, even in endemic areas, there is considerable apprehension around tick bites, and physicians tend to overprescribe antibiotic prophylaxis. More importantly, the patient should save the tick in any dry vessel for identification, and tick identification should be performed at a commercial laboratory or local health department. A large proportion of tick bites in Lyme disease–endemic areas are from non-*Ixodes* ticks (eg, *Amblyomma* and *Dermacentor* spp.) and therefore do not result in transmission of *B burgdorferi*. Tick analysis for *B burgdorferi* DNA should not be ordered because this testing is unreliable

Table 2
Estimated protection time against mosquitoes for DEET

DEET Concentration, %	Protection Time, Hours	
	Mean	Range
5	2	1.5–2.5
10	3.5	2.5–4.5
15	5	3.5–5.5
20	5.5	4–6.5
30	6.5	5–8

Data from Onyett H, Canadian Paediatric Society, Infectious Diseases and Immunization Committee. Preventing mosquito and tick bites: a Canadian update. Paediatr Child Health 2014;19(6):327.

and furthermore does not predict transmission risk. The duration of attachment of an *Ixodes* tick does predict transmission risk, because there is a 36- to 72-hour delay between the onset of feeding and the migration of spirochetes from the midgut to the salivary glands where transmission to the host can occur. The incidence of human infection is increased 20-fold from ticks attached less than 72 hours compared with those attached for 72 hours or longer.[57] Tick identification and assessment of engorgement can be used to help define a small, high-risk subset of people who should benefit from antibiotic prophylaxis. However, the expertise to assess tick engorgement is not usually available, so a "wait and watch" approach is appropriate, given the overall low risk of infection from an *Ixodes* tick bite, in the range of 1% to 4% in endemic areas.[58] A child who had an attached tick needs to be monitored closely for signs and symptoms of Lyme disease (and other tick-borne diseases) for up to 1 month. There is no clinical use to serologic testing in an asymptomatic child after a tick bite.

SUMMARY

Manifestations of Lyme disease in children are similar to those seen in adults, but there seems to be a greater risk of visual impairment in acute disseminated disease, based on observations made in children. In addition, the prognosis of late Lyme disease (arthritis) is notably better in children, with refractory arthritis a rare occurrence. Practitioners who see children need to be reminded of the potential consequences of indiscriminate serologic screening for Lyme disease.

REFERENCES

1. Steere AC, Malawista SE, Snydman DR, et al. Lyme arthritis: an epidemic of oligoarticular arthritis in children and adults in three Connecticut communities. Arthritis Rheum 1977;20(1):7–17.
2. Hazard GW, Leland K, Mathewson HO. Erythema chronicum migrans and "Lyme arthritis." JAMA 1976;236:2392.
3. Mast WE, Burrows WM. Erythema chronicum migrans and "Lyme arthritis." JAMA 1976;236:859–60.
4. Bacon RM, Kugeler KJ, Mead PS, Centers for Disease Control and Prevention (CDC). Surveillance for Lyme disease–United States, 1992-2006. MMWR Surveill Summ 2008;57(10):1–9.
5. Gerber MA, Shapiro ED, Burke GS, et al. Lyme disease in children in southeastern Connecticut. Pediatric Lyme Disease Study Group. N Engl J Med 1996;335(17):1270–4.
6. Christen HJ, Hanefeld F, Eiffert H, et al. Epidemiology and clinical manifestations of Lyme borreliosis in childhood. A prospective multicentre study with special regard to neuroborreliosis. Acta Paediatr Suppl 1993;386:1–75.
7. Sood SK. What we have learned about Lyme borreliosis from studies in children. Wien Klin Wochenschr 2006;118:638–42.
8. Mullegger RR. Dermatological manifestations of Lyme borreliosis. Eur J Dermatol 2004;14(5):296–309.
9. Shapiro ED. *Borrelia burgdorferi* (Lyme disease). Pediatr Rev 2014;35(12):500–9.
10. Sikand V, Mullegger R. Early Lyme borreliosis. In: Sood SK, editor. Lyme borreliosis in Europe and North America. Hoboken (NJ): John Wiley & Sons, Inc; 2011. p. 53–79.
11. Feder HM Jr, Hoss DM, Zemel L, et al. Southern tick-associated rash illness (STARI) in the North: STARI following a tick bite in Long Island, New York. Clin Infect Dis 2011;53(10):e142–6.

12. Arnez M, Pleterski-Rigler D, Luznik-Bufon T, et al. Solitary and multiple erythema migrans in children: comparison of demographic, clinical and laboratory findings. Infection 2003;31(6):404–9.

13. Arnez M, Pleterski-Rigler D, Luznik-Bufon T, et al. Children with multiple erythema migrans: are there any pre-treatment symptoms and/or signs suggestive for central nervous system involvement? Wien Klin Wochenschr 2002; 114(13–14):524–9.

14. Shapiro ED, Gerber MA. Lyme disease and facial nerve palsy. Arch Pediatr Adolesc Med 1997;151(12):1183–4.

15. Nigrovic LE, Thompson AD, Fine AM, et al. Clinical predictors of Lyme disease among children with a peripheral facial palsy at an emergency department in a Lyme disease-endemic area. Pediatrics 2008;122(5):e1080–5.

16. Shah SS, Zaoutis TE, Turnquist J, et al. Early differentiation of Lyme from enteroviral meningitis. Pediatr Infect Dis J 2005;24(6):542–5.

17. Avery RA, Frank G, Glutting JJ, et al. Prediction of Lyme meningitis in children from a Lyme disease-endemic region: a logistic-regression model using history, physical, and laboratory findings. Pediatrics 2006;117:e1–7.

18. Cohn KA, Thompson AD, Shah SS, et al. Validation of a clinical prediction rule to distinguish Lyme meningitis from aseptic meningitis. Pediatrics 2012;129(1): e46–53.

19. Kan L, Sood SK, Maytal J. Pseudotumor cerebri in Lyme disease: a case report and literature review. Pediatr Neurol 1998;18(5):439–41.

20. Rothermel H, Hedges TR III, Steere AC. Optic neuropathy in children with Lyme disease. Pediatrics 2001;108(2):477–81.

21. Christen HJ. Lyme neuroborreliosis in children. Ann Med 1996;28(3):235–40.

22. Adams WV, Rose CD, Eppes SC, et al. Cognitive effects of Lyme disease in children: a 4 year followup study. J Rheumatol 1999;26(5):1190–4.

23. Arav-Boger R, Crawford T, Steere AC, et al. Cerebellar ataxia as the presenting manifestation of Lyme disease. Pediatr Infect Dis J 2002;21(4):353–6.

24. Haddad FA, Nadelman RB. Lyme disease and the heart. Front Biosci 2003;8: s769–82.

25. Feder HM Jr, Gerber MA, Krause PJ, et al. Early Lyme disease: a flu-like illness without erythema migrans. Pediatrics 1993;91(2):456–9.

26. Krause PJ, McKay K, Thompson CA, et al. Deer-associated infection study group. Disease-specific diagnosis of coinfecting tickborne zoonoses: babesiosis, human granulocytic ehrlichiosis, and Lyme disease. Clin Infect Dis 2002;34(9):1184–91.

27. Szer IS, Taylor E, Steere AC. The long-term course of Lyme arthritis in children. N Engl J Med 1991;325(3):159–63.

28. Gerber MA, Zemel LS, Shapiro ED. Lyme arthritis in children: clinical epidemiology and long-term outcomes. Pediatrics 1998;102:905–8.

29. Deanehan JK, Nigrovic PA, Milewski MD, et al. Synovial fluid findings in children with knee monoarthritis in Lyme disease endemic areas. Pediatr Emerg Care 2014;30(1):16–9.

30. Sood SK, Rubin LG, Blader ME, et al. Positive Lyme disease serology in juvenile rheumatoid arthritis in a Lyme disease endemic area: analysis by immunoblot. J Rheumatol 1993;20:739–41.

31. Huppertz HI, Bentas W, Haubitz I, et al. Diagnosis of paediatric Lyme arthritis using a clinical score. Eur J Pediatr 1998;157(4):304–8.

32. Johnson BJ, Aguero-Rosenfeld ME, Wilske B. Serodiagnosis of Lyme borreliosis. In: Sood SK, editor. Lyme borreliosis in Europe and North America. Hoboken (NJ): John Wiley & Sons, Inc; 2011. p. 185–212.

33. Steere AC, Glickstein L. Elucidation of Lyme arthritis. Nat Rev Immunol 2004;4(2): 143–52.
34. Huppertz HI, Karch H, Suschke HJ, et al. Lyme arthritis in European children and adolescents. The Pediatric Rheumatology Collaborative Group. Arthritis Rheum 1995;38(3):361–8.
35. Daikh BE, Emerson FE, Smith RP, et al. Lyme arthritis: a comparison of presentation, synovial fluid analysis, and treatment course in children and adults. Arthritis Care Res 2013;65(12):1986–90.
36. Colli C, Leinweber B, Müllegger R, et al. Borrelia burgdorferi-associated lymphocytoma cutis: clinicopathologic, immunophenotypic, and molecular study of 106 cases. J Cutan Pathol 2004;31(3):232–40.
37. Nadal D, Gundelfinger R, Flueler U, et al. Acrodermatitis chronica atrophicans. Arch Dis Child 1988;63(1):72–4.
38. Zalaudek I, Leinweber B, Kerl H, et al. Acrodermatitis chronica atrophicans in a 15-year-ol girl misdiagnosed as venous insufficiency for 6 years. J Am Acad Dermatol 2005;52(6):1091–4.
39. Steere AC, Sikand VK, Schoen RT, et al. Asymptomatic infection with *Borrelia burgdorferi*. Clin Infect Dis 2003;37(4):528–32.
40. Markowitz LE, Steere AC, Benach JL, et al. Lyme disease during pregnancy. JAMA 1986;255(24):3394–6.
41. Elliott DJ, Eppes SC, Klein JD. Teratogen update: Lyme disease. Teratology 2001; 64:276–81.
42. Strobino B, Abid S, Gewitz M. Maternal Lyme disease and congenital heart disease: a case-control study in an endemic area. Am J Obstet Gynecol 1999; 180(3 Pt 1):711–6.
43. Gerber MA, Zalneraitis EL. Childhood neurologic disorders and Lyme disease during pregnancy. Pediatr Neurol 1994;11(1):41–3.
44. Arnež M, Ružić-Sabljić E. *Borrelia burgdorferi* sensu lato bacteremia in Slovenian children with solitary and multiple erythema migrans. Pediatr Infect Dis J 2011; 30(11):988–90.
45. Jain VK, Hilton E, Maytal J, et al. Immunoglobulin M immunoblot for diagnosis of *Borrelia burgdorferi* infection in patients with acute facial palsy. J Clin Microbiol 1996;34:2033–5.
46. Wormser GP, Dattwyler RJ, Shapiro ED, et al. The clinical assessment, treatment, and prevention of Lyme disease, human granulocytic anaplasmosis, and babesiosis: clinical practice guidelines by the Infectious Diseases Society of America. Clin Infect Dis 2006;43(9):1089–134 [Erratum appears in Clin Infect Dis 2007;45(7):941].
47. Tory HO, Zurakowski D, Sundel RP. Outcomes of children treated for Lyme arthritis: results of a large pediatric cohort. J Rheumatol 2010;37(5):1049–55.
48. Sood SK, Ilowite NT. Lyme arthritis in children: is chronic arthritis a common complication? J Rheumatol 2000;27(8):1836–8.
49. Salazar J, Gerber M, Goff C. Long-term outcome of Lyme disease in children given early treatment. J Pediatr 1993;122:591–3.
50. Skogman BH, Glimåker K, Nordwall M, et al. Long-term clinical outcome after Lyme neuroborreliosis in childhood. Pediatrics 2012;130(2):262–9.
51. Shapiro ED, Sood SK. Prognosis of persons with Lyme borreliosis. In: Sood SK, editor. Lyme borreliosis in Europe and North America. Hoboken (NJ): John Wiley & Sons, Inc; 2011. p. 213–23.
52. Feder HM Jr, Johnson BJ, O'Connell S, et al. A critical appraisal of "chronic Lyme disease." N Engl J Med 2007;357:1422–30.

53. Hayes EB, Piesman J. How can we prevent Lyme disease? N Engl J Med 2003; 348:2424–30.
54. Ross EA, Savage KA, Utley LJ, et al. Insect repellent [correction of repellant] interactions: sunscreens enhance DEET (N,N-diethyl-m-toluamide) absorption. Drug Metab Dispos 2004;32(8):783–5.
55. Katz TM, Miller JH, Hebert AA. Insect repellents: historical perspectives and new developments. J Am Acad Dermatol 2008;58(5):865–71.
56. Nadelman RB, Nowakowski J, Fish D, et al. Prophylaxis with single-dose doxycycline for the prevention of Lyme disease after an *Ixodes scapularis* tick bite. N Engl J Med 2001;345(2):79–84.
57. Sood SK, Salzman MB, Johnson BJ, et al. Duration of tick attachment as a predictor of the risk of Lyme disease in an area in which Lyme disease is endemic. J Infect Dis 1997;175(4):996–9.
58. Shapiro ED. Clinical practice. Lyme disease. N Engl J Med 2014;370(18): 1724–31.
59. American Academy of Pediatrics. Prevention of tickborne infections. In: Pickering LK, Baker CJ, Kimberlin DW, et al, editors. Red Book: 2012 Report of the Committee on Infectious Diseases. Elk Grove Village (IL): American Academy of Pediatrics; 2012. p. 207–9.
60. Onyett H, Canadian Paediatric Society, Infectious Diseases and Immunization Committee. Preventing mosquito and tick bites: a Canadian update. Paediatr Child Health 2014;19(6):326–32.

Laboratory Diagnosis of Lyme Disease

Advances and Challenges

Adriana R. Marques, MD

KEYWORDS

- Lyme disease • *Borrelia burgdorferi* • Laboratory diagnosis • Serology

KEY POINTS

- It is difficult to demonstrate *Borrelia burgdorferi* by direct techniques (culture and polymerase chain reaction [PCR]). The spirochete is more easily found in the skin and plasma samples of patients with early disease (erythema migrans), and in the synovial fluid of patients with Lyme arthritis (using PCR).
- The sensitivity of antibody-based tests increases with the duration of the infection. Less than 50% of patients with erythema migrans are positive at presentation. These patients should receive treatment based on the clinical diagnosis.
- Serologic tests are most helpful in patients with clinical findings indicating later stages of Lyme disease.
- Many tests for Lyme disease are being performed in patients with low likelihood to have the disease, a situation in which a positive result is more likely to be a false-positive.
- The current assays do not distinguish between active and past infection, and patients may continue to be seropositive for years.
- The use of nonvalidated Lyme diagnostic tests is not recommended.

OVERVIEW

Lyme disease, or Lyme borreliosis, is a multisystem illness caused by the spirochete *Borrelia burgdorferi* and it is the most common tick-borne illness in the United States and Europe. Newly revised estimates from the Centers for Disease Control and Prevention (CDC) suggest that there are likely to be around 300,000 new cases of

This research was supported by the Intramural Research Program National Institute of Allergy and Infectious Diseases, NIH.

Disclaimer: The findings and conclusions in this article are those of the author and do not necessarily represent the official views of the National Institute of Allergy and Infectious Diseases.

Laboratory of Clinical Infectious Diseases, National Institute of Allergy and Infectious Diseases, National Institutes of Health, 10/12C118 10 Center Drive, Bethesda, MD 20892, USA

E-mail address: amarques@niaid.nih.gov

Infect Dis Clin N Am 29 (2015) 295–307
http://dx.doi.org/10.1016/j.idc.2015.02.005
0891-5520/15/$ – see front matter Published by Elsevier Inc.

id.theclinics.com

Lyme disease per year in the United States.[1] *B burgdorferi* is transmitted by the bite of infected ticks of the *Ixodes ricinus* complex. In the United States, most cases of Lyme disease are caused by the blacklegged tick (*Ixodes scapularis*), occurring in the mid-Atlantic, northeast, and upper Midwest regions.

B burgdorferi is a gram-negative bacterium, and has the elongated and spiral shape of the spirochetes.[2] It varies from 10 to 30 μm in length and 0.2 to 0.5 μm in width. It has a linear chromosome and a variable number of circular and linear plasmids.[3] The *B burgdorferi* sensu lato group includes at least 20 genospecies.[4] Three genospecies are most commonly associated with human infections: *B burgdorferi* sensu stricto, which causes disease in North America and Europe; and *Borrelia afzelii* and *Borrelia garinii*, which occur in Europe and Asia.[5] Additional genospecies have been shown to at least occasionally cause human disease in Europe (eg, *Borrelia spielmanii* and *Borrelia valaisiana*).[5] There is some variation in the clinical presentation depending on the infecting genospecies, with *B burgdorferi* sensu stricto predominating in arthritis, *B garinii* in neurologic disease, and *B afzelii* in chronic skin manifestations.[6] Even within the same genospecies, there is variation in presentation and dissemination capability.[7,8]

For clinical purposes, Lyme disease is divided into early localized, early disseminated, and late stages. Lyme disease usually begins with the characteristic skin lesion, erythema migrans (EM), at the site of the tick bite.[9–11] After several days or weeks, the spirochete may disseminate and patients can develop neurologic, cardiac, and rheumatologic involvement.[12–15] The infection is characterized by low number of bacteria, which can persist in collagen-rich tissues. Although antibiotic therapy accelerates resolution of the disease, manifestations can spontaneously regress without antibiotic therapy. The resolution of disease is mediated by immune responses, which control the infection. However, without antibiotic therapy, it can recur and/or new manifestations can appear.[9,16,17]

The available laboratory methods for the diagnosis of Lyme disease are in 2 categories: direct methods to detect *B burgdorferi*, and indirect methods that detect the immune response against it (mainly the detection of antibodies against *B burgdorferi*). It is important to recognize that laboratory tests should be ordered and interpreted in the context of the clinical evaluation and the likelihood that the patient has Lyme disease. This article reviews the laboratory diagnostics for Lyme disease (with focus on the United States) and discusses current recommendations and new developments.

DIRECT METHODS FOR DETECTION OF *BORRELIA BURGDORFERI*

Laboratory tests for direct detection of *B burgdorferi* are hampered by very low numbers of spirochetes in most clinical samples. The lack of sensitive, easy, fast, direct tests for the presence of *B burgdorferi* is one of the main challenges in the laboratory diagnosis of Lyme disease. Although direct tests for *B burgdorferi* can sometimes be helpful, none are required for the diagnosis of the disease. The main direct test modalities used are culture and PCR. Histopathology has limited utility, being used mostly to exclude other diseases, and in the evaluation of suspected cases of borrelial lymphocytoma and acrodermatitis chronica atrophicans.[18,19] Detection of *B burgdorferi* is difficult and time consuming because of the extreme scarcity of organisms.[20–23] Warthin-Starry and modified Dieterle silver stains, focus-floating microscopy, as well as direct and indirect immunofluorescence assays with antiborrelial antibodies have been used, but can be difficult to interpret and require special expertise and careful use of controls.[24–26] At present, no antigen assays are recommended for the diagnosis of Lyme disease. A research test for detection of outer surface protein (Osp) A has been used in cerebrospinal fluid.[27] An assay to detect antigens in urine has been shown to be unreliable.[28]

CULTURE

Culture is not a routinely available diagnostic method for the diagnosis of Lyme disease in clinical practice, because of its relatively low sensitivity, long incubation, and the requirement of special media and expertise. However, the ability to isolate and culture *B burgdorferi* is essential in Lyme disease research, and culture remains the gold standard to confirm the diagnosis. Methods that would improve sensitivity and simplify the procedure are needed to allow it to be adopted more extensively.

B burgdorferi has a limited metabolic capacity and requires a complex growth medium for cultivation. Media used for culturing *B burgdorferi* include variations of the Barbour-Stoenner-Kelly medium[29] and the modified Kelly-Pettenkofer medium.[30] Cultures are examined using dark-field microscopy or fluorescent microscopy after staining aliquots with acridine orange, but sensitivity is improved by testing aliquots with PCR methods.[31] *B burgdorferi* replicates slowly and cultures are kept for 8 to 12 weeks before being considered negative.[31]

The probability of culturing *B burgdorferi* depends on the specimen, the stage of the disease, and the expertise of the laboratory. It may also depend on the genotype.[32] Antibiotic therapy with agents effective against *B burgdorferi* (even a single dose) significantly affects the recovery rate.[33,34]

Culture of skin biopsies from EM has a sensitivity of 40% to 60%.[30,34–41] In the United States, where disease is caused by *B burgdorferi* sensu stricto, positive cultures are associated with shorter duration of the disease and smaller lesions.[35,42] Positive skin biopsy cultures in central Europe (where most of the isolates were *B afzelii*) were associated with larger lesions (up to about 15 cm in diameter) and increased duration (up to 30 days).[43] These findings are likely related to the different *Borrelia* species and the host immune response that eventually controls the infection. *B afzelii* causes slow-growing EM lesions with few systemic symptoms, whereas *B burgdorferi* sensu stricto is associated with more rapidly expanding skin lesions and more systemic symptoms.[11] Culture is moderately successful in skin biopsies of acrodermatitis chronica atrophicans lesions.[34]

Culture of 9-mL plasma samples from untreated patients with early and early disseminated infection has a sensitivity of around 40%, which can be increased to 75% by frequently testing culture aliquots with a sensitive PCR. Blood cultures are more likely to be positive in patients with multiple EM.[31,36] *B burgdorferi* is seldom cultured from the blood of patients with Lyme disease with later manifestations of the disease.[44,45] Culture of cerebrospinal fluid is rarely positive.[41,46–48] *B burgdorferi* has not been reliably cultivated from synovial fluid.[49]

There are serious concerns[50] regarding a new serum culture assay that claims a high positivity rate[51] and further validation is needed. Results from another culture assays reported as having high positivity rates in patients with chronic disease[52] could not be replicated.[53,54]

POLYMERASE CHAIN REACTION

In general, sensitivity of PCR assays for detection of *B burgdorferi* DNA directly in skin or blood samples seems similar to culture, but there is more variation because of methodology, gene targets, and primer sets used.[34–38,42,45] When optimal culture methods are used, PCR seems to be less sensitive, particularly for plasma samples, which may relate to the smaller sample volume tested in PCR assays.[36] A new assay using broad-range PCR and electrospray ionization mass spectrometry seems promising.[55] At this point, the main use of PCR assays is for evaluating synovial fluid samples in patients with Lyme arthritis, in whom B burgdorferi DNA can be detected in up to 70% to 85% of patients.[42,56,57] A positive PCR does not necessarily mean an infection is active.[42] Sensitivity of PCR in cerebrospinal fluid samples of patients with early neuroborreliosis is low (10%–30%) and even lower in late disease.[58]

INDIRECT METHODS

Indirect methods detect the immune response of the host against the causative organism. Most laboratory tests performed for Lyme disease are based on detection of the antibody responses against B burgdorferi in serum. Antibody-based assays are the only type of diagnostic testing for Lyme disease approved by the US Food and Drug Administration.

A major problem in laboratory diagnostics of Lyme disease is the appropriate use of tests. About 3.4 million Lyme serologic tests are done in the United States every year,[59] which is vastly more than the estimated number of 300,000 cases of the disease. It is likely that tests are being used in situations for which they are not recommended, including ruling out Lyme disease in populations with a low probability of having the disease. The predictive value of a test is determined by its sensitivity, specificity, and the prevalence of the disease in the population to be tested. Consequently, in a patient with low probability of disease, a negative test rules out the disease, whereas a positive test is more likely to be a false-positive.

To improve the specificity of serologic testing for Lyme disease, a 2-tier approach (**Fig. 1**) was recommended in 1995 by the CDC.[60] The first step uses a sensitive enzyme immunoassay (EIA) or, rarely, an indirect immunofluorescence assay. If the test is negative, there is no further testing. If the test is borderline or positive, the sample is retested using separate immunoglobulin (Ig) M and IgG Western blots (WBs; also referred to as immunoblots in the literature) as the second step. The WB is interpreted using standardized criteria, requiring at least 2 of 3 signature bands for a positive IgM WB, and 5 of 10 signature bands for a positive IgG WB. The IgM WB results are used only for disease of less than 4 weeks' duration. These recommendations apply to infection acquired in the United States, because other species within the B burgdorferi sensu lato complex can cause disease in Europe and Asia.

The use of specialty laboratories offering nonvalidated Lyme diagnostic tests, including unique interpretation of WB results, is discouraged. They offer no documented advantage in terms of sensitivity, whereas there is a large decrease in specificity.[61] The use of antibody assays in synovial fluid is not recommended.[62] There is little published information about use of WBs in cerebrospinal fluid for the diagnosis of neuroborreliosis.

The current 2-tier algorithm works well when used as recommended, but there are many areas for improvement. Problems include the low sensitivity during early infection, subjective interpretation of bands, and confusion by health care providers and patients regarding how to interpret results.

Most assays are based on whole-cell sonicate (WCS) derived from cultured B burgdorferi. WCS-based assays can have a significant number of false-positive results because of the presence of cross-reactive antigens.[63] Also, proteins expressed in culture can differ from antigens expressed in vivo. An example is the Vmp-like sequence, expressed (VlsE) lipoprotein, which causes a rapid and strong humoral response during infection, whereas there is minimal VlsE expression in cultured B burgdorferi. Adding VlsE to both first-tier and second-tier tests has improved their

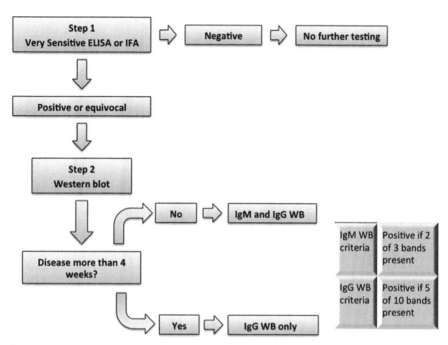

Fig. 1. Current CDC recommendations on serologic diagnosis of Lyme disease: 2-tier algorithm. Both immunoglobulin (Ig) G and IgM Western blot (WB) results are reported, but an IgM WB-positive result is only significant for patients who have been ill for less than a month. ELISA, enzyme-linked immunosorbent assay; IFA, immunofluorescence antibody assay. (*Adapted from* CDC. Recommendations for test performance and interpretation from the Second National Conference on Serologic Diagnosis of Lyme Disease. MMWR Morb Mortal Wkly Rep 1995;44:590–1.)

performance.[64] Tests using the C6 peptide (a 26-amino acid peptide derived from invariant region 6 of VlsE) have comparable sensitivity with WCS-based EIAs, with significantly improved specificity, most markedly in patients with other diseases.[64–72] The C6 enzyme-linked immunosorbent assay (ELISA) can also be used in patients who acquire the infection in Europe, because it is able to detect antibody responses elicited by other *B burgdorferi* sensu lato species, and can be used as a stand-alone diagnostic strategy when such cases are evaluated in the United States.[70,73] A variety of other recombinant and synthetic antigens have been evaluated for use in serodiagnosis of Lyme disease, including antigens combining portions of different proteins. Conserved regions of OspC, an antigen recognized early during the course of infection by *B burgdorferi*, have been explored to develop diagnostic peptides, which are used as single-peptide or as part of multipeptide assays.[66,68,74–77]

The sensitivity of antibody-based tests increases with the duration of the infection, and there is a lag from initial infection until the time when there are sufficient levels of antibodies to be detected. Patients who present very early in their illness are more likely to have a negative result. Less than 50% of patients with EM are positive at presentation, and these patients should receive treatment based on the clinical diagnosis. Serologic tests are most helpful in patients with clinical findings indicating later stages of Lyme disease.

Fig. 2 shows how the duration of illness substantially affects the results of antibody-based tests. In a large study comparing the C6 ELISA with a WCS ELISA and the 2-tier

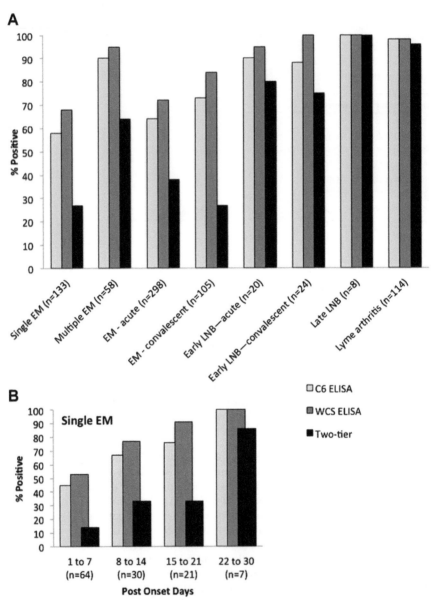

Fig. 2. Serologic results, clinical presentation and duration of illness. (*A*) Rates of seropositivity for the C6 ELISA, WCS ELISA, and 2-tier algorithm in relation to disease presentation and time of sample (acute and convalescent). (*B*) Rates of seropositivity in relation to duration of disease in patients with a single EM. LNB, Lyme neuroborreliosis. (*Data from* Wormser GP, Schriefer M, Aguero-Rosenfeld ME, et al. Single-tier testing with the C6 peptide ELISA kit compared with two-tier testing for Lyme disease. Diagn Microbiol Infect Dis 2013;75:9–15; and Wormser GP, Nowakowski J, Nadelman RB, et al. Impact of clinical variables on *Borrelia burgdorferi*-specific antibody seropositivity in acute-phase sera from patients in North America with culture-confirmed early Lyme disease. Clin Vaccine Immunol 2008;15:1519–22.)

algorithm,[69] patients with single EM lesions were less likely to be seropositive than patients with multiple EM, and patients in the convalescent phase were more likely to be positive than patients in the acute phase. Most patients with Lyme arthritis or late neuroborreliosis were positive (**Fig. 2**A). In another study,[78] less then 50% of patients with a single EM were positive by WCS ELISA or C6 ELISA and only 14% were positive by 2-tier testing when the patients were tested within the first week of illness, but the sensitivity of the tests increased with each weekly time point thereafter (see **Fig. 2**B).

As shown in many studies,[64,69,71,72,78] the additional IgM WB step decreases sensitivity in early disease, the only situation in which its use is indicated. Positive IgM results for *Borrelia* can occur in more than 40% of parvovirus B19 infections[79] and have been observed in patients with human granulocytic anaplasmosis,[80] Epstein-Barr virus infections, and patients with autoimmune diseases. In addition, false-positive IgM WBs are common in commercial laboratories,[81] and there is misinterpretation of positive IgM results in those patients with symptoms for longer than 4 weeks. Therefore, there is a need to change the testing algorithm for early Lyme disease, avoiding the use of the IgM WB. Possible strategies include the use of the WCS ELISA followed by the C6 ELISA,[71,82] the addition of the VlsE band,[64] and the use of multipeptide assays.[75,76]

Future developments that are needed include point-of-care tests. These tests would be particularly useful in evaluating patients with stage 2 manifestations of Lyme disease, like facial palsy or carditis. At present, if these patients do not have other manifestations of Lyme disease or a suggestive history, the diagnosis may depend on serologic tests results, resulting in a delay in appropriate therapy.

Current assays do not distinguish between active and inactive infection, and patients may continue to be seropositive for years, including an IgM response, even after adequate antibiotic treatment.[83,84] It is hoped that, with further studies using new, promising immunoassay techniques, a combination of multiple antigens can be developed that will help in early diagnosis, inform on the stage and disease manifestations, and on the presence of active versus past infection.[85–87]

INTRATHECAL ANTIBODY PRODUCTION

The concomitant analysis of serum and cerebrospinal fluid is used to show selective production of anti–*B burgdorferi* antibodies in the central nervous system. Measuring the antibody concentration only in the cerebrospinal fluid can be misleading, because a positive result may be caused by passive transfer of antibodies from the serum. Evidence of intrathecal antibody production is considered a gold standard for the diagnosis of Lyme neuroborreliosis in Europe, where most studies originate and where *B garinii* is the species most often associated with neurologic disease. There are many difficulties in the interpretation of results from these studies, because of the lack of a gold standard; the use of different case definitions, different assays, and interpretative criteria; retrospective evaluation; and little comparison among assays and among laboratories. Overall, the sensitivity of intrathecal antibody production in acute Lyme neuroborreliosis is around 50%.[41,46,88–95] Intrathecal antibody can persist after therapy.[96,97] Although there are few studies, positive intrathecal antibody production seems to be found less frequently in patients with neuroborreliosis in the United States.[14,27,93]

CXCL13

CXCL13 is a B lymphocyte chemoattractant chemokine that is increased in the cerebrospinal fluid of patients with acute Lyme neuroborreliosis and may be helpful in certain clinical settings, but its diagnostic value remains to be established.[46,98,99] At this point, this test is not routinely available to clinicians.

OTHER TESTS

The clinical usefulness of cell proliferation assays, Enzyme-Linked ImmunoSpot (ELISPOT) assays, cytokine measurements, complement split products, and lymphocyte transformation tests has not been established, and these tests should not be used for the diagnosis of Lyme disease. Natural killer cell measurements (CD57) are not helpful.[100]

Xenodiagnosis, using the natural tick vector (*I scapularis*) to detect evidence of infection in Lyme disease, is an experimental test, and its clinical applications depend on the results of future studies. Although xenodiagnosis is unlikely to be used in routine practice, it can offer researchers a tool to develop new tests for the disease.

SUMMARY

Major advances in laboratory testing for Lyme disease have occurred in recent years, but there is need for further progress. Improvements of several aspects of the currently recommended testing algorithm are needed. These aspects include making the algorithm simpler, possibly as a single test or procedure; using objective, quantitative data; having greater sensitivity in early disease; and being independent of disease duration. The use of the current IgM WBs should be avoided, because it decreases the sensitivity in the clinical situations for which it is recommended (early Lyme disease), and has lower specificity than tests for IgG antibody generally. There is a need to improve direct methods for detection of *B burgdorferi*, and to develop accurate, sensitive, and rapid diagnostic tests for early Lyme disease; preferably point-of-care tests. No current test can be used to follow the response to antibiotic therapy; the development of biomarkers for active infection would be a major advance.

REFERENCES

1. CDC. How many people get Lyme disease? 2013. Available at: http://www.cdc.gov/lyme/stats/humanCases.html. Accessed September 17, 2014.
2. Tilly K, Rosa PA, Stewart PE. Biology of infection with *Borrelia burgdorferi*. Infect Dis Clin North Am 2008;22:217–34, v.
3. Di L, Pagan PE, Packer D, et al. BorreliaBase: a phylogeny-centered browser of *Borrelia* genomes. BMC Bioinformatics 2014;15:233.
4. Radolf JD, Caimano MJ, Stevenson B, et al. Of ticks, mice and men: understanding the dual-host lifestyle of Lyme disease spirochaetes. Nat Rev Microbiol 2012;10:87–99.
5. Franke J, Hildebrandt A, Dorn W. Exploring gaps in our knowledge on Lyme borreliosis spirochaetes–updates on complex heterogeneity, ecology, and pathogenicity. Ticks Tick Borne Dis 2013;4:11–25.
6. Stanek G, Wormser GP, Gray J, et al. Lyme borreliosis. Lancet 2012;379:461–73.
7. Wormser GP, Brisson D, Liveris D, et al. *Borrelia burgdorferi* genotype predicts the capacity for hematogenous dissemination during early Lyme disease. J Infect Dis 2008;198:1358–64.
8. Hanincova K, Mukherjee P, Ogden NH, et al. Multilocus sequence typing of *Borrelia burgdorferi* suggests existence of lineages with differential pathogenic properties in humans. PLoS One 2013;8:e73066.
9. Steere AC, Bartenhagen NH, Craft JE, et al. The early clinical manifestations of Lyme disease. Ann Intern Med 1983;99:76–82.

10. Nadelman RB, Nowakowski J, Forseter G, et al. The clinical spectrum of early Lyme borreliosis in patients with culture-confirmed erythema migrans. Am J Med 1996;100:502–8.
11. Strle F, Nadelman RB, Cimperman J, et al. Comparison of culture-confirmed erythema migrans caused by Borrelia burgdorferi sensu stricto in New York State and by Borrelia afzelii in Slovenia. Ann Intern Med 1999;130:32–6.
12. Kindstrand E, Nilsson BY, Hovmark A, et al. Peripheral neuropathy in acrodermatitis chronica atrophicans - a late Borrelia manifestation. Acta Neurol Scand 1997;95:338–45.
13. Halperin JJ, Logigian EL, Finkel MF, et al. Practice parameters for the diagnosis of patients with nervous system Lyme borreliosis (Lyme disease).Quality Standards Subcommittee of the American Academy of Neurology. Neurology 1996;46:619–27.
14. Logigian EL, Kaplan RF, Steere AC. Chronic neurologic manifestations of Lyme disease. N Engl J Med 1990;323:1438–44.
15. Steere AC, Schoen RT, Taylor E. The clinical evolution of Lyme arthritis. Ann Intern Med 1987;107:725–31.
16. Steere AC, Malawista SE, Hardin JA, et al. Erythema chronicum migrans and Lyme arthritis. The enlarging clinical spectrum. Ann Intern Med 1977;86:685–98.
17. Steere AC, Malawista SE, Snydman DR, et al. Lyme arthritis: an epidemic of oligoarticular arthritis in children and adults in three Connecticut communities. Arthritis Rheum 1977;20:7–17.
18. Tee SI, Martínez-Escanamé M, Zuriel D, et al. Acrodermatitis chronica atrophicans with pseudolymphomatous infiltrates. Am J Dermatopathol 2013;35:338–42.
19. Mullegger RR, Glatz M. Skin manifestations of Lyme borreliosis: diagnosis and management. Am J Clin Dermatol 2008;9:355–68.
20. De Koning J, Bosma RB, Hoogkamp-Korstanje JA. Demonstration of spirochaetes in patients with Lyme disease with a modified silver stain. J Med Microbiol 1987;23:261–7.
21. de Koning J, Tazelaar DJ, Hoogkamp-Korstanje JA, et al. Acrodermatitis chronica atrophicans: a light and electron microscopic study. J Cutan Pathol 1995;22:23–32.
22. Johnston YE, Duray PH, Steere AC, et al. Lyme arthritis. Spirochetes found in synovial microangiopathic lesions. Am J Pathol 1985;118:26–34.
23. Duray PH. Clinical pathologic correlations of Lyme disease. Rev Infect Dis 1989;11(Suppl 6):S1487–93.
24. Eisendle K, Grabner T, Zelger B. Focus floating microscopy: "gold standard" for cutaneous borreliosis? Am J Clin Pathol 2007;127:213–22.
25. Aberer E, Kersten A, Klade H, et al. Heterogeneity of Borrelia burgdorferi in the skin. Am J Dermatopathol 1996;18:571–9.
26. Aberer E, Klade H, Hobisch G. A clinical, histological, and immunohistochemical comparison of acrodermatitis chronica atrophicans and morphea. Am J Dermatopathol 1991;13:334–41.
27. Coyle PK, Schutzer SE, Deng Z, et al. Detection of Borrelia burgdorferi-specific antigen in antibody-negative cerebrospinal fluid in neurologic Lyme disease. Neurology 1995;45:2010–5.
28. Klempner MS, Schmid CH, Hu L, et al. Intralaboratory reliability of serologic and urine testing for Lyme disease. Am J Med 2001;110:217–9.
29. Pollack RJ, Telford SR 3rd, Spielman A. Standardization of medium for culturing Lyme disease spirochetes. J Clin Microbiol 1993;31:1251–5.

30. Ruzic-Sabljic E, Lotric-Furlan S, Maraspin V, et al. Comparison of isolation rate of *Borrelia burgdorferi* sensu lato in MKP and BSK-II medium. Int J Med Microbiol 2006;296(Suppl 40):267–73.
31. Liveris D, Schwartz I, Bittker S, et al. Improving the yield of blood cultures from patients with early Lyme disease. J Clin Microbiol 2011;49:2166–8.
32. Xu G, Wesker J, White C, et al. Detection of heterogeneity of *Borrelia burgdorferi* in *Ixodes* ticks by culture-dependent and culture-independent methods. J Clin Microbiol 2013;51:615–7.
33. Nadelman RB, Nowakowski J, Forseter G, et al. Failure to isolate *Borrelia burgdorferi* after antimicrobial therapy in culture-documented Lyme borreliosis associated with erythema migrans: report of a prospective study. Am J Med 1993;94:583–8.
34. Picken MM, Picken RN, Han D, et al. A two year prospective study to compare culture and polymerase chain reaction amplification for the detection and diagnosis of Lyme borreliosis. Mol Pathol 1997;50:186–93.
35. Liveris D, Wang G, Girao G, et al. Quantitative detection of *Borrelia burgdorferi* in 2-millimeter skin samples of erythema migrans lesions: correlation of results with clinical and laboratory findings. J Clin Microbiol 2002;40:1249–53.
36. Liveris D, Schwartz I, McKenna D, et al. Comparison of five diagnostic modalities for direct detection of *Borrelia burgdorferi* in patients with early Lyme disease. Diagn Microbiol Infect Dis 2012;73:243–5.
37. O'Rourke M, Traweger A, Lusa L, et al. Quantitative detection of *Borrelia burgdorferi* sensu lato in erythema migrans skin lesions using internally controlled duplex real time PCR. PLoS One 2013;8:e63968.
38. Cerar T, Ruzic-Sabljic E, Glinsek U, et al. Comparison of PCR methods and culture for the detection of *Borrelia* spp. in patients with erythema migrans. Clin Microbiol Infect 2008;14:653–8.
39. Ruzic-Sabljic E, Maraspin V, Cimperman J, et al. Comparison of isolation rate of *Borrelia burgdorferi* sensu lato in two different culture media, MKP and BSK-H. Clin Microbiol Infect 2014;20:636–41.
40. Coulter P, Lema C, Flayhart D, et al. Two-year evaluation of *Borrelia burgdorferi* culture and supplemental tests for definitive diagnosis of Lyme disease. J Clin Microbiol 2005;43:5080–4.
41. Ogrinc K, Lotrič-Furlan S, Maraspin V, et al. Suspected early Lyme neuroborreliosis in patients with erythema migrans. Clin Infect Dis 2013;57:501–9.
42. Li X, McHugh GA, Damle N, et al. Burden and viability of *Borrelia burgdorferi* in skin and joints of patients with erythema migrans or Lyme arthritis. Arthritis Rheum 2011;63:2238–47.
43. Strle F, Lusa L, Ružić-Sabljić E, et al. Clinical characteristics associated with *Borrelia burgdorferi* sensu lato skin culture results in patients with erythema migrans. PLoS One 2013;8:e82132.
44. Maraspin V, Ogrinc K, Ruzic-Sabljic E, et al. Isolation of *Borrelia burgdorferi* sensu lato from blood of adult patients with borrelial lymphocytoma, Lyme neuroborreliosis, Lyme arthritis and acrodermatitis chronica atrophicans. Infection 2011;39:35–40.
45. Nowakowski J, McKenna D, Nadelman RB, et al. Blood cultures for patients with extracutaneous manifestations of Lyme disease in the United States. Clin Infect Dis 2009;49:1733–5.
46. Cerar T, Ogrinc K, Lotric-Furlan S, et al. Diagnostic value of cytokines and chemokines in Lyme neuroborreliosis. Clin Vaccine Immunol 2013;20:1578–84.

47. Strle F, Ruzic-Sabljic E, Cimperman J, et al. Comparison of findings for patients with *Borrelia garinii* and *Borrelia afzelii* isolated from cerebrospinal fluid. Clin Infect Dis 2006;43:704–10.

48. Cerar T, Ogrinc K, Cimperman J, et al. Validation of cultivation and PCR methods for diagnosis of Lyme neuroborreliosis. J Clin Microbiol 2008;46: 3375–9.

49. Wormser GP, Nadelman RB, Schwartz I. The amber theory of Lyme arthritis: initial description and clinical implications. Clin Rheumatol 2012;31:989–94.

50. Johnson BJ, Pilgard MA, Russell TM. Assessment of new culture method for detection of *Borrelia* species from serum of Lyme disease patients. J Clin Microbiol 2014;52:721–4.

51. Sapi E, Pabbati N, Datar A, et al. Improved culture conditions for the growth and detection of *Borrelia* from human serum. Int J Med Sci 2013;10:362–76.

52. Phillips SE, Mattman LH, Hulinska D, et al. A proposal for the reliable culture of *Borrelia burgdorferi* from patients with chronic Lyme disease, even from those previously aggressively treated. Infection 1998;26:364–7.

53. Marques AR, Stock F, Gill V. Evaluation of a new culture medium for *Borrelia burgdorferi*. J Clin Microbiol 2000;38:4239–41.

54. Tilton RC, Barden D, Sand M. Culture *Borrelia burgdorferi*. J Clin Microbiol 2001; 39:2747.

55. Eshoo MW, Crowder CC, Rebman AW, et al. Direct molecular detection and genotyping of *Borrelia burgdorferi* from whole blood of patients with early Lyme disease. PLoS One 2012;7:e36825.

56. Nocton JJ, Dressler F, Rutledge BJ, et al. Detection of *Borrelia burgdorferi* DNA by polymerase chain reaction in synovial fluid from patients with Lyme arthritis. N Engl J Med 1994;330:229–34.

57. Persing DH, Rutledge BJ, Rys PN, et al. Target imbalance: disparity of *Borrelia burgdorferi* genetic material in synovial fluid from Lyme arthritis patients. J Infect Dis 1994;169:668–72.

58. Mygland A, Ljøstad U, Fingerle V, et al. EFNS guidelines on the diagnosis and management of European Lyme neuroborreliosis. Eur J Neurol 2010;17:8–16 e1–4.

59. Hinckley AF, Connally NP, Meek JI, et al. Lyme disease testing by large commercial laboratories in the United States. Clin Infect Dis 2014;59:676–81.

60. CDC. Recommendations for test performance and interpretation from the Second National Conference on Serologic Diagnosis of Lyme Disease. MMWR Morb Mortal Wkly Rep 1995;44:590–1.

61. Fallon BA, Pavlicova M, Coffino SW, et al. A comparison of Lyme disease serologic test results from four laboratories in patients with persistent symptoms after antibiotic treatment. Clin Infect Dis 2014;59(12):1705–10.

62. Barclay SS, Melia MT, Auwaerter PG. Misdiagnosis of late-onset Lyme arthritis by inappropriate use of *Borrelia burgdorferi* immunoblot testing with synovial fluid. Clin Vaccin Immunol 2012;19:1806–9.

63. Gomes-Solecki MJ, Dunn JJ, Luft BJ, et al. Recombinant chimeric *Borrelia* proteins for diagnosis of Lyme disease. J Clin Microbiol 2000;38:2530–5.

64. Branda JA, Aguero-Rosenfeld ME, Ferraro MJ, et al. 2-tiered antibody testing for early and late Lyme disease using only an immunoglobulin G blot with the addition of a VlsE band as the second-tier test. Clin Infect Dis 2010;50:20–6.

65. Marques AR, Martin DS, Philipp MT. Evaluation of the C6 peptide enzyme-linked immunosorbent assay for individuals vaccinated with the recombinant OspA vaccine. J Clin Microbiol 2002;40:2591–3.

66. Bacon RM, Biggerstaff BJ, Schriefer ME, et al. Serodiagnosis of Lyme disease by kinetic enzyme-linked immunosorbent assay using recombinant VlsE1 or peptide antigens of *Borrelia burgdorferi* compared with 2-tiered testing using whole-cell lysates. J Infect Dis 2003;187:1187–99.

67. Philipp MT, Marques AR, Fawcett PT, et al. C6 test as an indicator of therapy outcome for patients with localized or disseminated Lyme borreliosis. J Clin Microbiol 2003;41:4955–60.

68. Burbelo PD, Issa AT, Ching KH, et al. Rapid, simple, quantitative, and highly sensitive antibody detection for Lyme disease. Clin Vaccine Immunol 2010;17:904–9.

69. Wormser GP, Schriefer M, Aguero-Rosenfeld ME, et al. Single-tier testing with the C6 peptide ELISA kit compared with two-tier testing for Lyme disease. Diagn Microbiol Infect Dis 2013;75:9–15.

70. Branda JA, Strle F, Strle K, et al. Performance of United States serologic assays in the diagnosis of Lyme borreliosis acquired in Europe. Clin Infect Dis 2013;57:333–40.

71. Branda JA, Linskey K, Kim YA, et al. Two-tiered antibody testing for Lyme disease with use of 2 enzyme immunoassays, a whole-cell sonicate enzyme immunoassay followed by a VlsE C6 peptide enzyme immunoassay. Clin Infect Dis 2011;53:541–7.

72. Steere AC, McHugh G, Damle N, et al. Prospective study of serologic tests for Lyme disease. Clin Infect Dis 2008;47:188–95.

73. Wormser GP, Tang AT, Schimmoeller NR, et al. Utility of serodiagnostics designed for use in the United States for detection of Lyme borreliosis acquired in Europe and vice versa. Med Microbiol Immunol 2014;203:65–71.

74. Gomes-Solecki MJ, Wormser GP, Schriefer M, et al. Recombinant assay for serodiagnosis of Lyme disease regardless of OspA vaccination status. J Clin Microbiol 2002;40:193–7.

75. Porwancher RB, Hagerty CG, Fan J, et al. Multiplex immunoassay for Lyme disease using VlsE1-IgG and pepC10-IgM antibodies: improving test performance through bioinformatics. Clin Vaccine Immunol 2011;18:851–9.

76. Arnaboldi PM, Seedarnee R, Sambir M, et al. Outer surface protein C peptide derived from *Borrelia burgdorferi* sensu stricto as a target for serodiagnosis of early Lyme disease. Clin Vaccine Immunol 2013;20:474–81.

77. Mathiesen MJ, Christiansen M, Hansen K, et al. Peptide-based OspC enzyme-linked immunosorbent assay for serodiagnosis of Lyme borreliosis. J Clin Microbiol 1998;36:3474–9.

78. Wormser GP, Nowakowski J, Nadelman RB, et al. Impact of clinical variables on *Borrelia burgdorferi*-specific antibody seropositivity in acute-phase sera from patients in North America with culture-confirmed early Lyme disease. Clin Vaccine Immunol 2008;15:1519–22.

79. Tuuminen T, Hedman K, Soderlund-Venermo M, et al. Acute parvovirus B19 infection causes nonspecificity frequently in *Borrelia* and less often in *Salmonella* and *Campylobacter* serology, posing a problem in diagnosis of infectious arthropathy. Clin Vaccine Immunol 2011;18:167–72.

80. Wormser GP, Horowitz HW, Nowakowski J, et al. Positive Lyme disease serology in patients with clinical and laboratory evidence of human granulocytic ehrlichiosis. Am J Clin Pathol 1997;107:142–7.

81. Seriburi V, Ndukwe N, Chang Z, et al. High frequency of false positive IgM immunoblots for *Borrelia burgdorferi* in clinical practice. Clin Microbiol Infect 2012;18:1236–40.

82. Wormser GP, Levin A, Soman S, et al. Comparative cost-effectiveness of two-tiered testing strategies for serodiagnosis of Lyme disease with noncutaneous manifestations. J Clin Microbiol 2013;51:4045–9.

83. Kalish RA, McHugh G, Granquist J, et al. Persistence of immunoglobulin M or immunoglobulin G antibody responses to Borrelia burgdorferi 10–20 years after active Lyme disease. Clin Infect Dis 2001;33:780–5.

84. Peltomaa M, McHugh G, Steere AC. Persistence of the antibody response to the VlsE sixth invariant region (IR6) peptide of Borrelia burgdorferi after successful antibiotic treatment of Lyme disease. J Infect Dis 2003;187:1178–86.

85. Chandra A, Wormser GP, Marques AR, et al. Anti-Borrelia burgdorferi antibody profile in post-Lyme disease syndrome. Clin Vaccine Immunol 2011;18:767–71.

86. Chandra A, Latov N, Wormser GP, et al. Epitope mapping of antibodies to VlsE protein of Borrelia burgdorferi in post-Lyme disease syndrome. Clin Immunol 2011;141:103–10.

87. Philipp MT, Wormser GP, Marques AR, et al. A decline in C6 antibody titer occurs in successfully treated patients with culture-confirmed early localized or early disseminated Lyme Borreliosis. Clin Diagn Lab Immunol 2005;12:1069–74.

88. Djukic M, Schmidt-Samoa C, Lange P, et al. Cerebrospinal fluid findings in adults with acute Lyme neuroborreliosis. J Neurol 2012;259:630–6.

89. Stanek G, Lusa L, Ogrinc K, et al. Intrathecally produced IgG and IgM antibodies to recombinant VlsE, VlsE peptide, recombinant OspC and whole cell extracts in the diagnosis of Lyme neuroborreliosis. Med Microbiol Immunol 2013;203(2):125–32.

90. Henningsson AJ, Christiansson M, Tjernberg I, et al. Laboratory diagnosis of Lyme neuroborreliosis: a comparison of three CSF anti-Borrelia antibody assays. Eur J Clin Microbiol Infect Dis 2013;33(5):797–803.

91. van Burgel ND, Brandenburg A, Gerritsen HJ, et al. High sensitivity and specificity of the C6-peptide ELISA on cerebrospinal fluid in Lyme neuroborreliosis patients. Clin Microbiol Infect 2011;17:1495–500.

92. Cerar T, Ogrinc K, Strle F, et al. Humoral immune responses in patients with Lyme neuroborreliosis. Clin Vaccine Immunol 2010;17:645–50.

93. Steere AC, Berardi VP, Weeks KE, et al. Evaluation of the intrathecal antibody response to Borrelia burgdorferi as a diagnostic test for Lyme neuroborreliosis. J Infect Dis 1990;161:1203–9.

94. Halperin JJ, Golightly M. Lyme borreliosis in Bell's palsy. long island neuroborreliosis collaborative study group. Neurology 1992;42:1268–70.

95. Smouha EE, Coyle PK, Shukri S. Facial nerve palsy in Lyme disease: evaluation of clinical diagnostic criteria. Am J Otol 1997;18:257–61.

96. Martin R, Martens U, Sticht-Groh V, et al. Persistent intrathecal secretion of oligoclonal, Borrelia burgdorferi-specific IgG in chronic meningoradiculomyelitis. J Neurol 1988;235:229–33.

97. Hammers-Berggren S, Hansen K, Lebech AM, et al. Borrelia burgdorferi-specific intrathecal antibody production in neuroborreliosis: a follow-up study. Neurology 1993;43:169–75.

98. Bremell D, Mattsson N, Edsbagge M, et al. Cerebrospinal fluid CXCL13 in Lyme neuroborreliosis and asymptomatic HIV infection. BMC Neurol 2013;13:2.

99. Schmidt C, Plate A, Angele B, et al. A prospective study on the role of CXCL13 in Lyme neuroborreliosis. Neurology 2011;76:1051–8.

100. Marques A, Brown MR, Fleisher TA. Natural killer cell counts are not different between patients with post-Lyme disease syndrome and controls. Clin Vaccine Immunol 2009;16:1249–50.

Posttreatment Lyme Disease Syndrome

John N. Aucott, MD

KEYWORDS

- Posttreatment Lyme disease syndrome • Persistent symptoms • Fatigue
- Fibromyalgia • Musculoskeletal pain

KEY POINTS

- Overall, prognosis following appropriate antibiotic treatment of early or late Lyme disease is favorable but can be complicated by persistent symptoms of unknown cause.
- Posttreatment Lyme disease syndrome (PTLDS) is characterized by fatigue, musculoskeletal pain, and cognitive complaints that persist for 6 months or longer after completion of antibiotic therapy.
- PTLDS can vary markedly in disease severity from mild to severe symptoms with diminished health-related quality of life.
- Two-tier serologic testing is neither sensitive nor specific for diagnosis of PTLDS because of variability in convalescent serologic responses after treatment of early Lyme disease.
- Recommended treatment of PTLDS is largely symptom-based. There are currently no FDA-approved treatments for patients with PTLDS.

INTRODUCTION: NATURE OF THE PROBLEM

In general, the prognosis after treatment of uncomplicated infection with *Borrelia burgdorferi*, the causative agent of Lyme disease, is favorable. However, the clinical management of early or late-stage Lyme disease may in some cases be complicated by persistent fatigue, musculoskeletal, and cognitive symptoms after completion of standard antibiotic therapy. This documented constellation of patient-reported symptoms, which may be intermittent or constant,[1] can be called posttreatment Lyme disease syndrome (PTLDS) when symptoms are prolonged for a period of 6 months or greater.[2,3] Although objective findings, such as persistence of the erythema migrans rash (EM), cranial nerve palsy, meningitis, or radiculitis, may occasionally occur after treatment of early Lyme disease, these objective physical findings or laboratory manifestations more typical of untreated Lyme disease are not part of the clinical spectrum

Division of Rheumatology, Department of Medicine, Johns Hopkins University School of Medicine, 5200 Eastern Avenue, Baltimore, MD 21224, USA
E-mail address: jaucott2@jhmi.edu

Infect Dis Clin N Am 29 (2015) 309–323
http://dx.doi.org/10.1016/j.idc.2015.02.012
0891-5520/15/$ – see front matter © 2015 Elsevier Inc. All rights reserved.

id.theclinics.com

of PTLDS. Similarly, persistent joint synovitis may occur after repeated courses of antibiotic therapy for late Lyme arthritis and is also considered a distinct process, termed antibiotic-refractory late Lyme arthritis.[4]

Early investigators observed that patients with early or late-stage Lyme disease may have lingering symptoms after completion of antibiotic therapy, despite prompt administration of effective antibiotic therapy and resolution of the physical findings of infection.[5–7] The frequency of PTLDS among such patients has been found to differ between 0% and 50% in published studies, and is likely related to variability of study design and enrollment criteria of the sample populations used.[5,8] Reports of long-term follow-up in patients with early presentation and treatment of EM have generally shown excellent long-term outcomes.[1] In the most recent treatment trials of EM conducted in North America, rates of PTLDS are approximately 10% to 20%.[3] However, rates may be 50% in the community practice of medicine, where delayed diagnosis and treatment may be more common and classification of symptoms attributed to Lyme disease less certain.[9,10] In addition, persistent symptoms may be more common among patients with sensory symptoms or frank neurologic involvement. In one series, patients who presented with facial palsy and were not treated for neuroborreliosis were more likely to have long-term symptoms and a diminished health-related quality of life on 10- to 20-year follow-up.[11]

In all stages of Lyme disease, clinical response to therapy may be delayed, with continued improvement over a period of weeks to months beyond the initial treatment duration. Minor lingering symptoms usually resolve spontaneously and do not necessarily indicate continued infection requiring further antibiotic therapy.[12] Occasionally, however, patients may have an unsatisfactory response to initial therapy with the onset of new, worsening, or persistent symptoms, which may prompt a defined course of an alternative antibiotic.[13] Occasionally, the coexistence of a second tick-borne pathogen, such as *Babesia*, may explain ongoing illness after treatment of Lyme disease.[14] Biomarkers to identify patients at risk for PTLDS, or for distinguishing minor, resolving symptoms from an unsatisfactory response to initial therapy, are not currently available, but is an area of active research.[15] Therefore, PTLDS remains a diagnosis of exclusion and should not be made when other, specific diagnoses can explain the patient's symptoms and laboratory findings. These factors, in the context of an unknown cause and insensitive and nonspecific symptoms, laboratory studies, and other clinical tools, render the diagnosis and clinical management of PTLDS challenging for physicians.

RISK FACTORS AND SEVERITY OF DISEASE

Box 1 shows a list of identified risk factors for PTLDS. A delay in diagnosis and subsequent treatment has been identified as the primary risk factor for PTLDS.[9,16] Other reported risk factors include a larger number of symptoms and a greater symptom severity at the time of treatment.[1,5] Fever, headache, photosensitivity, or neck stiffness during the acute illness have also been reported as risk factors for the persistent symptoms after initial antibiotic therapy.[17] Initial treatment with antibiotics other than first-line agents, such as azithromycin, may be more likely to occur in the community setting where misdiagnosis rates are higher.[10] Such situations may also be associated with a higher risk of PTLDS.[6] A negative posttreatment serology was found to be more common in patients with posttreatment symptoms in one study,[6] but baseline and convalescent serostatus was not associated with outcomes in another study.[1] Early studies among patients diagnosed with acute Lyme disease found that duration of antibiotic therapy does not predict risk of PTLDS.[18,19]

Box 1
Risk factors for PTLDS

Probable

- Delay in diagnosis
- Overall severity of symptoms at treatment
- Presence of neurologic symptoms at time of initial treatment

Possible

- Presence of fever, headache, photosensitivity, or neck stiffness during acute illness
- Initial treatment with nonrecommended antibiotics
- Lack of antibody seroconversion

PTLDS may also be more common after treatment of acute neuroborreliosis. The presence of sensory neurologic symptoms and frank neurologic involvement at the time of diagnosis and treatment may be another risk factor for the development of PTLDS. Patients treated for acute and subacute neuroborreliosis in Europe have reported rates of PTLDS ranging from 25% to 50%,[20–22] generally higher than in North American studies of patients with EM. Some North American investigators have also suggested that facial palsy at initial presentation may be a risk factor for PTLDS.[11]

There is a large spectrum of illness severity in PTLDS, from minor symptoms to a more severe illness that has been characterized by declines in health-related quality of life and mild to moderate cognitive deficits in some patients.[23–25] In antibiotic treatment trials of ideally diagnosed and treated early Lyme disease, only 10% of patients were found to have low health-related quality of life,[26] which may be related to fatigue.[27] However, in patients identified after treatment in the community setting, the impact of PTLDS on health-related quality of life was much higher.[24] The more severe end of this illness spectrum has been described in population-based studies, where patients often had delayed treatment, initial misdiagnosis, or nonideal initial therapy.[9,11,16]

UNDERLYING MECHANISMS

Despite extensive study of Lyme disease, PTLDS remains an enigmatic condition, because the underlying pathogenesis of the syndrome is not understood. The clinical validity of PTLDS as the sequelae of an infectious disease continues to be debated. One explanation is that the apparent association of symptoms after treatment of Lyme disease represents anchoring bias, incorrectly linking common nonspecific symptoms to an antecedent episode of Lyme disease.[28] However, there is precedent for postinfectious syndromes of persistent fatigue following other infectious diseases, such as Epstein-Barr virus, Q fever, and Ross River virus. In one large study from Australia, 12% of those infected with these agents had persistent symptoms at 6 months. The investigators found that the presence of fatigue was predicted by the severity of initial symptoms, and was not predicted by psychological factors.[29] Although PTLDS-defining symptoms, such as fatigue and pain, are common in the general population, a meta-analysis of studies using non–Lyme infected control subjects has shown an increased prevalence of many symptoms in patients with PTDLS compared with control subjects.[30] A subsequent prospective controlled clinical trial has provided additional evidence that symptoms are more severe after treatment of

Lyme disease than in healthy matched control subjects, and are not primarily caused by pre-existing depression.[25,26]

In addition, evidence is emerging regarding the possible immune pathophysiology of PTLDS. *Borrelia* lipoprotein antigens are highly inflammatory, and retained antigens after killing of *Borrelia* has been shown in the mouse model and hypothesized in human illness.[31,32] Evidence for specific immune response patterns and autoimmunity is also emerging as a potential mechanism for PTLDS.[33] In one study of patients treated for EM in Europe, elevated interleukin-23 levels during acute disease were associated with the subsequent development of PTLDS.[15] Antineural antibodies and certain antiborrelial antibodies have also been reported in PTLDS.[34,35]

Genetic predisposition to autoimmunity in Lyme disease is best described in late Lyme arthritis, where HLA-DR4 predisposes to the development of persistent inflammatory Lyme arthritis in a subset of patients that does not respond to further courses of antibiotic treatment.[36] Patients who are HLA-DR4 positive and who have treatment-resistant Lyme arthritis have also been shown to have a strong immune response to an epitope on OspA that cross-reacts with human lymphocyte function antigen 1, which may serve as an autoantigen.[37] In addition, a polymorphism in the TLRI gene (1805GG), which is present in 50% of whites, has been implicated in persistent autoimmune arthritis after antibiotic treatment.[38]

Certain genotypes of *B burgdorferi* in North America have been found to be more inflammatory and more likely to disseminate at the time of initial infection.[39] These genotypes of *B burgdorferi* are associated with more symptomatic initial infection, which may be a risk factor for later PTLDS. Finally, recent animal studies have demonstrated residual organisms and the possibility of persistence of *B burgdorferi* DNA in mice and primates previously treated with antibiotics.[40–42] Whether antibiotic-tolerant "persister" organisms play a role in human PTLDS remains unknown, although results from a small xenodiagnoses study report the identification of *B burgdorferi* DNA by polymerase chain reaction in a single patient with PTLDS.[43]

PATIENT HISTORY

The proposed case definition for PTLDS published in the 2006 practice guidelines of the Infectious Diseases Society of America is based on identifying individuals with persistent, otherwise unexplained symptoms after treatment of documented Lyme disease (**Box 2**).[2] The central feature of this case definition is the presence of persistent or recurrent symptoms that began within the 6 months following completion of a regimen of currently recommended antibiotic therapy for physician-documented early or late Lyme disease (and subsequently persist for a period of 6 months or greater).[2] A detailed past medical history and record review may be necessary to document a prior history of previously treated Lyme disease. The most commonly recognized symptoms reported by patients with PTLDS are fatigue, musculoskeletal pain, and cognitive complaints. However, a range of other symptoms have also been reported, such as sensory symptoms, sleep disruption, and emotional symptoms, as shown in **Table 1**.[16,17,44,45]

PHYSICAL EXAMINATION

Objective findings have been difficult to document in PLTDS. Unlike patients with persistent arthritis after treatment of late Lyme disease, patients with PTLDS have arthralgias and musculoskeletal pain, but rare evidence of joint synovitis.[17] Objective neurologic signs have also been difficult to document.[17] PTLDS is distinct from the residual, slowly resolving, or incomplete resolution of neurologic deficits that may occur

Box 2
Proposed definition of post–Lyme disease syndrome

Inclusion criteria

An adult or child with a documented episode of early or late Lyme disease fulfilling the case definition of the Centers for Disease Control and Prevention.[46] If based on erythema migrans, the diagnosis must be made and documented by an experienced health care practitioner.

After treatment of the episode of Lyme disease with a generally accepted treatment regimen[47] there is resolution or stabilization of the objective manifestations of Lyme disease.

Onset of any of the following subjective symptoms within 6 months of the diagnosis of Lyme disease and persistence of continuous or relapsing symptoms for at least a 6-month period after completion of antibiotic therapy: fatigue, widespread musculoskeletal pain, complaints of cognitive difficulties.

Subjective symptoms are of such severity that, when present, they result in substantial reduction in previous levels of occupational, educational, social, or personal activities.

Exclusion criteria

An active, untreated, well-documented coinfection, such as babesiosis.

The presence of objective abnormalities on physical examination or on neuropsychologic testing that may explain the patient's complaints. For example, a patient with antibiotic-refractory Lyme arthritis would be excluded. A patient with late neuroborreliosis associated with encephalopathy, who has recurrent or refractory objective cognitive dysfunction, would be excluded.

A diagnosis of fibromyalgia or chronic fatigue syndrome before the onset of Lyme disease.

A prolonged history of undiagnosed or unexplained somatic complaints, such as musculoskeletal pains or fatigue, before the onset of Lyme disease.

A diagnosis of an underlying disease or condition that might explain the patient's symptoms (eg, morbid obesity, with a body mass index [calculated as weight in kilograms divided by the square of height in meters] $\geq$45; sleep apnea and narcolepsy; side effects of medications; autoimmune diseases; uncontrolled cardiopulmonary or endocrine disorders; malignant conditions within 2 years, except for uncomplicated skin cancer; known current liver disease; any past or current diagnosis of a major depressive disorder with psychotic or melancholic features; bipolar affective disorders; schizophrenia of any subtype; delusional disorders of any subtype; dementias of any subtype; anorexia nervosa or bulimia nervosa; and active drug abuse or alcoholism at present or within 2 years).

Laboratory or imaging abnormalities that might suggest an undiagnosed process distinct from post–Lyme disease syndrome, such as a highly elevated erythrocyte sedimentation rate (150 mm/h); abnormal thyroid function; a hematologic abnormality; abnormal levels of serum albumin, total protein, globulin, calcium, phosphorus, glucose, urea nitrogen, electrolytes, or creatinine; significant abnormalities on urine analysis; elevated liver enzyme levels; or a test result suggestive of the presence of a collagen vascular disease.

Although testing by either culture or polymerase chain reaction for evidence of *Borrelia burgdorferi* infection is not required, should such testing be done by reliable methods, a positive result would be an exclusion.

From Wormser GP, Dattwyler RJ, Shapiro ED, et al. The clinical assessment, treatment, and prevention of Lyme disease, human granulocytic anaplasmosis, and babesiosis: clinical practice guidelines by the Infectious Diseases Society of America. Clin Infect Dis 2006;43(9):1089–134; with permission.

Table 1	
Symptoms found to be more common in PTLDS than control subjects	
Author	**Symptoms**
Shadick et al,[16] 1994	Arthralgia
	Numbness, tingling, burning pain
	Coordination difficulties
	Fatigue
	Concentration difficulties
	Emotional irritability
Shadick et al,[17] 1999	Joint pain
	Symptoms of memory impairment
Seltzer et al,[44] 2000	Joint or muscle pain
	Ability to formulate ideas
Vázquez et al,[45] 2003	Neck pain
	Changes in behavior
	Joint or muscle pain
	Numbness or funny sensations in nerves
	Problems with memory

after treatment of acute or subacute neuroborreliosis meningitis, radiculitis, or cranial palsy.[20] For instance, the resolution of pain after treatment of radiculopathy or neuropathy may be very gradual and with chronic involvement, this response may be incomplete. Some patients may develop chronic radicular pain, similar to patients with postherpetic neuroalgia. In one report, only one-half of patients who had late neurologic symptoms showed either resolution or sustained improvement after 6 months of follow-up after a 2-week course of ceftriaxone.[48] Facial palsy itself resolves completely or almost completely in nearly all patients (121 of 122 patients in one series).[49] In contrast to slowly or incompletely resolving neurologic signs, the syndrome of PTLDS is defined by patient-reported symptoms after treatment of neuroborreliosis.

A complete neurologic examination with attention to evaluation of the peripheral nerves is indicated, and findings of decreased vibratory sensation may be most sensitive to damage from Lyme disease.[16] Case reports of PTLDS have suggested that small fiber sensory neuropathy and autonomic neuropathy may play a role in these neurologic symptoms, and as a result they are difficult to document.[50] Physical examination findings of orthostatic intolerance may be elicited on vital signs, because there is some evidence that postural orthostatic tachycardia syndrome is one possible mechanism for the symptoms of fatigue in PTLDS.[51,52]

IMAGING AND ADDITIONAL TESTING

Two-tier serologic testing at the time of clinical evaluation of PTLDS is alone neither sensitive nor specific to confirm prior treated Lyme disease nor to evaluate the clinical response to initial therapy because seroevolution after treatment of early Lyme disease is unpredictable in any given patient.[53,54] Prior appropriate treatment is required to make the diagnosis of PTLDS; consequently, it would be predicted that patients with PTLDS may be seronegative or may have IgM or IgG antibodies on Western blot testing that are insufficient to meet diagnostic criteria, despite historical documentation of a definite case of Lyme disease.[9,53–55] Similarly, declines in B burgdorferi C6 antibody titers do not correlate with recovery from PTLDS symptoms.[56] Serologic testing is also limited by the persistence of antibodies decades after resolution of all clinical symptoms attributed to Lyme disease in many patients. In one study of patients diagnosed 10 to 20 years earlier with early Lyme disease or late Lyme arthritis, the IgM remained positive in 10% of those initially diagnosed with early Lyme disease and 15% of those diagnosed with late Lyme arthritis. IgG western blots remained positive in 25% with remote early Lyme disease and 62% with remote late Lyme disease.[55] This may lead to the misattribution of later nonspecific symptoms of a different cause to previous Lyme disease. Similarly, immunologic memory of other remote infections is common; therefore, extensive serologic testing for other bacterial infections is rarely helpful and likely to be confusing to patients and physicians unfamiliar with such limitations. There is very little evidence for the role of coinfection with other tick-borne pathogens in the risk for or pathophysiology of symptoms that represent PTLDS.[57,58]

MRI has not shown convincing evidence for specific focal brain abnormalities among patients with PTLDS.[59] Central nervous system imaging with single-photon emission computed tomography scanning has been investigated in the context of PTLDS and posttreatment encephalopathy, and has been reported to show nonspecific white matter abnormalities.[60] In patients with symptoms of abnormal or diminished sensation, nerve conduction studies or skin biopsy for small fiber nerve evaluation are important to document the presence of large or small fiber neuropathy, respectively.

Patients with posttreatment symptoms may be difficult to separate clinically from patients with untreated late Lyme encephalopathy. The use of cognitive testing and lumbar puncture can be useful in these cases. In untreated late Lyme encephalopathy, subtle cerebrospinal fluid abnormalities including elevated protein or slightly elevated cell count are often but not universally present.[61] In addition, neurocognitive testing in patients with late Lyme encephalopathy is abnormal, showing objective manifestations of cognitive dysfunction. Patients with prominent cognitive complaints caused by PTLDS are sometimes said to have posttreatment encephalopathy,[27] a condition in which cognitive complaints and evidence of central nervous system inflammation are often difficult to quantify by current techniques, if they exist.

DIFFERENTIAL DIAGNOSIS

The lack of specific biomarkers to establish the cause of nonspecific symptoms in many patients has led to the appearance of the term "chronic Lyme disease," which is applied by some practitioners to describe a more heterogeneous, diverse group of patients. The diagnosis of chronic Lyme disease may mean different things to different patients and different medical practitioners.[62] This may lead to confusion and suggests the need for a more precise taxonomy of the illnesses related to Lyme disease; those related to other tick-borne infections; and those that remain syndromic, such as fibromyalgia or chronic fatigue syndrome or idiopathic causes. Many patients who seek evaluation for chronic Lyme disease are not found to have past evidence of Lyme disease and do not meet the case definition of PTLDS or untreated late Lyme disease (**Box 3**).[62,63] The frequency of PTLDS in referral settings seeing patients for evaluation of chronic Lyme disease ranges from less than 5% in nonendemic regions[64] to 15% to 20% in endemic regions of the United States.[65,66] Studies from tertiary referral clinics suggest that women may be more likely than men to be referred or self-referred for evaluation of long-standing symptoms thought to be caused by Lyme disease.[63,66,67] The range of Lyme disease and non–Lyme disease related diagnoses present in this heterogeneous group of patients has been described by several investigators.[63,65,67]

Others seeking evaluation for chronic Lyme disease may not fit neatly into any specifically defined disease category,[62,65] or meet criteria for fibromyalgia, chronic fatigue

> **Box 3**
> **Categories of chronic Lyme disease**
>
> *Category 1*
> Symptoms of unknown cause, with no evidence of *Borrelia burgdorferi* infection
>
> *Category 2*
> A well-defined illness unrelated to *B burgdorferi* infection
>
> *Category 3*
> Symptoms of unknown cause, with antibodies against *B burgdorferi* but no history of objective clinical findings that is consistent with Lyme disease
>
> *Category 4*
> Post–Lyme disease syndrome
>
> *From* Feder HM Jr, Johnson BJ, O'Connell S, et al. A critical appraisal of chronic Lyme disease. N Engl J Med 2007;357(14):1422–30.

syndrome, or other medically unexplained syndromes of unknown cause.[63,68–70] Close examination of referral populations show a group with well-documented Lyme disease who have onset of fibromyalgia after initial treatment of well documented Lyme disease. In this group of post–Lyme disease fibromyalgia, a sex-based difference is seen with woman outnumbering men by a ratio of 2:1.[63,68] In those individuals diagnosed with fibromyalgia, the concept of central sensitization may be hypothesized as part of the pathophysiology of the continued pain.[71]

PTLDS is a diagnosis of exclusion and should not be made when other, specific diagnoses can explain symptoms and laboratory findings. Patients seeking evaluation for chronic Lyme disease are often found to have an alternative diagnosis, such as degenerative arthritis.[67] Occasionally, Lyme disease may be associated with the development of a specific autoimmune illness, such as rheumatoid arthritis.[67] The pathophysiologic relationship of neurologic diagnoses, such as Parkinson disease, amyotrophic lateral sclerosis, and multiple sclerosis, to previous Lyme disease has been hypothesized, but is unproved.[72] Most cases may be hypothesized to be coincidental or caused by autoimmunity or possibly other pathophysiologies triggered by infection.[73]

TREATMENT OF POSTTREATMENT LYME DISEASE SYNDROME

There is no Food and Drug Administration–approved treatment of PTLDS. Previous controlled clinical trials with intravenous antibiotics have failed to provide convincing evidence that antibiotics provide sustained improvement in fatigue or other symptoms, although design and interpretation of these studies have been debated.[23,24,70,74] Current Infectious Diseases Society of America guidelines recommend against intravenous or prolonged oral antibiotic therapy for cases of PTLDS without objective evidence for active *B burgdorferi* infection.[2]

Patients with PTLDS who also meet diagnostic criteria for fibromyalgia could be candidates for treatment with agents, such as pregabalin and milnacipran, which have been shown to provide symptomatic improvement. In some cases PTLDS may be associated with postural orthostatic tachycardia syndrome in which treatment of orthostatic intolerance may improve symptoms of fatigue.[51] Pharmacologic treatment tailored toward symptoms of pain, sleep disruption, attention-deficit disorder, and fatigue may be considered, but has never been subject to controlled trials to test effectiveness in the PTLDS population.

Although there is a lack of consensus in the literature for identifying and treating possible physiologic causes for persisting symptoms, there are clinical care options for targeting symptom management and reducing the impact of symptoms on daily life functioning. There are validated behavioral symptoms management interventions for pain,[75–77] symptoms of cognitive decline,[78,79] and fatigue[80–82] to facilitate maximal participation in life activities. Other nonpharmacologic modalities to consider include low-impact exercise and sleep hygiene interventions. All of these interventions are currently available, and individuals who are suffering with symptoms of PTLDS can be referred for appropriate interventions based on individual symptom presentation.

The treatment of antibiotic-refractory late Lyme arthritis, based on the initial "adequate" therapy of B burgdorferi infection and including up to two to three defined courses of antibiotics,[83] may be one model for further investigation. Experience suggests that this management approach results in few if any cases of residual infection, as measured by B burgdorferi polymerase chain reaction of synovectomy samples in those who remain symptomatic.[84,85] In those who remain symptomatic, the mechanism of persistent synovitis has been extensively investigated and includes evidence for autoimmune arthritis.[86,87] Primary treatment of this autoimmune phase has been with disease-modifying anti-inflammatory drugs, such as hydroxychloroquine and methotrexate.[88] Future research into the role of other anti-inflammatory agents includes oral antibiotics with anti-inflammatory properties.[89,90] Doxycycline has shown benefit in other illness, such as rosacea, thought to be inflammatory in origin.[91,92]

If persistent infection is found to contribute to the pathogenesis of PTLDS, new antibiotic regimens will need to be developed that are directed toward the latent and persisting stage of the organism.[93] Further research to elucidate the mechanisms underlying persistent symptoms after Lyme disease and controlled trials of new approaches to the treatment and management of these patients are needed.[3]

SUMMARY

Overall, prognosis following appropriate antibiotic treatment of early or late Lyme disease is favorable but can be complicated by persistent symptoms of unknown cause. PTLDS is characterized by fatigue, musculoskeletal pain, and cognitive complaints that persist for 6 months or longer after completion of antibiotic therapy. PTLDS can vary markedly in disease severity from mild to severe symptoms with diminished health-related quality of life. The pathophysiology and mechanisms of persistent illness in PTLDS are not understood and there are little data on the effectiveness of nonantibiotic interventions. Risk factors for PTLDS include delayed diagnosis, increased severity of symptoms, and presence of neurologic symptoms at time of initial treatment. Two-tier serologic testing is neither sensitive nor specific for diagnosis of PTLDS because of variability in convalescent serologic responses after treatment of early Lyme disease. Recommended treatment of PTLDS is largely symptom-based because there are currently no Food and Drug Administration–approved treatments for patients with PTLDS.

REFERENCES

1. Nowakowski J, Nadelman RB, Sell R, et al. Long-term follow-up of patients with culture-confirmed Lyme disease. Am J Med 2003;115(2):91–6.
2. Wormser GP, Dattwyler RJ, Shapiro ED, et al. The clinical assessment, treatment, and prevention of Lyme disease, human granulocytic anaplasmosis, and

babesiosis: clinical practice guidelines by the Infectious Diseases Society of America. Clin Infect Dis 2006;43(9):1089–134.

3. Marques A. Chronic Lyme disease: a review. Infect Dis Clin North Am 2008;22(2): 341–60.

4. Kalish RA, Leong JM, Steere AC. Association of treatment-resistant chronic Lyme arthritis with HLA-DR4 and antibody reactivity to OspA and OspB of *Borrelia burgdorferi*. Infect Immun 1993;61(7):2774–9. Available at: http://www.pubmedcentral. nih.gov/articlerender.fcgi?artid=280920&tool=pmcentrez&rendertype=abstract. Accessed July 14, 2014.

5. Steere AC, Hutchinson GJ, Rahn DW, et al. Treatment of the early manifestations of Lyme disease. Ann Intern Med 1983;99(1):22–6. Available at: http://www.ncbi. nlm.nih.gov/pubmed/6407378. Accessed September 18, 2014.

6. Luft B, Dattwyler R, Johnson RC, et al. Azithromycin compared with amoxicillin in the treatment of erythema migrans: a double-blind, randomized, controlled trial. Ann Intern Med 1996;124:785–92. Available at: http://annals.org/article.aspx? articleid=709606. Accessed January 30, 2015.

7. Dattwyler RJ, Wormser GP, Rush TJ, et al. A comparison of two treatment regimens of ceftriaxone in late Lyme disease. Wien Klin Wochenschr 2005; 117(11–12):393–7. Available at: http://www.ncbi.nlm.nih.gov/pubmed/16053194. Accessed July 17, 2014.

8. Cerar D, Cerar T, Ruzić-Sabljić E, et al. Subjective symptoms after treatment of early Lyme disease. Am J Med 2010;123(1):79–86.

9. Asch ES, Bujak DI, Weiss M, et al. Lyme disease: an infectious and postinfectious syndrome. J Rheumatol 1994;21(3):454–61. Available at: http://www.ncbi.nlm.nih. gov/pubmed/8006888. Accessed June 17, 2014.

10. Aucott J, Morrison C, Munoz B, et al. Diagnostic challenges of early Lyme disease: lessons from a community case series. BMC Infect Dis 2009;9:79.

11. Kalish R, Kaplan R, Taylor E, et al. Evaluation of study patients with Lyme disease, 10-20-year follow-up. J Infect Dis 2001;183(3):453–60.

12. Dattwyler RJ, Volkman DJ, Conaty SM, et al. Amoxycillin plus probenecid versus doxycycline for treatment of erythema migrans borreliosis. Lancet 1990; 336(8728):1404–6. Available at: http://www.ncbi.nlm.nih.gov/pubmed/1978873. Accessed June 2, 2014.

13. Nadelman RB, Luger SW, Frank E, et al. Comparison of cefuroxime axetil and doxycycline in the treatment of early Lyme disease. Ann Intern Med 1992; 117(4):273–80. Available at: http://www.ncbi.nlm.nih.gov/pubmed/1637021. Accessed March 28, 2014.

14. Krause PJ, Telford SR, Spielman A, et al. Concurrent Lyme disease and babesiosis. Evidence for increased severity and duration of illness. JAMA 1996;275(21): 1657–60. Available at: http://www.ncbi.nlm.nih.gov/pubmed/8637139. Accessed July 29, 2014.

15. Strle K, Stupica D, Drouin EE, et al. Elevated levels of IL-23 in a subset of patients with post-Lyme disease symptoms following erythema migrans. Clin Infect Dis 2014;58(3):372–80.

16. Shadick NA, Phillips CB, Logigian EL, et al. The long-term clinical outcomes of Lyme disease. A population-based retrospective cohort study. Ann Intern Med 1994;121(8):560–7. Available at: http://www.ncbi.nlm.nih.gov/pubmed/8085687.

17. Shadick NA, Phillips CB, Sangha O, et al. Musculoskeletal and neurologic outcomes in patients with previously treated Lyme disease. Ann Intern Med 1999;131(12):919–26. Available at: http://www.ncbi.nlm.nih.gov/pubmed/ 10610642.

18. Wormser GP, Ramanathan R, Nowakowski J, et al. Duration of antibiotic therapy for early Lyme disease. A randomized, double-blind, placebo-controlled trial. Ann Intern Med 2003;138(9):697–704. Available at: http://www.ncbi.nlm.nih.gov/pubmed/12729423.
19. Kowalski TJ, Tata S, Berth W, et al. Antibiotic treatment duration and long-term outcomes of patients with early Lyme disease from a Lyme disease-hyperendemic area. Clin Infect Dis 2010;50(4):512–20.
20. Berglund J, Stjernberg L, Ornstein K, et al. 5-y Follow-up study of patients with neuroborreliosis. Scand J Infect Dis 2002;34(6):421–5.
21. Treib J, Fernandez A, Haass A, et al. Clinical and serologic follow-up in patients with neuroborreliosis. Neurology 1998;51(5):1489–91. Available at: http://www.ncbi.nlm.nih.gov/pubmed/9818893. Accessed July 17, 2014.
22. Ljøstad U, Mygland A. Remaining complaints 1 year after treatment for acute Lyme neuroborreliosis; frequency, pattern and risk factors. Eur J Neurol 2010; 17(1):118–23.
23. Fallon BA, Keilp JG, Corbera KM, et al. A randomized, placebo-controlled trial of repeated IV antibiotic therapy for Lyme encephalopathy. Neurology 2008;70(13): 992–1003.
24. Klempner MS, Hu LT, Evans J, et al. Two controlled trials of antibiotic treatment in patients with persistent symptoms and a history of Lyme disease. N Engl J Med 2001;345(2):85–92.
25. Aucott JN, Rebman AW, Crowder LA, et al. Post-treatment Lyme disease syndrome symptomatology and the impact on life functioning: is there something here? Qual Life Res 2013;22(1):75–84.
26. Aucott JN, Crowder LA, Kortte KB. Development of a foundation for a case definition of post-treatment Lyme disease syndrome. Int J Infect Dis 2013;17(6): e443–9.
27. Chandra AM, Keilp JG, Fallon BA. Correlates of perceived health-related quality of life in post-treatment Lyme encephalopathy. Psychosomatics 2013;54(6): 552–9.
28. Halperin JJ. Lyme disease: neurology, neurobiology, and behavior. Clin Infect Dis 2014;58(9):1267–72.
29. Hickie I, Davenport T, Wakefield D, et al. Post-infective and chronic fatigue syndromes precipitated by viral and non-viral pathogens: prospective cohort study. BMJ 2006;333(7568):575.
30. Cairns V, Godwin J. Post-lyme borreliosis syndrome: a meta-analysis of reported symptoms. Int J Epidemiol 2005;34(6):1340–5.
31. Bockenstedt LK, Gonzalez DG, Haberman AM, et al. Spirochete antigens persist near cartilage after murine Lyme borreliosis therapy. J Clin Invest 2012;122(7): 2652–60.
32. Wormser GP, Nadelman RB, Schwartz I. The amber theory of Lyme arthritis: initial description and clinical implications. Clin Rheumatol 2012;31(6):989–94.
33. Jacek E, Fallon BA, Chandra A, et al. Increased IFNα activity and differential antibody response in patients with a history of Lyme disease and persistent cognitive deficits. J Neuroimmunol 2013;255(1–2):85–91.
34. Chandra A, Wormser GP, Klempner MS, et al. Anti-neural antibody reactivity in patients with a history of Lyme borreliosis and persistent symptoms. Brain Behav Immun 2010;24(6):1018–24.
35. Chandra A, Wormser GP, Marques AR, et al. Anti-*Borrelia burgdorferi* antibody profile in post-Lyme disease syndrome. Clin Vaccine Immunol 2011;18(5): 767–71.

36. Steere AC, Dwyer E, Winchester R. Association of chronic Lyme arthritis with HLA-DR4 and HLA-DR2 alleles. N Engl J Med 1990;323(4):219–23.
37. Gross DM, Forsthuber T, Tary-Lehmann M, et al. Identification of LFA-1 as a candidate autoantigen in treatment-resistant Lyme arthritis. Science 1998; 281(5377):703–6. Available at: http://www.ncbi.nlm.nih.gov/pubmed/9685265. Accessed June 2, 2014.
38. Strle K, Shin JJ, Glickstein LJ, et al. Association of a Toll-like receptor 1 polymorphism with heightened Th1 inflammatory responses and antibiotic-refractory Lyme arthritis. Arthritis Rheum 2012;64(5):1497–507.
39. Strle K, Jones KL, Drouin EE, et al. *Borrelia burgdorferi* RST1 (OspC type A) genotype is associated with greater inflammation and more severe Lyme disease. Am J Pathol 2011;178(6):2726–39.
40. Embers ME, Barthold SW, Borda JT, et al. Persistence of *Borrelia burgdorferi* in rhesus macaques following antibiotic treatment of disseminated infection. PLoS One 2012;7(1):e29914.
41. Hodzic E, Feng S, Holden K, et al. Persistence of *Borrelia burgdorferi* following antibiotic treatment in mice. Antimicrob Agents Chemother 2008;52(5):1728–36.
42. Bockenstedt LK, Mao J, Hodzic E, et al. Detection of attenuated, noninfectious spirochetes in *Borrelia burgdorferi*-infected mice after antibiotic treatment. J Infect Dis 2002;186(10):1430–7.
43. Marques AR, Telford SR, Turk SP, et al. Xenodiagnosis to detect *Borrelia burgdorferi* infection: a first-in-human study. Clin Infect Dis 2014;58(7):937–45.
44. Seltzer EG, Gerber MA, Cartter ML, et al. Long-term outcomes of persons with Lyme disease. JAMA 2000;283(5):609–16.
45. Vázquez M, Sparrow SS, Shapiro ED. Long-term neuropsychologic and health outcomes of children with facial nerve palsy attributable to Lyme disease. Pediatrics 2003;112(2):e93–7. Available at: http://www.ncbi.nlm.nih.gov/pubmed/12897313. Accessed July 17, 2014.
46. Case definitions for infectious conditions under public health surveillance. Centers for Disease Control and Prevention. MMWR Recomm Rep 1997;46(RR-10): 1–55. Available at: http://www.ncbi.nlm.nih.gov/pubmed/9148133. Accessed June 2, 2014.
47. Medical Letter. Treatment of Lyme disease. Med Lett Drugs Ther 2005;47(1209): 41–3. Available at: http://www.ncbi.nlm.nih.gov/pubmed/15912123. Accessed November 25, 2014.
48. Logigian EL, Kaplan RF, Steere AC. Chronic neurologic manifestations of Lyme disease. N Engl J Med 1990;323(21):1438–44.
49. Clark JR, Carlson RD, Sasaki CT, et al. Facial paralysis in Lyme disease. Laryngoscope 1985;95(11):1341–5. Available at: http://www.ncbi.nlm.nih.gov/pubmed/4058212. Accessed June 2, 2014.
50. Younger DS, Orsher S. Lyme neuroborreliosis: preliminary results from an urban referral center employing strict CDC criteria for case selection. Neurol Res Int 2010;2010:525206.
51. Kizilbash SJ, Ahrens SP, Bruce BK, et al. Adolescent fatigue, POTS, and recovery: a guide for clinicians. Curr Probl Pediatr Adolesc Health Care 2014;44(5): 108–33.
52. Kanjwal K, Karabin B, Kanjwal Y, et al. Postural orthostatic tachycardia syndrome following Lyme disease. Cardiol J 2011;18(1):63–6. Available at: http://www.ncbi.nlm.nih.gov/pubmed/21305487.
53. Aguero-Rosenfeld ME, Nowakowski J, Bittker S, et al. Evolution of the serologic response to *Borrelia burgdorferi* in treated patients with culture-confirmed erythema

migrans. J Clin Microbiol 1996;34(1):1–9. Available at: http://www.pubmedcentral. nih.gov/articlerender.fcgi?artid=228718&tool=pmcentrez&rendertype=abstract.
54. Aguero-Rosenfeld ME, Wang G, Schwartz I, et al. Diagnosis of Lyme borreliosis. Clin Microbiol Rev 2005;18(3):484–509.
55. Kalish RA, McHugh G, Granquist J, et al. Persistence of immunoglobulin M or immunoglobulin G antibody responses to *Borrelia burgdorferi* 10-20 years after active Lyme disease. Clin Infect Dis 2001;33(6):780–5.
56. Fleming RV, Marques AR, Klempner MS, et al. Pre-treatment and post-treatment assessment of the C(6) test in patients with persistent symptoms and a history of Lyme borreliosis. Eur J Clin Microbiol Infect Dis 2004;23(8):615–8.
57. Ramsey A, Belongia E. Outcomes of treated human granulocytic ehrlichiosis cases. Emerg Infect Dis 2002;8(4):398–401. Available at: http://citeseerx.ist. psu.edu/viewdoc/download?doi=10.1.1.392.743&rep=rep1&type=pdf. Accessed January 30, 2015.
58. Wang TJ, Liang MH, Sangha O, et al. Coexposure to *Borrelia burgdorferi* and *Babesia microti* does not worsen the long-term outcome of Lyme disease. Clin Infect Dis 2000;31(5):1149–54.
59. Hildenbrand P, Craven DE, Jones R, et al. Lyme neuroborreliosis: manifestations of a rapidly emerging zoonosis. AJNR Am J Neuroradiol 2009;30(6):1079–87.
60. Fallon BA, Lipkin RB, Corbera KM, et al. Regional cerebral blood flow and metabolic rate in persistent Lyme encephalopathy. Arch Gen Psychiatry 2009;66(5):554–63.
61. Logigian EL, Kaplan RF, Steere AC. Successful treatment of Lyme encephalopathy with intravenous ceftriaxone. J Infect Dis 1999;180(2):377–83.
62. Feder H Jr, Johnson BJ, O'Connell S, et al. A critical appraisal of "chronic Lyme disease". N Engl J Med 2007;357:1422–30. Available at: http://www.nejm.org/doi/full/10.1056/NEJMra072023.
63. Sigal LH. Summary of the first 100 patients seen at a Lyme disease referral center. Am J Med 1990;88(6):577–81. Available at: http://www.ncbi.nlm.nih.gov/pubmed/2346158. Accessed April 4, 2014.
64. Burdge DR, O'Hanlon DP. Experience at a referral center for patients with suspected Lyme disease in an area of nonendemicity: first 65 patients. Clin Infect Dis 1993;16(4):558–60. Available at: http://www.ncbi.nlm.nih.gov/pubmed/8513065. Accessed July 17, 2014.
65. Aucott J, Seifter A, Rebman A. Probable late Lyme disease: a variant manifestation of untreated *Borrelia burgdorferi* infection. BMC Infect Dis 2012;12(1):173.
66. Reid MC, Schoen RT, Evans J, et al. The consequences of overdiagnosis and overtreatment of Lyme disease: an observational study. Ann Intern Med 1998; 128(5):354–62. Available at: http://www.ncbi.nlm.nih.gov/pubmed/9490595.
67. Steere AC, Taylor E, McHugh GL, et al. The overdiagnosis of Lyme disease. JAMA 1993;269(14):1812–6. Available at: http://www.ncbi.nlm.nih.gov/pubmed/8459513. Accessed June 2, 2014.
68. Dinerman H, Steere AC. Lyme disease associated with fibromyalgia. Ann Intern Med 1992;117(4):281–5. Available at: http://www.ncbi.nlm.nih.gov/pubmed/1637022.
69. Gaudino EA, Coyle PK, Krupp LB. Post-lyme syndrome and chronic fatigue syndrome. Neuropsychiatric similarities and differences. Arch Neurol 1997;54(11): 1372–6. Available at: http://www.ncbi.nlm.nih.gov/pubmed/9362985. Accessed July 17, 2014.
70. Krupp LB, Hyman LG, Grimson R, et al. Study and treatment of post Lyme disease (STOP-LD): a randomized double masked clinical trial. Neurology 2003; 60(12):1923–30.

71. Batheja S, Nields JA, Landa A, et al. Post-treatment Lyme syndrome and central sensitization. J Neuropsychiatry Clin Neurosci 2013;25(3):176–86.
72. Auwaerter PG, Bakken JS, Dattwyler RJ, et al. Antiscience and ethical concerns associated with advocacy of Lyme disease. Lancet Infect Dis 2011;11(9):713–9.
73. Halperin JJ. Nervous system Lyme disease: is there a controversy? Semin Neurol 2011;31(3):317–24.
74. Fallon BA, Petkova E, Keilp JG, et al. Ongoing discussion about the US clinical Lyme trials. Am J Med 2014;127(2):e7.
75. Carbonell-Baeza A, Aparicio VA, Chillón P, et al. Effectiveness of multidisciplinary therapy on symptomatology and quality of life in women with fibromyalgia. Clin Exp Rheumatol 2011;29(6 Suppl 69):S97–103. Available at: http://www.ncbi.nlm.nih.gov/pubmed/22243556. Accessed March 26, 2014.
76. Okifuji A, Ackerlind S. Behavioral medicine approaches to pain. Med Clin North Am 2007;91(1):45–55.
77. Stanos S, Houle TT. Multidisciplinary and interdisciplinary management of chronic pain. Phys Med Rehabil Clin N Am 2006;17(2):435–50, vii.
78. Cicerone KD, Langenbahn DM, Braden C, et al. Evidence-based cognitive rehabilitation: updated review of the literature from 2003 through 2008. Arch Phys Med Rehabil 2011;92(4):519–30.
79. Li H, Li J, Li N, et al. Cognitive intervention for persons with mild cognitive impairment: a meta-analysis. Ageing Res Rev 2011;10(2):285–96.
80. Bakshi R. Fatigue associated with multiple sclerosis: diagnosis, impact and management. Mult Scler 2003;9(3):219–27. Available at: http://www.ncbi.nlm.nih.gov/pubmed/12814166. Accessed March 28, 2014.
81. Staud R. Treatment of fibromyalgia and its symptoms. Expert Opin Pharmacother 2007;8(11):1629–42.
82. Mitchell SA, Beck SL, Hood LE, et al. Putting evidence into practice: evidence-based interventions for fatigue during and following cancer and its treatment. Clin J Oncol Nurs 2007;11(1):99–113.
83. Steere AC, Angelis SM. Therapy for Lyme arthritis: strategies for the treatment of antibiotic-refractory arthritis. Arthritis Rheum 2006;54(10):3079–86.
84. Carlson D, Hernandez J, Bloom BJ, et al. Lack of *Borrelia burgdorferi* DNA in synovial samples from patients with antibiotic treatment-resistant Lyme arthritis. Arthritis Rheum 1999;42(12):2705–9.
85. Li X, McHugh GA, Damle N, et al. Burden and viability of *Borrelia burgdorferi* in skin and joints of patients with erythema migrans or Lyme arthritis. Arthritis Rheum 2011;63(8):2238–47.
86. Londoño D, Cadavid D, Drouin EE, et al. Antibodies to endothelial cell growth factor and obliterative microvascular lesions in synovia of patients with antibiotic-refractory Lyme arthritis. Arthritis Rheumatol 2014;66:2124–33.
87. Drouin EE, Seward RJ, Strle K, et al. A novel human autoantigen, endothelial cell growth factor, is a target of T and B cell responses in patients with Lyme disease. Arthritis Rheum 2013;65(1):186–96.
88. Schoen RT, Aversa JM, Rahn DW, et al. Treatment of refractory chronic Lyme arthritis with arthroscopic synovectomy. Arthritis Rheum 1991;34(8):1056–60. Available at: http://www.ncbi.nlm.nih.gov/pubmed/1859481. Accessed June 2, 2014.
89. Amsden GW. Anti-inflammatory effects of macrolides: an underappreciated benefit in the treatment of community-acquired respiratory tract infections and chronic inflammatory pulmonary conditions? J Antimicrob Chemother 2005;55(1):10–21.

90. Su W, Wan Q, Han L, et al. Doxycycline exerts multiple anti-allergy effects to attenuate murine allergic conjunctivitis and systemic anaphylaxis. Biochem Pharmacol 2014;91(3):359–68.

91. Pfeffer I, Borelli C, Zierhut M, et al. Treatment of ocular rosacea with 40 mg doxycycline in a slow release form. J Dtsch Dermatol Ges 2011;9(11):904–7.

92. Korting HC, Schöllmann C. Tetracycline actions relevant to rosacea treatment. Skin Pharmacol Physiol 2009;22(6):287–94.

93. Feng J, Wang T, Shi W, et al. Identification of novel activity against *Borrelia burgdorferi* persisters using an FDA approved drug library. Emerg Microbes Infect 2014;3(7):e49.

Chronic Lyme Disease

Paul M. Lantos, MD

KEYWORDS

- Lyme disease • Chronic Lyme disease • *Borrelia burgdorferi* • Chronic fatigue
- Chronic pain • Antibiotics

KEY POINTS

- There is no accepted clinical definition for chronic Lyme disease.
- Most patients with a diagnosis of chronic Lyme disease have no evidence of Lyme disease.
- Persistent subjective symptoms during recovery from Lyme disease are not active infection.
- Prolonged antibiotic courses are ineffective and unsafe patients for patients with prolonged symptoms after Lyme disease.

THE CHRONIC LYME DISEASE CONTROVERSY

Chronic Lyme disease (CLD) is a poorly defined term that describes the attribution of various atypical syndromes to protracted *Borrelia burgdorferi* infection. These syndromes are atypical for Lyme disease in their lack of the objective clinical abnormalities that are well-recognized in Lyme disease and, in many cases, the absence of serologic evidence of Lyme disease as well as the absence of plausible exposure to the infection. The syndromes usually diagnosed as CLD include chronic pain, fatigue, neurocognitive, and behavioral symptoms, as well as various alternative medical diagnoses—most commonly neurologic and rheumatologic diseases. Perhaps the most recognized and contentious facet of this debate is whether it is effective, appropriate, or even acceptable to treat patients with protracted antibiotic courses based on a clinical diagnosis of CLD.

The dialogue over CLD provokes strong feelings, and has been more acrimonious than any other aspect of Lyme disease. Many patients who have been diagnosed

Financial Disclosures/Conflicts of Interest: None.
Dr P.M. Lantos is supported by the National Center for Advancing Translational Sciences of the National Institutes of Health under Award Number KL2TR001115. The content is solely the responsibility of the author and does not necessarily represent the official views of the National Institutes of Health.
Divisions of Pediatric Infectious Diseases and General Internal Medicine, Duke University School of Medicine, DUMC 100800, Durham, NC 27710, USA
E-mail address: paul.lantos@duke.edu

Infect Dis Clin N Am 29 (2015) 325–340
http://dx.doi.org/10.1016/j.idc.2015.02.006
0891-5520/15/$ – see front matter © 2015 Elsevier Inc. All rights reserved.
id.theclinics.com

with CLD have experienced great personal suffering; this is true regardless of whether *B burgdorferi* infection is responsible for their experience. On top of this, many patients with a CLD diagnosis share the perception that the medical community has failed to effectively explain or treat their illnesses. In support of this patient base is a community of physicians and alternative treatment providers as well as a politically active advocacy community. This community promotes legislation that has attempted to shield CLD specialists from medical board discipline and medicolegal liability for unorthodox practices, to mandate insurance coverage of extended parenteral antibiotics, and most visibly to challenge legally a Lyme disease practice guideline. The advocacy community commonly argues that Lyme disease is grossly underdiagnosed and is responsible for an enormous breadth of illness; they also argue that the general scientific and public health establishments ignore or even cover up evidence to this effect. A large body of information about CLD has emerged on the Internet and other media, mostly in the forms of patient testimonials and promotional materials by CLD providers. For a medical consumer and for the physician unfamiliar with this subject, this volume of information can be confusing and difficult to navigate.

The CLD controversy does not, however, straddle a simple divide between 2 opposed scientific factions. Within the scientific community, the concept of CLD has for the most part been rejected. Clinical practice guidelines from numerous North American and European medical societies discourage the diagnosis of CLD and recommend against treating patients with prolonged or repeated antibiotic courses.[1–21] Neither national nor state public health bodies depart from these recommendations. Within the medical community, only a small minority of physicians have accepted this diagnosis: 1 study found that only 6 of 285 (2.1%) randomly surveyed primary care physicians in Connecticut, among the most highly endemic regions for Lyme disease, diagnosed patients with CLD and still fewer were willing to prescribe long courses of antibiotics.[22,23]

THE CONFUSING TERMINOLOGY OF CHRONIC LYME DISEASE

The mere name "chronic Lyme disease" is in itself a source of confusion. Lyme disease, in conventional use, specifically describes infection with the tick-borne spirochete *B burgdorferi* sensu lato. The diagnosis "chronic Lyme disease," by incorporating that terminology, connotes a similar degree of microbiologic specificity; the addition of the word "chronic" further implies that there is some distinction between "chronic" Lyme disease and other manifestations of the infection. This distinction in itself is problematic because several manifestations of Lyme disease may indeed present subacutely or chronically, including Lyme arthritis, acrodermatitis chronicum atrophicans, borrelial lymphocytoma, and late Lyme encephalopathy.

"Chronic Lyme disease," however, has no clinical definition and is not characterized by any objective clinical findings. The only published attempt to define CLD provisionally produced a description too broad to distinguish CLD from myriad other medical conditions, and the case definition did not mention evidence of *B burgdorferi* infection (**Box 1**).[24] The absence of a definition makes it impossible to investigate whether a patient population with putative CLD has evidence of infection with *B burgdorferi*; this would seem to be a basic requirement to include a syndrome within the term "Lyme disease." It stands to reason that it is impossible to even posit a well-designed antibiotic trial when the study population is undefined.

In the absence of a definition, it is instructive to examine the circumstances under which patients receive a diagnosis of CLD. These circumstances can be

---

Box 1
Working definition of chronic Lyme disease proposed by ILDAS

For the purpose of the ILADS guidelines, 'chronic Lyme disease' is inclusive of persistent symptomatologies including fatigue, cognitive dysfunction, headaches, sleep disturbance and other neurologic features, such as demyelinating disease, peripheral neuropathy and sometimes motor neuron disease, neuropsychiatric presentations, cardiac presentations (including electrical conduction delays and dilated cardiomyopathy), and musculoskeletal problems.

Abbreviation: ILADS, International Lyme and Associated Diseases Society.
   From Cameron D, Gaito A, Harris N, et al. Evidence-based guidelines for the management of Lyme disease. Expert Rev Anti Infect Ther 2004;2(Suppl 1):S4.

---

inferred from the breakdown of patients referred for suspected Lyme disease. In 7 studies conducted in endemic areas, comprising a total of 1902 patients referred for suspected Lyme disease, 7% to 31% had active Lyme disease and 5% to 20% had previous Lyme disease, based on concordance of their clinical presentations with recognized manifestations of Lyme disease.[25–31] The remaining 50% to 88%, however, had no evidence of ever having had Lyme disease. Most of these patients had either alternative medical diagnoses or had medically unexplained symptoms, such as chronic fatigue syndrome or fibromyalgia. Lyme disease was in many cases diagnosed simply for lack of an alternative diagnosis—referred to in 1 paper as a "diagnosis of Lyme disease by exclusion."[30] Two studies documented that many of the referred patients had psychiatric diagnoses and/or maladaptive psychological traits, such as catastrophization and negative affect.[26,28] Many patients had symptoms of long duration and had received multiple courses of antibiotics.

A common reason for referral was a positive Lyme disease serologic test. On clinical review, however, the patients lacked clinical findings concordant with a Lyme disease diagnosis. This is certainly a side effect of a great volume of Lyme disease testing conducted in the United States—more than 3 million tests are thought to be ordered annually.[32] Most such tests are ordered with a very low pretest probability in settings such as chronic nonspecific fatigue, based on patient request, after a tick bite (when even an infected patient would be most likely seronegative), or as part as a general neurologic or rheumatologic evaluation. In the absence of specific clinical findings, however, Lyme disease testing has a very low positive predictive value.[33] Patients may have positive Lyme serology for a variety of reasons, including asymptomatic seroconversion, cross-reactive antibodies generated by other infectious or inflammatory diseases, or a previous treated episode of Lyme disease; asymptomatic seropositivity is well-described in endemic areas.[25,29,30,33–40] Thus, the misattribution of chronic symptoms to Lyme disease is an inevitable consequence of high-volume, low-probability testing.

THE MISDIAGNOSIS OF CHRONIC LYME DISEASE

Many patients referred for Lyme disease are ultimately found to have a rheumatologic or neurologic diagnosis. Rheumatologic diagnoses commonly misdiagnosed as Lyme disease include osteoarthritis, rheumatoid arthritis, degenerative diseases of the spine, and spondyloarthropathies.[26,27,41] Some patients are found to have neurologic diseases, including multiple sclerosis, demyelinating diseases, amyotrophic lateral sclerosis, neuropathies, and dementia.[27] Some CLD advocates have argued that these various conditions are simply manifestations of Lyme disease,[24,42–44] but these hypotheses are untenable. Lyme disease is transmitted quite focally,[45] and there is no epidemiologic evidence that these alternative diagnoses cluster in regions with high Lyme disease transmission. There has been no association between diagnoses such as multiple sclerosis, amyotrophic lateral sclerosis, or rheumatoid arthritis and antecedent Lyme disease, these diagnoses do not arise concurrently with other recognized manifestations of disseminated Lyme disease (such as Lyme arthritis), and there is no quality evidence associating any of these diagnoses with seroconversion to *B burgdorferi*. Although there can certainly be clinical overlap between Lyme disease and other conditions, objective findings and studies will generally allow them to be differentiated.

Medically unexplained symptoms, whether resulting in entities such as fibromyalgia and chronic fatigue syndrome or syndromes with a less distinct pattern, account for most of the remaining patients who are diagnosed with CLD. Unlike Lyme disease, these frustrating conditions generally lack objective clinical or other objective abnormalities, and they are dominated by subjective complaints and functional impairment.[46–48] No evidence suggests that these clinical entities geographically cluster in regions with *B burgdorferi* transmission. Fibromyalgia has been found to follow Lyme disease temporally in some cases: in a prospective study of 287 patients treated for confirmed Lyme disease, 22 (8%) went on to develop fibromyalgia within 5 months of treatment.[49] Additional antibiotics were not beneficial. This finding, however, is contradicted by a prospective cohort study in which only 1 of 100 patients treated for culture-confirmed Lyme disease developed fibromyalgia during the subsequent 11 to 20 years.[50] Severe fatigue was found in 9 of these patients, but it was attributable in all cases to other causes.[51] Many patients experience prolonged symptoms during convalescence from systemic infections, including symptoms of fibromyalgia and chronic fatigue.[49,52] Such symptoms, however, do not seem to be associated particularly with antecedent Lyme disease; in fact, the prevalence of fatigue and fibromyalgia among patients with past Lyme disease is similar to their prevalence in the general population.

BIOLOGICAL EXPLANATIONS FOR CHRONIC LYME DISEASE

Several arguments have been made to support the biological plausibility of CLD and to justify its treatment with lengthy courses of antibiotics. One is that *B burgdorferi* localizes intracellularly in the infected host, and that the antibiotics typically chosen to treat it do not penetrate cells effectively. Aside from the fact that *B burgdorferi* predominantly occupies the extracellular matrix,[53] the antibiotics currently recommended to treat Lyme disease are well-established to treat a variety of intracellular infections. For example, doxycycline and azithromycin are first-line drugs for the treatment of *Mycoplasma*, *Chlamydia*, and *Legionella*, and doxycycline is the drug of choice for *Rickettsia* and related species. Ceftriaxone is effective against *Salmonella* and *Neisseria*, both of which are predominantly intracellular; amoxicillin is effective against *Listeria*.

Another commonly voiced argument is that *B burgdorferi* assumes a round morphology, variously described as "cyst forms," "spheroplasts," "L-forms," and "round bodies." These variants are said to be resistant to antibiotic treatment and require alternative antibiotics and dosing strategies. On close review of the literature there is little evidence that these variants arise in vivo in humans, let alone that they are associated with CLD-like symptom complexes or that they require treatment.[54]

MICROBIOLOGIC INVESTIGATIONS INTO CHRONIC LYME DISEASE

There is very little microbiologic evidence that supports persistent *B burgdorferi* infection in patients who lack objective manifestations of Lyme disease, such as erythema migrans, arthritis, meningitis, and neuropathies. Advocates for CLD contend that our ability to detect *B burgdorferi* is hampered by current technology and an incomplete scientific understanding of *B burgdorferi*, and that conventional diagnostic testing misses patients with CLD.[55,56] Naturally, this raises the question of why we should assume that chronic *B burgdorferi* infection exists at all if we are so ill-equipped to detect it. Even when chronically symptomatic patients have a well-documented history of treated Lyme disease, investigators have been unable to document persistent infection.[57–59] A recent study in which ticks were allowed to feed on persistently symptomatic posttreatment patients yielded molecular evidence of *B burgdorferi* in 1 of 16 patients and no patient had cultivatable organisms.[60]

Studies reporting the retrieval of *B burgdorferi* from antibiotic-treated animals are indirect and have limited generalizability to human disease. First, it is impossible to create an animal model of CLD when this diagnosis is usually based on symptoms described by a patient. Second, rodents serve as reservoir species for *B burgdorferi* in nature and may tolerate persistent asymptomatic infection. Third, some experimental studies use large inocula of *B burgdorferi* that have been grown to stationary phase; the organism assumes a more drug-resistant phenotype under these growth conditions and this may not reflect natural infection.

Because validated testing methods fail to support the connection between *B burgdorferi* and clinically diagnosed CLD, physicians who specialize in CLD often turn to alternative tests. This has included the use of novel culture techniques, detection of *B burgdorferi* DNA in urine specimens, and enumeration of CD57-positive lymphocytes.[61–65] Independent investigations, however, have repudiated the validity of these tests.[66–70]

COINFECTIONS

Some CLD advocates emphasize that CLD is a polymicrobial infection in which patients suffer from multiple tick-borne coinfections.[71,72] In practice, patients with a diagnosis of CLD are often diagnosed with and treated for numerous superimposed infections, including *Babesia* spp and *Anaplasma phagocytophilum* (well-described tick-borne pathogens), *Bartonella henselae* (which is not known to be transmitted by ticks), pathogens of unclear clinical relevance such as the xenotropic murine leukemia virus-related virus, and even completely fictitious pathogens such as "*Protomyxozoa rheumatica.*" There is no evidence to support chronic anaplasmosis; chronic symptomatic babesiosis when present invariably is associated with fever and molecular or microscopic evidence of parasitemia. *Bartonella* species are readily identified in ticks, but there is virtually no quality evidence of tick-borne transmission to humans or of simultaneous Lyme disease and bartonellosis.[73] It is important to recognize that, in the context of CLD, a diagnosis of coinfection may be just as spurious.

PERSISTENT SYMPTOMS AFTER TREATMENT FOR LYME DISEASE

It is well-recognized that some patients experience prolonged symptoms during convalescence from Lyme disease, and a subset suffer significant functional impairment.[57–59,74–78] The most common complaints among such patients are arthralgias, myalgias, headache, neck and backache, fatigue, irritability, and cognitive dysfunction (particularly perceived difficulty with memory and concentration).[57–59]

A working definition was developed to categorize patients with 'post-Lyme disease symptoms' (PLDS), those patients with persistent clinical symptoms after treatment for Lyme disease, but who lack objective evidence of treatment failure, reinfection, or relapse (**Box 2**).[20] PLDS is not strictly speaking a coherent clinical diagnosis; its primary value has been to define a patient cohort for further study. Nonetheless, it is worth considering how it conceptually differs from CLD. To meet criteria for PLDS, patients must have unequivocal documentation of appropriately treated Lyme disease, lack objective manifestations of Lyme disease, and have persistent symptoms that cannot be explained by other medical illnesses. Thus, of patients with chronic symptoms that have been *attributed* to Lyme disease, those meeting criteria for PLDS are those for whom infection with *B burgdorferi* is most plausible. This makes the studies of PLDS paradigmatic for the understanding of CLD.

The frequency of PLDS is difficult to estimate, but as a function of patients with a known history of Lyme disease, it seems to be rare. This is exemplified by the great difficulty 3 investigative teams had in recruiting subjects for clinical trials investigating this condition.[57–59] Of 5846 patients screened over several years, only 222 (3.8%) could be randomized ultimately, which is striking considering that between 30,000 and 300,000 Americans are thought to contract Lyme disease annually. PLDS also seems to be uncommon among subjects in clinical trials. In 10 prospective studies of erythema migrans and early disseminated Lyme disease, fewer than 10% of subjects described persistent symptoms such as myalgias and fatigue after 9 or more months (range, 0%–23%), and the prevalence of severe symptoms was 0% to 2.8%.[79–88] One trial found that, after 12 months, patients treated for erythema migrans were no more likely to have subjective symptoms than an uninfected control group.[80]

If PLDS is rare among patients with a history of Lyme disease, in the general population it becomes impossible to discern from the high background rate of similar symptoms among adults. Up to 20% of surveyed adults report chronic fatigue.[89,90] In 1 report, 3.75% to 12.1% of the general population suffered severe pain and 36.4% to 45.1% moderate pain, whereas only 42.5% to 59.1% of the general population was pain free.[91] In a separate study, 11.2% of respondents suffered chronic, widespread pain.[92] One-quarter to one-third of the general population describe chronic cognitive dysfunction.[91] These symptoms often coincide with anxiety or depression, which in their own right are common in the general population. Interestingly, many who complain of cognitive dysfunction are found to be normal when formally tested.[59,75,79,93–96] In all likelihood, subjective post-Lyme symptoms are not unique to Lyme disease but rather are common to the recovery from many systemic illnesses. Bacterial pneumonia, for example, can be followed by months of nonspecific symptoms that impair quality of life.[97]

RISK FACTORS FOR PERSISTENT SYMPTOMS AFTER TREATMENT FOR LYME DISEASE

Patients with the most severe symptoms on clinical presentation are the most likely to have persistent symptoms during convalescence.[98–100] Severe headache, arthritis, arthralgias, and fatigue at presentation predicted persistent symptoms in a retrospectively examined cohort of 215 patients.[101] In a prospective treatment trial for early Lyme disease, persistent symptoms at several late follow-up visits (6 months through 5 years) were more common in patients who had more symptoms, higher symptom scores and multiple (vs solitary) erythema migrans lesions.[85] Patients with a longer duration of symptoms may also be at greater risk of persistent symptoms: a review of 38 subjects who had been previously treated for Lyme disease found that persistent

Box 2
Proposed definition of post-Lyme disease syndromes from the Infectious Disease Society of America

Inclusion criteria

- An adult or child with a documented episode of early or late Lyme disease fulfilling the case definition of the Centers for Disease Control and Prevention. If based on erythema migrans, the diagnosis must be made and documented by an experienced health care practitioner.

- After treatment of the episode of Lyme disease with a generally accepted treatment regimen, there is resolution or stabilization of the objective manifestation(s) of Lyme disease.

- Onset of any of the following subjective symptoms within 6 months of the diagnosis of Lyme disease and persistence of continuous or relapsing symptoms for at least a 6-month period after completion of antibiotic therapy:

  ○ Fatigue

  ○ Widespread musculoskeletal pain

  ○ Complaints of cognitive difficulties

- Subjective symptoms are of such severity that, when present, they result in substantial reduction in previous levels of occupational, educational, social or personal activities.

Exclusion criteria

- An active, untreated, well-documented coinfection, such as babesiosis.

- The presence of objective abnormalities on physical examination or on neuropsychologic testing that may explain the patient's complaints. For example, a patient with antibiotic-refractory Lyme arthritis would be excluded. A patient with late neuroborreliosis associated with encephalopathy, who has recurrent or refractory objective cognitive dysfunction, would be excluded.

- A diagnosis of fibromyalgia or chronic fatigue syndrome before the onset of Lyme disease.

- A prolonged history of undiagnosed or unexplained somatic complaints, such as musculoskeletal pains or fatigue, before the onset of Lyme disease.

- A diagnosis of an underlying disease or condition that might explain the patient's symptoms (eg, morbid obesity, with a body mass index [calculated as weight in kilograms divided by the square of height in meters] of 45 kg/m^2 or greater; sleep apnea and narcolepsy; side effects of medications; autoimmune diseases; uncontrolled cardiopulmonary or endocrine disorders; malignant conditions within 2 years, except for uncomplicated skin cancer; known current liver disease; any past or current diagnosis of a major depressive disorder with psychotic or melancholic features; bipolar affective disorders; schizophrenia of any subtype; delusional disorders of any subtype; dementias of any subtype; anorexia nervosa or bulimia nervosa; and active drug abuse or alcoholism at present or within 2 years).

- Laboratory or imaging abnormalities that might suggest an undiagnosed process distinct from post-Lyme disease syndrome, such as a highly elevated erythrocyte sedimentation rate (150 mm/h); abnormal thyroid function; a hematologic abnormality; abnormal levels of serum albumin, total protein, globulin, calcium, phosphorus, glucose, urea nitrogen, electrolytes or creatinine; significant abnormalities on urine analysis; elevated liver enzyme levels; or a test result suggestive of the presence of a collagen vascular disease.

- Although testing by either culture or polymerase chain reaction for evidence of *Borrelia burgdorferi* infection is not required, should such testing be done by reliable methods, a positive result would be an exclusion.

From Wormser GP, Dattwyler RJ, Shapiro ED, et al. The clinical assessment, treatment, and prevention of Lyme disease, human granulocytic anaplasmosis, and babesiosis: clinical practice guidelines by the Infectious Diseases Society of America. Clin Infect Dis 2006;43(9):1121; with permission.

somatic and neuropsychological sequelae were strongly associated with prolonged illness before treatment.[77]

On the other hand, the duration of antibiotic therapy does not influence the persistence of subjective symptoms after treatment. In a prospective trial of therapy for 180 patients with early Lyme disease, neuropsychologic deficits were equally common among patients treated for 10 versus 20 days at follow-up 30 months later.[87] In a retrospective study of 607 patients treated for early Lyme disease, 99 ± 0.2% of patients were well after 2 years of follow-up, regardless of whether they had received fewer than 10, 11 to 14, or more than 14 days of therapy.[88] In a randomized, open-label trial of therapy for late Lyme disease, patients treated for 14 days were no more likely to have severe symptoms than those treated for 28 days, even though objective treatment failures were significantly more likely in the 14-day arm.[102] After 3 weeks of parenteral ceftriaxone, an additional 100 days of oral amoxicillin was no better than placebo at improving cognitive and somatic outcomes.[103]

We have an incomplete picture as to why some patients are left with chronic symptoms after Lyme disease whereas the majority does well. Genetic variability among B burgdorferi isolates and its significance for clinical disease is an important emerging area of research. This is difficult to link with clinical outcomes, however, because different strains of the organism cannot be discriminated by standard clinical testing. Anti-Borrelia antibody titers are higher among patients with PLDS compared with those with an uncomplicated post-Lyme disease course; antibody profiles are different between these 2 groups as well.[104] Patients with neurologic Lyme disease have elevated cerebrospinal fluid biomarkers, including CXCL13 and neopterin.[105] These return to normal after antibiotic therapy, and are not increased in patients with PLDS. Further research is needed to better characterize the biology of PLDS.

EXTENDED ANTIBIOTICS FOR THE TREATMENT OF POST-LYME DISEASE SYNDROMES

Three research groups have examined prospectively the effectiveness of prolonged antibiotic courses for post-Lyme disease syndromes.[57–59,75] All trials had strict entrance criteria similar to the aforementioned definition of PLDS. The Klempner and colleagues[58] study reported 2 parallel trials in which their cohort of 129 subjects was divided into seropositive (n = 78) and seronegative (n = 51) arms. Subjects randomized to treatment groups received 30 days of intravenous (IV) ceftriaxone followed by 60 days of oral doxycycline. Those randomized to the placebo arm received IV placebo for 30 days, followed by an oral placebo for 60 days. The primary outcome was health-related quality of life as assessed by standardized instruments (the Medical Outcomes Study 36-item Short-Form General Health Survey [SF-36] and the Fibromyalgia Impact Questionnaire). These instruments were administered at baseline, and then 30, 90, and 180 days. There was no difference in any outcome measure between placebo and treatment groups in either the seropositive or seronegative arm, or in a detailed battery of neuropsychological tests that was published subsequently.[75] Although all patients had complained of cognitive dysfunction at baseline (and this was the primary complaint in >70%), objective measures of cognitive function, such as memory and attention, were normal compared with age-referenced normative data. Depression, anxiety, and somatic complaints improved in both the antibiotic and placebo arms groups between baseline and day 180.

In a separate trial, Krupp and colleagues[59] investigated the effect of antibiotics for persistent severe fatigue after treatment for Lyme disease. Twenty-eight patients were randomized to receive 28 days of IV ceftriaxone and 24 received IV placebo. The primary outcome measure was score on the Fatigue Severity Scale (FSS-11). Additional outcomes were visual analog scales (VAS) of fatigue and pain, the SF-36, the Center for Epidemiologic Studies Depression Scale, and a comprehensive battery of cognitive function. Outcomes were measured at baseline and at 6 months. At follow-up, there was a significant but partial improvement on the FSS-11 in the ceftriaxone arm compared with placebo, with 18 of 26 (69%) versus 5 of 22 (23%) patients showing improvement from baseline ($P = .001$). The fatigue VAS, although not significant, corroborated a benefit for the treatment arm ($P = .08$). No measure of mood or cognitive function differed at the 6-month follow-up. It was noted that a much higher proportion of patients on ceftriaxone correctly guessed their treatment assignment. Whether this was a failure of masking, and whether this would have affected the outcome of a subjective measure like fatigue, is difficult to discern. The commonality and nonspecificity of fatigue, and the observation that antibiotics may improve chronic fatigue in noninfectious or other postinfectious illnesses, raise doubts as to whether it was the elimination of *B burgdorferi* that resulted in this outcome.[106–108]

Fallon and colleagues[57] investigated a more prolonged IV treatment course. In this cohort, 23 patients were randomized to receive IV ceftriaxone and 14 patients to receive IV placebo for 10 weeks, followed by 14 weeks of observation off of therapy. Six domains of cognitive function were tested and compiled to produce a composite 'cognitive index' score. The primary outcome of interest was cognitive index compared with baseline and between groups at week 24. An interim evaluation at week 12 demonstrated significant improvement over baseline in the ceftriaxone group ($P<.01$), whereas this was not the case for the placebo group. A between-group comparison at week 12 approached statistical significance ($P = .053$) as well. At week 24, however, these differences had disappeared: both groups had improved over their within-group baseline, but there was no difference between groups ($P = .76$). Five of the randomized patients withdrew from the study owing to adverse events, leaving only 20 drug and 12 placebo patients available for statistical analysis. An additional 4 ceftriaxone patients remained in the study despite adverse events that truncated their therapy. The patients who dropped out were not analyzed by intention to treat, which, given the small sample size in this trial, might have affected the published statistics.

Adverse events were common in these studies, particularly catheter-associated venous thromboembolism, catheter-associated bacteremia, allergic reactions, and ceftriaxone-induced gallbladder toxicity. In the Klempner and colleagues[58] trial, 1 patient on ceftriaxone suffered a pulmonary embolism and 1 experienced a syndrome of fever, anemia, and gastrointestinal bleeding that was felt to be an allergic phenomenon. In the Krupp and colleagues[59] trial, 3 patients on IV placebo developed line sepsis and 1 patient on ceftriaxone had an anaphylactic reaction. In the Fallon and colleagues[57] trial, 6 patients on ceftriaxone had adverse events: 2 venous thromboembolic events, 3 allergic reactions, and 1 case of ceftriaxone-induced cholecystitis (requiring cholecystectomy), in addition to a placebo patient who developed line sepsis. Other studies reiterate the frequency of adverse events in persons with prolonged exposure to IV catheters and antibiotics. In an observational study by Stricker and colleagues,[109] there were 19 potentially life-threatening adverse events among 200 patients on long-term IV antibiotics for the treatment of CLD. These included 4 cases of venous thromboembolic disease, 6 cases of suspected line sepsis, 7 patients with allergic reactions, and 2 who developed ceftriaxone-induced gallbladder disease (both necessitating cholecystectomy). The mean duration of antibiotic therapy in this cohort was 118 days, and the adverse events reported occurred after a mean of 81 days from initiation of therapy. Although no deaths occurred in these studies, there have indeed been documented fatalities and near fatalities owing to prolonged IV antibiotic therapy for the treatment of Lyme disease.[110–112]

CLINICAL APPROACH TO PATIENTS WITH A CHRONIC LYME DISEASE DIAGNOSIS

Even if CLD lacks biological legitimacy, its importance as a phenomenon can be monumental to the individual patient. This is because many if not most patients who believe they have this condition are suffering, in many cases for years. Many have undergone frustrating, expensive, and ultimately fruitless medical evaluations, and many have become quite disaffected with a medical system that has failed to provide answers, let alone relief.

Beyond this generalization, patients referred for CLD have heterogeneous medical, social, and educational backgrounds. Furthermore, there is great variation in their "commitment" to a CLD diagnosis. Some patients are entirely convinced they have CLD, they request specific types of therapy, and they are not interested in adjudicating the CLD diagnosis. By contrast, others are not particularly interested in CLD per se, and are content to move on to a broader evaluation. In the author's experience most patients fall somewhere in between—a certain amount of time must be spent reviewing past experiences and past laboratory tests, then explaining why Lyme disease may not account for their illnesses.

Several strategies are generally helpful in approaching CLD in the clinic. First, the physician needs to suppress preconceptions or biases about such patients. Some encounters are long, some are short, some are tense, and some are congenial—but this is hardly unique to Lyme disease. Second, the process of clinical information gathering in medicine, that is, complaint, history, physical examination, and diagnostic testing, is no different in the context of CLD. Even if much discussion is centered on CLD, the goal of the encounter should still be to evaluate the patient and make the soundest assessment and plan.

Finally, it is of utmost importance to not seem to be impatient, dismissive, or rushed. Many patients who seek care for CLD already have accumulated frustration if not outright disaffection with the medical community. Subtle cues like body language, tone of voice, and affect can be critical to gaining or losing a patient's trust. Furthermore, each patient's clinical story and personal history is unique and valid, even if one concludes that they do not have Lyme disease.

SUMMARY

A limitation of modern medicine is our ability to explain and treat chronic pain, fatigue, and other disabling symptoms. It should come as no surprise that patients suffering from these symptoms have placed their hope in treatable conditions. Over time, a number of infectious diseases have been hypothesized as responsible, including *Candida*, *Brucella*, Epstein–Barr virus, xenotropic murine leukemia virus-related virus, and *B burgdorferi*. The scientific community has largely rejected chronic, treatment-refractory *B burgdorferi* infection, usually termed CLD, based on the absence of a defined patient population, the failure to detect cultivatable, clinically relevant organisms after standard treatment. Because the label CLD is applied to a highly heterogeneous spectrum of patients, the term CLD is better thought of as describing a phenomenon of attribution rather than a single disease. Even the subset of chronically symptomatic patients with a well-documented history of Lyme disease, usually termed PLDS, have little evidence of active infection, and their symptoms do not respond to antibiotics any better than to placebo. Controversies such as that over CLD are likely to persist for as long as patients suffer from poorly explained, disabling symptoms. We must hope that future research will provide better explanations and safe, effective treatments.

REFERENCES

1. Société de pathologie infectieuse de langue française. Lyme borreliose: diagnostic, therapeutic and preventive approaches–long text. Med Mal Infect 2007;37(Suppl 3):S153–74 [in French].
2. Neuroborreliose. Leitlinien der Deutschen Gesellschaft für Neurologie. [Neuroborreliosis: Guidelines of the German Society for Neurology]. Leitlinien-Register. 2008;Nr 030/071.
3. Läkemedelsbehandling av borreliainfektion – ny rekommendation. Drug treatment of Lyme disease: new recommendation. Inf Från Läkemedelsverket 2009;4:12–7.
4. Kutane Manifestationen der Lyme Borreliose. Leitlinien der Deutschen Dermatologischen Gesellschaft, Arbeitsgemeinschaft für Dermatologische Infektiologie [Cutaneous manifestations of Lyme borreliosis. Guidelines of the German Society of Dermatology, Dermatologic Association for Infectious Diseases]. Leitlinien-Register. 2009;Nr 013/044.
5. Pickering LK, Kimberlin DW, Long MD. Red Book 2012 report of the committee on infectious diseases. 29th edition. Elk Grove Village (IL): American Academy of Pediatrics; 2012.
6. Dessau RB, Bangsborg JM, Jensen TP, et al. Laboratory diagnosis of infection caused by Borrelia burgdorferi. Ugeskr Laeger 2006;168(34):2805–7 [in Danish].
7. Evison J, Aebi C, Francioli P, et al. Lyme disease part I: epidemiology and diagnosis. Rev Med Suisse 2006;2(60):919–24 [in French].
8. Evison J, Aebi C, Francioli P, et al. Lyme disease part 2: clinic and treatment. Rev Med Suisse 2006;2(60):925–8, 930-4. [in French].
9. Evison J, Aebi C, Francioli P, et al. Lyme disease part 3: prevention, pregnancy, immunodeficient state, post-Lyme disease syndrome. Rev Med Suisse 2006; 2(60):935–6, 8-40. [in French].
10. Flisiak R, Pancewicz S, Polish Society of Epidemiology and Infectious Diseases. Diagnostics and treatment of Lyme borreliosis. Recommendations of Polish Society of Epidemiology and Infectious Diseases. Przegl Epidemiol 2008;62(1): 193–9 [in Polish].
11. Halperin JJ, Shapiro ED, Logigian E, et al. Practice parameter: treatment of nervous system Lyme disease (an evidence-based review): report of the Quality Standards Subcommittee of the American Academy of Neurology. Neurology 2007;69(1):91–102.
12. Lantos PM, Charini WA, Medoff G, et al. Final report of the Lyme disease review panel of the Infectious Diseases Society of America. Clin Infect Dis 2010;51(1):1–5.
13. Ljostad U, Mygland A. Lyme borreliosis in adults. Tidsskr Nor Laegeforen 2008; 128(10):1175–8 [in Norwegian].
14. Mygland A, Ljostad U, Fingerle V, et al. EFNS guidelines on the diagnosis and management of European Lyme neuroborreliosis. Eur J Neurol 2010;17(1): 8–16 e1-4.
15. O'Connell S, editor. Recommendations for the diagnosis and treatment of Lyme borreliosis: guidelines and consensus papers from specialist societies and expert groups in Europe and North America. Federation of Infections Societies (FIS) "Infection 2009". Birmingham (United Kingdom): 2009.
16. Oksi J. Diagnostics and treatment of Lyme borreliosis. Duodecim 2000;116(6): 605–12 [in Finnish].

17. Speelman P, de Jongh BM, Wolfs TF, et al. Guideline 'Lyme borreliosis'. Ned Tijdschr Geneeskd 2004;148(14):659–63.
18. Strle F. Principles of the diagnosis and antibiotic treatment of Lyme borreliosis. Wien Klin Wochenschr 1999;111(22–23):911–5.
19. Vanousova D, Hercogova J. Lyme borreliosis treatment. Dermatol Ther 2008; 21(2):101–9.
20. Wormser GP, Dattwyler RJ, Shapiro ED, et al. The clinical assessment, treatment, and prevention of Lyme disease, human granulocytic anaplasmosis, and babesiosis: clinical practice guidelines by the Infectious Diseases Society of America. Clin Infect Dis 2006;43(9):1089–134.
21. Stanek G, O'Connell S, Cimmino M, et al. European Union Concerted Action on Risk Assessment in Lyme Borreliosis: clinical case definitions for Lyme borreliosis. Wien Klin Wochenschr 1996;108(23):741–7.
22. Johnson M, Feder HM Jr. Chronic Lyme disease: a survey of Connecticut primary care physicians. J Pediatr 2010;157(6):1025–9.e1–2.
23. Murray T, Feder HM Jr. Management of tick bites and early Lyme disease: a survey of Connecticut physicians. Pediatrics 2001;108(6):1367–70.
24. Cameron D, Gaito A, Harris N, et al. Evidence-based guidelines for the management of Lyme disease. Expert Rev Anti Infect Ther 2004;2(Suppl 1): S1–13.
25. Reid MC, Schoen RT, Evans J, et al. The consequences of overdiagnosis and overtreatment of Lyme disease: an observational study. Ann Intern Med 1998; 128(5):354–62.
26. Sigal LH. Summary of the first 100 patients seen at a Lyme disease referral center. Am J Med 1990;88(6):577–81.
27. Steere AC, Taylor E, McHugh GL, et al. The overdiagnosis of Lyme disease. JAMA 1993;269(14):1812–6.
28. Hassett AL, Radvanski DC, Buyske S, et al. Psychiatric comorbidity and other psychological factors in patients with "chronic Lyme disease". Am J Med 2009;122(9):843–50.
29. Qureshi MZ, New D, Zulqarni NJ, et al. Overdiagnosis and overtreatment of Lyme disease in children. Pediatr Infect Dis J 2002;21(1):12–4.
30. Rose CD, Fawcett PT, Gibney KM, et al. The overdiagnosis of Lyme disease in children residing in an endemic area. Clin Pediatr 1994;33(11):663–8.
31. Djukic M, Schmidt-Samoa C, Nau R, et al. The diagnostic spectrum in patients with suspected chronic Lyme neuroborreliosis–the experience from one year of a university hospital's Lyme neuroborreliosis outpatients clinic. Eur J Neurol 2011;18(4):547–55.
32. Hinckley AF, Connally NP, Meek JI, et al. Lyme disease testing by large commercial laboratories in the United States. Clin Infect Dis 2014;59(5):676–81.
33. Tugwell P, Dennis DT, Weinstein A, et al. Laboratory evaluation in the diagnosis of Lyme disease. Ann Intern Med 1997;127(12):1109–23.
34. Smith HV, Gray JS, McKenzie G. A Lyme borreliosis human serosurvey of asymptomatic adults in Ireland. Zentralbl Bakteriol 1991;275(3):382–9.
35. Zhioua E, Gern L, Aeschlimann A, et al. Longitudinal study of Lyme borreliosis in a high risk population in Switzerland. Parasite 1998;5(4):383–6.
36. Steere AC, Sikand VK, Meurice F, et al. Vaccination against Lyme disease with recombinant Borrelia burgdorferi outer-surface lipoprotein A with adjuvant. Lyme Disease Vaccine Study Group. N Engl J Med 1998;339(4):209–15.
37. Steere AC, Sikand VK, Schoen RT, et al. Asymptomatic infection with Borrelia burgdorferi. Clin Infect Dis 2003;37(4):528–32.

38. Fahrer H, van der Linden SM, Sauvain MJ, et al. The prevalence and incidence of clinical and asymptomatic Lyme borreliosis in a population at risk. J Infect Dis 1991;163(2):305–10.
39. Gustafson R, Svenungsson B, Gardulf A, et al. Prevalence of tick-borne encephalitis and Lyme borreliosis in a defined Swedish population. Scand J Infect Dis 1990;22(3):297–306.
40. Steere AC, Taylor E, Wilson ML, et al. Longitudinal assessment of the clinical and epidemiological features of Lyme disease in a defined population. J Infect Dis 1986;154(2):295–300.
41. Seidel MF, Domene AB, Vetter H. Differential diagnoses of suspected Lyme borreliosis or post-Lyme-disease syndrome. Eur J Clin Microbiol Infect Dis 2007;26(9):611–7.
42. Savely V. Lyme disease: a diagnostic dilemma. Nurse Pract 2010;35(7):44–50.
43. Stricker RB, Johnson L. 'Rare' infections mimicking multiple sclerosis: consider Lyme disease. Clin Neurol Neurosurg 2011;113(3):259–60.
44. Fritzsche M. Chronic Lyme borreliosis at the root of multiple sclerosis–is a cure with antibiotics attainable? Med Hypotheses 2005;64(3):438–48.
45. Bacon RM, Kugeler KJ, Mead PS, Centers for Disease Control and Prevention. Surveillance for Lyme disease–United States, 1992-2006. MMWR Surveill Summ 2008;57(10):1–9.
46. Barsky AJ, Borus JF. Functional somatic syndromes. Ann Intern Med 1999; 130(11):910–21.
47. Hatcher S, Arroll B. Assessment and management of medically unexplained symptoms. BMJ 2008;336(7653):1124–8.
48. Smith RC, Dwamena FC. Classification and diagnosis of patients with medically unexplained symptoms. J Gen Intern Med 2007;22(5):685–91.
49. Dinerman H, Steere AC. Lyme disease associated with fibromyalgia. Ann Intern Med 1992;117(4):281–5.
50. Wormser GP, Weitzner E, McKenna D, et al. Long-term assessment of fibromyalgia in patients with culture-confirmed Lyme disease. Arthritis Rheum 2014. [Epub ahead of print].
51. Wormser GP, Weitzner E, McKenna D, et al. Long-term assessment of fatigue in patients with culture-confirmed Lyme disease. Am J Med 2014;128(2):181–4.
52. Hickie I, Davenport T, Wakefield D, et al. Post-infective and chronic fatigue syndromes precipitated by viral and non-viral pathogens: prospective cohort study. BMJ 2006;333(7568):575.
53. Cabello FC, Godfrey HP, Newman SA. Hidden in plain sight: Borrelia burgdorferi and the extracellular matrix. Trends Microbiol 2007;15(8):350–4.
54. Lantos PM, Auwaerter PG, Wormser GP. A systematic review of Borrelia burgdorferi morphologic variants does not support a role in chronic Lyme disease. Clin Infect Dis 2014;58(5):663–71.
55. Stricker RB, Johnson L. The Lyme disease chronicles, continued. Chronic Lyme disease: in defense of the patient enterprise. FASEB J 2010;24(12):4632–3 [author reply: 4633–4].
56. Stricker RB, Johnson L. Lyme wars: let's tackle the testing. BMJ 2007;335(7628): 1008.
57. Fallon BA, Keilp JG, Corbera KM, et al. A randomized, placebo-controlled trial of repeated IV antibiotic therapy for Lyme encephalopathy. Neurology 2008; 70(13):992–1003.
58. Klempner MS, Hu LT, Evans J, et al. Two controlled trials of antibiotic treatment in patients with persistent symptoms and a history of Lyme disease. N Engl J Med 2001;345(2):85–92.

59. Krupp LB, Hyman LG, Grimson R, et al. Study and Treatment Of Post Lyme Disease (STOP-LD): a randomized double masked clinical trial. Neurology 2003;60(12):1923–30.

60. Marques A, Telford SR 3rd, Turk SP, et al. Xenodiagnosis to detect Borrelia burgdorferi infection: a first-in-human study. Clin Infect Dis 2014;58(7):937–45.

61. Stricker RB, Burrascano J, Winger E. Longterm decrease in the CD57 lymphocyte subset in a patient with chronic Lyme disease. Ann Agric Environ Med 2002;9(1):111–3.

62. Stricker RB, Winger EE. Decreased CD57 lymphocyte subset in patients with chronic Lyme disease. Immunol Lett 2001;76(1):43–8.

63. Phillips SE, Mattman LH, Hulinska D, et al. A proposal for the reliable culture of Borrelia burgdorferi from patients with chronic Lyme disease, even from those previously aggressively treated. Infection 1998;26(6):364–7.

64. Bayer ME, Zhang L, Bayer MH. Borrelia burgdorferi DNA in the urine of treated patients with chronic Lyme disease symptoms. A PCR study of 97 cases. Infection 1996;24(5):347–53.

65. Sapi E, Pabbati N, Datar A, et al. Improved culture conditions for the growth and detection of Borrelia from human serum. Int J Med Sci 2013;10(4):362–76.

66. Marques A, Brown MR, Fleisher TA. Natural killer cell counts are not different between patients with post-Lyme disease syndrome and controls. Clin Vaccine Immunol 2009;16(8):1249–50.

67. Rauter C, Mueller M, Diterich I, et al. Critical evaluation of urine-based PCR assay for diagnosis of Lyme borreliosis. Clin Diagn Lab Immunol 2005;12(8):910–7.

68. Marques AR, Stock F, Gill V. Evaluation of a new culture medium for Borrelia burgdorferi. J Clin Microbiol 2000;38(11):4239–41.

69. Tilton RC, Barden D, Sand M. Culture Borrelia burgdorferi. J Clin Microbiol 2001;39(7):2747.

70. Johnson BJ, Pilgard MA, Russell TM. Assessment of new culture method for detection of Borrelia species from serum of Lyme disease patients. J Clin Microbiol 2014;52(3):721–4.

71. Owen DC. Is Lyme disease always poly microbial?–The jigsaw hypothesis. Med Hypotheses 2006;67(4):860–4.

72. Stricker RB, Gaito A, Harris NS, et al. Coinfection in patients with Lyme disease: how big a risk? Clin Infect Dis 2003;37(9):1277–8 [author reply: 1278–9].

73. Lantos PM, Wormser GP. Chronic coinfections in patients diagnosed with chronic Lyme disease: a systematic literature review. Am J Med 2014;127(11):1105–10.

74. Logigian EL, Kaplan RF, Steere AC. Chronic neurologic manifestations of Lyme disease. N Engl J Med 1990;323(21):1438–44.

75. Kaplan RF, Trevino RP, Johnson GM, et al. Cognitive function in post-treatment Lyme disease: do additional antibiotics help? Neurology 2003;60(12):1916–22.

76. Steere AC, Levin RE, Molloy PJ, et al. Treatment of Lyme arthritis. Arthritis Rheum 1994;37(6):878–88.

77. Shadick NA, Phillips CB, Logigian EL, et al. The long-term clinical outcomes of Lyme disease. A population-based retrospective cohort study. Ann Intern Med 1994;121(8):560–7.

78. Sigal LH. Persisting complaints attributed to chronic Lyme disease: possible mechanisms and implications for management. Am J Med 1994;96(4):365–74.

79. Seltzer EG, Gerber MA, Cartter ML, et al. Long-term outcomes of persons with Lyme disease. JAMA 2000;283(5):609–16.

80. Cerar D, Cerar T, Ruzic-Sabljic E, et al. Subjective symptoms after treatment of early Lyme disease. Am J Med 2010;123(1):79–86.
81. Barsic B, Maretic T, Majerus L, et al. Comparison of azithromycin and doxycycline in the treatment of erythema migrans. Infection 2000;28(3): 153–6.
82. Dattwyler RJ, Luft BJ, Kunkel MJ, et al. Ceftriaxone compared with doxycycline for the treatment of acute disseminated Lyme disease. N Engl J Med 1997; 337(5):289–94.
83. Gerber MA, Shapiro ED, Burke GS, et al. Lyme disease in children in southeastern Connecticut. Pediatric Lyme Disease Study Group. N Engl J Med 1996;335(17):1270–4.
84. Nadelman RB, Luger SW, Frank E, et al. Comparison of cefuroxime axetil and doxycycline in the treatment of early Lyme disease. Ann Intern Med 1992; 117(4):273–80.
85. Nowakowski J, Nadelman RB, Sell R, et al. Long-term follow-up of patients with culture-confirmed Lyme disease. Am J Med 2003;115(2):91–6.
86. Smith RP, Schoen RT, Rahn DW, et al. Clinical characteristics and treatment outcome of early Lyme disease in patients with microbiologically confirmed erythema migrans. Ann Intern Med 2002;136(6):421–8.
87. Wormser GP, Ramanathan R, Nowakowski J, et al. Duration of antibiotic therapy for early Lyme disease. A randomized, double-blind, placebo-controlled trial. Ann Intern Med 2003;138(9):697–704.
88. Kowalski TJ, Tata S, Berth W, et al. Antibiotic treatment duration and long-term outcomes of patients with early Lyme disease from a Lyme disease-hyperendemic area. Clin Infect Dis 2010;50(4):512–20.
89. Buchwald D, Umali P, Umali J, et al. Chronic fatigue and the chronic fatigue syndrome: prevalence in a Pacific Northwest health care system. Ann Intern Med 1995;123(2):81–8.
90. Chen MK. The epidemiology of self-perceived fatigue among adults. Prev Med 1986;15(1):74–81.
91. Luo N, Johnson JA, Shaw JW, et al. Self-reported health status of the general adult U.S. population as assessed by the EQ-5D and Health Utilities Index. Med Care 2005;43(11):1078–86.
92. Croft P, Rigby AS, Boswell R, et al. The prevalence of chronic widespread pain in the general population. J Rheumatol 1993;20(4):710–3.
93. Kalish RA, Kaplan RF, Taylor E, et al. Evaluation of study patients with Lyme disease, 10-20-year follow-up. J Infect Dis 2001;183(3):453–60.
94. Shadick NA, Phillips CB, Sangha O, et al. Musculoskeletal and neurologic outcomes in patients with previously treated Lyme disease. Ann Intern Med 1999; 131(12):919–26.
95. Ravdin LD, Hilton E, Primeau M, et al. Memory functioning in Lyme borreliosis. J Clin Psychiatry 1996;57(7):282–6.
96. Kaplan RF, Jones-Woodward L. Lyme encephalopathy: a neuropsychological perspective. Semin Neurol 1997;17(1):31–7.
97. El Moussaoui R, Opmeer BC, de Borgie CA, et al. Long-term symptom recovery and health-related quality of life in patients with mild-to-moderate-severe community-acquired pneumonia. Chest 2006;130(4):1165–72.
98. Steere AC, Hutchinson GJ, Rahn DW, et al. Treatment of the early manifestations of Lyme disease. Ann Intern Med 1983;99(1):22–6.
99. Steere AC, Malawista SE, Newman JH, et al. Antibiotic therapy in Lyme disease. Ann Intern Med 1980;93(1):1–8.

100. Weber K, Preac-Mursic V, Wilske B, et al. A randomized trial of ceftriaxone versus oral penicillin for the treatment of early European Lyme borreliosis. Infection 1990;18(2):91–6.
101. Asch ES, Bujak DI, Weiss M, et al. Lyme disease: an infectious and postinfectious syndrome. J Rheumatol 1994;21(3):454–61.
102. Dattwyler RJ, Wormser GP, Rush TJ, et al. A comparison of two treatment regimens of ceftriaxone in late Lyme disease. Wien Klin Wochenschr 2005; 117(11–12):393–7.
103. Oksi J, Nikoskelainen J, Hiekkanen H, et al. Duration of antibiotic treatment in disseminated Lyme borreliosis: a double-blind, randomized, placebo-controlled, multicenter clinical study. Eur J Clin Microbiol Infect Dis 2007; 26(8):571–81.
104. Chandra A, Wormser GP, Marques AR, et al. Anti-Borrelia burgdorferi antibody profile in post-Lyme disease syndrome. Clin Vaccine Immunol 2011;18(5): 767–71.
105. Hytonen J, Kortela E, Waris M, et al. CXCL13 and neopterin concentrations in cerebrospinal fluid of patients with Lyme neuroborreliosis and other diseases that cause neuroinflammation. J Neuroinflammation 2014;11:103.
106. Arashima Y, Kato K, Komiya T, et al. Improvement of chronic nonspecific symptoms by long-term minocycline treatment in Japanese patients with Coxiella burnetii infection considered to have post-Q fever fatigue syndrome. Intern Med 2004;43(1):49–54.
107. Caperton EM, Heim-Duthoy KL, Matzke GR, et al. Ceftriaxone therapy of chronic inflammatory arthritis. A double-blind placebo controlled trial. Arch Intern Med 1990;150(8):1677–82.
108. Vermeulen RC, Scholte HR. Azithromycin in chronic fatigue syndrome (CFS), an analysis of clinical data. J Transl Med 2006;4:34.
109. Stricker RB, Green CL, Savely VR, et al. Safety of intravenous antibiotic therapy in patients referred for treatment of neurologic Lyme disease. Minerva Med 2010;101(1):1–7.
110. Nadelman RB, Arlin Z, Wormser GP. Life-threatening complications of empiric ceftriaxone therapy for 'seronegative Lyme disease'. South Med J 1991; 84(10):1263–5.
111. Holzbauer SM, Kemperman MM, Lynfield R. Death due to community-associated Clostridium difficile in a woman receiving prolonged antibiotic therapy for suspected Lyme disease. Clin Infect Dis 2010;51(3):369–70.
112. Patel R, Grogg KL, Edwards WD, et al. Death from inappropriate therapy for Lyme disease. Clin Infect Dis 2000;31(4):1107–9.

Human Granulocytic Anaplasmosis

Johan S. Bakken, MD, PhD[a,b], J. Stephen Dumler, MD[c,d],*

KEYWORDS

- Anaplasmosis • Human • Granulocytic • Diagnosis • Management

KEY POINTS

- The clinical presentation of human granulocytic anaplasmosis is an acute, febrile, nonspecific, viral-like illness. Leukopenia, thrombocytopenia, and increased hepatic transaminase levels are commonly seen early in the disease.
- A history of a tick bite or exposure is important, but its absence and lack of a diagnostic test result should not mitigate clinical consideration.
- Early treatment with doxycycline for adults and children (including those younger than 8 years of age) should be instituted on clinical suspicion alone.
- Although hospitalization occurs in 36% of cases, and life-threatening disease occurs in 3%, the case fatality rate is low (0.6%) and most patients resolve infections without complications.
- Persistent infection has not been shown, and evidence to support a role in chronic illness is lacking. Acute coinfections with other tick-transmitted pathogens can occur.

INTRODUCTION

Tick-borne infections in humans have been recognized in the United States for more than a century. Following the description of the agent of Rocky Mountain spotted fever in 1906,[1] several clinically important tick-associated human infectious syndromes have been characterized.[2–10] One tick-borne infection, human granulocytic anaplasmosis (HGA) caused by the rickettsial bacterium *Anaplasma phagocytophilum*, is transmitted by *Ixodes scapularis* ticks in the United States and can be sometimes

This work was supported by NIH R01AI44102.
[a] Department of Family Medicine, University of Minnesota School of Medicine, Duluth, MN, USA; [b] St. Luke's Infectious Disease Associates, 1001 East Superior Street, Suite L201, Duluth, MN 55802, USA; [c] Department of Pathology, University of Maryland School of Medicine, 685 West Baltimore Street, HSF1 322D, Baltimore, MD 21201, USA; [d] Department of Microbiology & Immunology, University of Maryland School of Medicine, Baltimore, MD 21201, USA
* Corresponding author. Department of Pathology, University of Maryland School of Medicine, 685 West Baltimore Street, HSF1 322D, Baltimore, MD 21201.
E-mail address: sdumler@som.umaryland.edu

Infect Dis Clin N Am 29 (2015) 341–355
http://dx.doi.org/10.1016/j.idc.2015.02.007
0891-5520/15/$ – see front matter © 2015 Elsevier Inc. All rights reserved.

id.theclinics.com

confused with or complicate Lyme disease. A compilation of data published by the US Centers for Disease Control and Prevention (CDC) and in *Morbidity and Mortality Weekly Reports* since HGA became reportable includes at least 15,952 cases since 1995 (**Fig. 1**). The incidence of HGA increased 12-fold between 2001 and 2011, and the disease can cause severe illness and occasionally death in otherwise healthy individuals. Although many patients with competent immune systems resolve their illnesses spontaneously even without antibiotic treatment, most symptomatic patients benefit from specific antibiotic therapy. As with most rickettsial infections, poor outcomes can occur without early identification and specific treatment, usually with doxycycline. The major difficulty with HGA is that the early symptoms and signs are nonspecific, often mimicking a viral illness, and rapid sensitive tests for diagnosis early in infection are not widely available. Thus, it is difficult to arrive at a specific diagnosis early in the course of the illness when antibiotic therapy is most likely to be successful. This article focuses on current practice for the diagnosis and management of HGA.[11,12]

PATIENT HISTORY

Most cases of HGA develop in individuals exposed to or bitten by *Ixodes* ticks.[13–16] Thus, a history of a tick bite or well-established exposure to ticks is an important clue. Ticks in the *Ixodes persulcatus* complex serve as competent vectors for multiple pathogens that can infect humans, including *A phagocytophilum*,[11] *Borrelia burgdorferi* (the agent of Lyme borreliosis),[17] *Babesia microti* (the agent of babesiosis),[18]

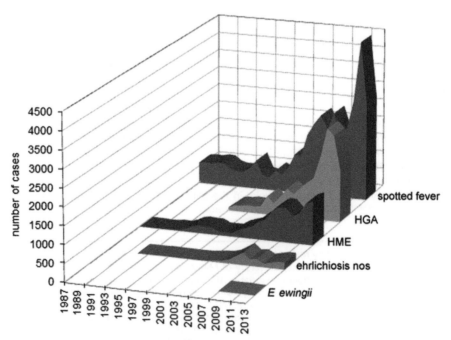

Fig. 1. Reported cases of tick-borne rickettsial infections in the United States, 1987 to 2013. The cumulative area plots show the overall burden of infection during this time interval. *E ewingii*, *Ehrlichia ewingii*; HME, human monocytic ehrlichiosis; nos, not otherwise specified; spotted fever, spotted fever group rickettsioses (including Rocky Mountain spotted fever). (*Data from* Morbidity and Mortality Weekly Reports, 1987–2014.)

Ehrlichia muris–like agent,[19] *Borrelia miyamotoi*,[3] and Powassan virus.[20] Vector ticks in North American endemic habitats include *I scapularis* in the northeastern and upper Midwest regions of the United States, and *Ixodes pacificus* along the northern Pacific coast. Despite its wide distribution, most HGA cases are reported from the upper Midwest and northeastern United States, overlapping the endemic regions for *I scapularis* (the black-legged deer tick).[21] Recent epidemiologic studies of tick habitats show that the endemic areas have expanded, and as such it is anticipated that so will the range where HGA will be found in humans.[22–24] However, at least 25% of patients with proven HGA do not report exposure to ticks and thus it should not be used as an absolute criterion for diagnosis or clinical suspicion.

Seroprevalence and incidence vary directly with age, suggesting that the principal risk factor for contracting HGA is duration of residence in endemic areas.[25,26] *I scapularis* ticks, although widespread, transmit infections to human in a limited geographic range. Therefore, understanding the ranges of endemic risk is also a critical component for patient evaluation. Serosurveys among individuals bitten by ticks in the United States show *A phagocytophilum* seroprevalence rates ranging between 8.9% and 36%.[25] Bakken and colleagues[26] reported a seroprevalence of 14.9% among healthy residents from northwestern Wisconsin who had no history of a recent tick bite. The highest annual US average HGA incidence rates between 2000 and 2007 were reported in Rhode Island (32.1 per million), Minnesota (30.2 per million), Connecticut (13.1 per million), Wisconsin (8.2 per million), New York State (7.7 per million), and Massachusetts (6.5 per million).[21] However, HGA incidence rates exceeding 650 cases per million are also reported in some northwestern Wisconsin counties.[14,21,27] HGA also occurs at a much lower incidence in Europe and Scandinavia and it is increasingly described in eastern parts of Asia, especially China, South Korea, and Japan.

Despite the strong association with tick bite, HGA can be acquired through alternate exposures to *A phagocytophilum*. Horowitz and colleagues[28] described HGA in a woman during pregnancy. The infant developed HGA 8 days after being born, and the investigators argued that transplacental transmission of *A phagocytophilum* occurred. Several butchers from northwestern Wisconsin acquired HGA after butchering large quantities of white-tailed deer carcasses during the hunting season.[29] None of the butchers had noted a preceding tick bite, raising the query as to whether they acquired HGA by direct exposure to infected deer blood through skin cuts, through inhalation of aerosolized blood, or through infected blood splashed directly on mucous membranes. A cluster of HGA cases associated with a severely hemorrhagic febrile illness occurred after nosocomial exposure in a Chinese hospital, ostensibly associated with exposure to the index patient's blood or respiratory secretions.[30] *A phagocytophilum* remains viable and infectious in refrigerated, stored blood for as long as 18 days.[31] A seroprevalence study of 992 blood donors from Connecticut and Wisconsin showed that 0.4% to 0.9% of the blood donors had *A phagocytophilum* antibodies.[32] There is no US mandate to screen blood products for *A phagocytophilum* infection, and at least 8 cases of HGA acquired via transfusions of infected leukoreduced blood products have been reported since 2007.[33]

Beyond *A phagocytophilum*, *Ixodes* ticks are often coinfected with other human pathogens.[34,35] Coinfections also occur frequently in the white-footed mouse (*Peromyscus leucopus*),[36,37] and serologic investigations and prospective studies of humans who had Lyme borreliosis show that between 1% and 9% of individuals living in Wisconsin[38] or western Sweden[39] have serologic evidence of prior *A phagocytophilum* infection. In a subsequent surveillance study of HGA in Wisconsin, 7 of 142 patients (5%) had erythema migrans and serologic evidence of recent *B burgdorferi* infection,[27] and both pathogens have been recovered in culture from coinfected individuals on several occasions.[40] Thus, sequential or simultaneous infections caused by multiple human pathogens could occur after 1 or multiple tick bites, and physicians who diagnose and treat patients with HGA must always consider the possibility of coinfection with other tick-borne agents.

Presentations and Complications

Patients with HGA frequently present with a nonspecific febrile illness. The clinical range of HGA spans from asymptomatic infection to fatal disease and there is a direct correlation between patient age and/or comorbid illnesses and the severity.[41] Most symptomatic patients report exposure to ticks 1 to 2 weeks before the onset of illness and often complain of fever/sweating/rigors, headache, myalgia, and arthralgia (**Table 1**), although the physical examination is often otherwise unrevealing. HGA can be severe, with 36% of patients requiring hospitalization and 3% with life-threatening complications[21]; in one report, up to 17% of hospitalized patients required admission to an intensive care unit.[14] Even though many patients present with severe headache or stiff neck prompting lumbar puncture, spinal fluid analysis is usually unremarkable.[42] Only a single patient with defined meningitis had *A phagocytophilum* documented in the CSF.[43] Among 2040 cases reported to the CDC between 2000 and 2007, 5 (0.2%) had reports of meningitis or encephalitis.[21]

Serious opportunistic infections can occur in immunocompromised patients during the course of HGA, and fatal cases of herpes simplex esophagitis, *Candida albicans* pneumonitis/esophagitis, and invasive pulmonary aspergillosis are described.[14,44,45] Even though the case fatality rate is less than or equal to 1%, significant complications can occur, including septic or toxic shock–like syndrome; acute respiratory distress

Table 1		
Published signs, symptoms, and key laboratory abnormalities (%) reported among laboratory-confirmed HGA in the USA, Europe, and in Asia (N = 68 to 794 across features)		
Frequency of Complaint	**Symptom, Sign, or Laboratory Abnormality (Number of Patients Evaluated)**	**Median % (IQR)**
Common	Fever (794)	100 (90–100)
	Malaise (391)	97 (90–98)
	Headache (648)	82 (64–93)
	Myalgia (789)	76 (67–87)
	Arthralgia (661)	56 (27–69)
	Increased serum ALT or AST level (397)	83 (63–98)
	Thrombocytopenia (566)	75 (61–91)
	Leukopenia (566)	55 (47–71)
Less common	Stiff neck (64)	45 (34–48)
	Nausea (521)	39 (35–49)
	Cough (523)	29 (20–30)
	Increased serum creatinine level (199)	49 (25–71)
	Anemia (198)	28 (6–44)
Uncommon	Diarrhea (317)	21 (13–28)
	Vomiting (312)	20 (19–29)
	Confusion (470)	17 (17–18)
	Rash[a] (489)	6 (3–10)

Abbreviations: ALT, alanine aminotransferase; AST, aspartate aminotransferase; IQR, interquartile range.
[a] Erythema migrans where described.

syndrome; invasive opportunistic infections with both viral and fungal agents; rhabdo-myolysis; pancarditis; acute renal failure; hemorrhage; and neurologic diseases such as brachial plexopathy, demyelinating polyneuropathy, and acute transient sensori-neural hearing loss.[21,45–48]

Most patients present with nonspecific changes in routine hematologic and chem-istry blood tests. Permutations of leukopenia, a left shift (sometimes reaching 50% or even higher), thrombocytopenia, and mild to moderate increase of hepatic transami-nase activities are present in most patients and provide suggestive clues to the diag-nosis.[41,49] Although both leukopenia and thrombocytopenia are present in many patients at the initial presentation, these abnormalities usually normalize by the end of the second week. Thus, normal white blood cell and platelet concentrations should not dissuade medical providers from including HGA in the differential diagnosis if the patient reports illness for more than 1 week. In contrast, patients who present with nonspecific fever of less than 7 days' duration and either leukocytosis or thrombocy-tosis have a low probability of having HGA.[49]

Diagnostic Testing and Imaging

HGA can be laboratory confirmed at the point of care by examination of a Wright-stained or Giemsa-stained peripheral blood smear during the early stage of infection (**Fig. 2**).[41,49,50] At least 20%, and in some studies up to 100%, of patients present with morulae in the cytoplasm of peripheral blood neutrophils in the first week of illness.[15,50,51] Polymerase chain reaction (PCR) amplification of A phagocytophi-lum–specific DNA from acute phase blood[14,15,52] or isolation of A phagocytophilum in HL-60 promyelocytic leukemia cell cultures inoculated with acute phase blood[13,41,53] can also confirm the diagnosis during the early stage of infection, but these test modalities are available in only a limited number of public health and com-mercial reference laboratories. Acute and convalescent serologic testing using an in-direct fluorescent antibody method for A phagocytophilum immunoglobulin (Ig) G with demonstration of 4-fold change or seroconversion is the most sensitive confir-matory laboratory test, and has been used most commonly to confirm HGA.[25,38,54–56]

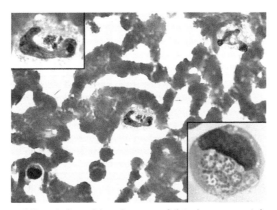

Fig. 2. A phagocytophilum–infected band neutrophil in human peripheral blood (Wright stain; original magnification, ×260). The top left inset shows the same band neutrophil and shows several morulae with a stippled basophilic appearance corresponding with individual bacteria (magnification, ×520). The bottom right insert shows A phagocytophilum cultivated in vitro in the human promyelocytic leukemia cell line HL-60. The individual basophilic bacteria are easily visualized within vacuoles of the infected cell (LeukoStat stain; magnification, ×520).

Specific IgM tests are only reactive during the first 40 days after infection, and are less sensitive than those that detect IgG antibodies, even during this early interval.[57] Once a patient becomes seroreactive, antibodies can persist for months or years in the absence of any clinical or laboratory-based evidence for ongoing infection; thus, reductions in antibody titers cannot be used as monitors of effective treatment.[25,55] Patients infected by A phagocytophilum often develop antibodies that concurrently react with Ehrlichia chaffeensis, the causative agent of human monocytic ehrlichiosis. In some regions, the distinct ticks that transmit these bacteria are both abundant. Thus, the definitive diagnosis must include antibody titers for both pathogens.

The minimal presumptive diagnostic criteria for HGA are unexplained fever and nonspecific symptoms such as headache, generalized myalgias, and rigors accompanied by suggestive changes in routine laboratory tests.[11,12,14,41,56] Probable and laboratory-confirmed HGA require a nonspecific febrile illness and laboratory confirmation by PCR, culture of blood, and/or detection of specific A phagocytophilum antibodies in serum (Table 2). Patients who present with an acute clinical illness compatible with HGA should always be considered for specific antibiotic treatment.[12,14,41,56] HGA is a reportable illness and all confirmed cases must be reported to the CDC or to the local state health department in the state where the diagnosis was made. The tabular list of the International Classification of Diseases, Ninth Revision (ICD-9), has categorized HGA under the subheading tick-borne rickettsioses/other ehrlichiosis with the numerical code 082.49 (ICD-10 code A77.49).[58]

It is important to remember that bites by infected Ixodes ticks may lead to simultaneous infections caused by multiple pathogens. The reported frequency of Lyme disease and HGA coinfection varies between 2% and 11.7%,[59] and patients who have a positive blood culture for A phagocytophilum and/or a 4-fold increase in antibody titer to at least 640 have significantly more symptoms in total than patients with early Lyme disease defined by the presence of erythema migrans only.[60]

Imaging studies play little additional role in the specific diagnosis of HGA but can be useful for evaluation of the extent of disease and specific organ/tissue involvement.

Table 2 Modified case definitions for HGA	
Case Definition	Laboratory Test Result
Supportive HGA	Morulae present in peripheral blood-smear neutrophils,[a] or Single serum A phagocytophilum IgG titer by IFA[b] ≥640
Confirmed HGA	A phagocytophilum IFA IgG seroconversion,[c] or Positive A phagocytophilum PCR[d] of blood, or Isolation of A phagocytophilum from blood,[e] or A phagocytophilum antigen present in tissue sample by immunohistochemistry

Definitions depend on a presentation with manifestations clinically consistent with HGA.
Abbreviation: IFA, immunofluorescent antibody test.
[a] Light microscopy of Wright-stained peripheral acute phase blood.
[b] Indirect immunofluorescent antibody test with A phagocytophilum antigen.
[c] At least 4-fold change in serum antibody titer.
[d] PCR with specific A phagocytophilum primers.
[e] Isolation of A phagocytophilum from blood incubated in HL-60 human promyelocytic cell line.
From Ehrlichiosis and anaplasmosis 2008 case definition. Centers for Disease Control and Prevention, 2008. 2014. Available at: http://wwwn.cdc.gov/nndss/script/casedef.aspx?CondYrID=667&DatePub=1/1/2008. Accessed September 19, 2014.

DIFFERENTIAL DIAGNOSIS

Owing to the undifferentiated presentation of HGA, the differential diagnosis can be vast. With the common manifestations of fever, headache, myalgia and malaise, viral syndromes such as enterovirus infection, Epstein-Barr virus infection, human herpes virus-6 infection, human parvovirus B19 infection, viral hepatitis, West Nile fever, and chikungunya fever should be included on the list of differential diagnoses. Other tick-borne infections must also be kept in mind, including Lyme disease, *B miyamotoi* infection, babesiosis, *E muris*–like agent infection, Powassan virus infection, and *Borrelia hermsii* relapsing fever. Acute bacterial infections to consider include disseminated gonococcal infection, endocarditis, meningococcemia, *Mycoplasma pneumoniae* infection, group A streptococcal postinfectious syndrome, secondary syphilis, septic shock syndromes, and typhoid fever (**Table 3**). Inflammatory illnesses of a possible infectious or noninfectious origin include allergic drug reactions,

Table 3
Differential diagnosis of HGA

Exposure Type	Viral Syndromes	Bacterial Agents/ Syndromes	Parasitic Agents/ Syndromes	Noninfectious Syndromes
History of vector exposure	Powassan virus disease/ tick-borne encephalitis	Lyme disease	Babesiosis	
	West Nile virus disease	*B miyamotoi* infection	Malaria	
	Dengue virus fever	*B hermsii* infection		
	Colorado tick fever	*E chaffeensis* infection		
	Heartland virus fever	*E ewingii* infection		
	Severe fever with thrombocytopenia virus infection	*E muris*–like agent infection		
	Chikungunya virus disease	Rocky Mountain spotted fever		
		Murine typhus		
		African tick-bite fever		
		Scrub typhus		
		Bartonellosis		
		Tularemia		
		Leptospirosis		
No vector exposure	EBV infection	Acute bacterial endocarditis		Kawasaki syndrome
	Human herpes virus-6 infection	Secondary syphilis		ITP
	Parvovirus B19 infection	*Neisseria gonorrhea* sepsis		TTP
	Viral hepatitis A, B, C	*Neisseria meningitidis* sepsis		Hemophagocytic syndrome
	Enterovirus infection	Group A *Streptococcal* infection		Immune-complex illness
	Hantaan virus infection	Leptospirosis		Allergic drug reaction
		Typhoid fever		Acute leukemia Lymphoma

Abbreviations: EBV, Epstein-Barr virus; ITP, idiopathic thrombocytopenic purpura; TTP, thrombotic thrombocytopenic purpura.

idiopathic thrombocytopenic purpura, immune complex–mediated illnesses, Kawasaki disease, thrombotic thrombocytopenic purpura, and hemophagocytic and macrophage activation syndromes.

Patients with HGA typically present during the warm seasons when ticks are known to be active, and up to 75% report tick bite or exposure to ticks in known tick-infested regions. Other vector-borne infections and zoonoses should be considered for patients who have had recent documented insect or arthropod bites, including babesiosis, Colorado tick fever, human monocytic ehrlichiosis, leptospirosis, Lyme disease, murine typhus, Q fever, rat-bite fever, Rocky Mountain spotted fever, and tularemia. In travelers, the list could be expanded to include dengue fever, malaria, and tick-borne encephalitis. Occasionally the major manifestation is reflected in hematologic laboratory abnormalities when the differential diagnosis should also include malignancies such as leukemia and lymphoma, especially when intracytoplasmic structures such as Auer rods may be identified and confused with morulae.

TREATMENT

In vitro investigations indicate that *A phagocytophilum* is uniformly susceptible to the tetracycline antibiotics.[61–64] Doxycycline hyclate has traditionally been the agent of choice because of its good patient tolerance and favorable pharmacokinetic properties compared with other tetracycline derivatives. For the most part, HGA is a mild illness, but there is a known direct relationship between serious infection, including cases with a fatal outcome, and patient variables such as advanced age, ongoing immunosuppressive therapy, predisposing chronic inflammatory illnesses, or underlying malignant diseases.[42,51] Because of the potential for serious or even fatal infection it is therefore recommended that all patients with suspected or documented HGA should undergo treatment with oral or intravenous doxycycline hyclate in the absence of specific contraindications to tetracycline drugs (**Table 4**).

The recommended therapy for adults is doxycycline 100 mg given orally at 12-hour intervals.[42,65] Children older than 8 years should also be treated with doxycycline given in divided doses with dosage adjusted to the patient's weight (4.4 mg/kg/24 hours, maximum dose 100 mg).[65,66] Doxycycline is also the drug of choice for children who are seriously ill regardless of age.[66] Doxycycline therapy typically leads to

Table 4
Recommended antibiotic treatment of HGA

Antibiotic Drug	Patient Age (y)	Antibiotic Dose	Duration (d)
Doxycycline hyclate	≤8	2.2 mg/kg 2 times daily IV or PO	4–5[a]
	>8	100 mg 2 times daily IV or PO	10–14[b]
Tetracycline HCl	>8	500 mg 4 times daily PO	10–14
Rifampin	Pediatric[c]	20 mg/kg/d (maximum 600 mg) in 2 divided doses PO	5–7[d]
	Adult[e]	300 mg 2 times daily PO	5–7

Abbreviations: IV, intravenous; PO, orally.
[a] Until fever has resolved and 3 additional days.
[b] If coincubating *B burgdorferi* infection is suspected, 14 days are recommended.
[c] Individuals aged 16 years or less.
[d] Short duration because therapy not directed toward coincubating *B burgdorferi* infection.
[e] Individuals aged 18 years or older.
Data from Refs.[11,12,65,66]

clinical improvement in 24 to 48 hours.[14,41,65,66] Thus, patients who fail to respond to treatment within this time frame should be reevaluated for alternative diagnoses and treatment.

The optimal duration of doxycycline therapy has not been established. Patients who have been treated for 7 to 10 days resolve their infections completely, and relapse or chronic infection has never been reported, even for those patients who were never treated with an active antibiotic. However, adult patients who are considered at risk for coinfection with *B burgdorferi* should continue doxycycline therapy for a full 14 days. A shorter course of doxycycline (5–7 days) has been advocated for pediatric patients because of the potential risk for adverse effects (dental staining) seen occasionally in young children.[65–67]

Rifamycins also have excellent in vitro activity against *A phagocytophilum*.[61–63] A few pregnant women and pediatric patients have been treated successfully with rifampin.[68–70] Thus, patients who have HGA and who are unsuited for tetracycline treatment because of a history of drug allergy or pregnancy, and children younger than 8 years of age who are not seriously ill, should be considered for rifampin therapy. Studies with levofloxacin show some activity in vitro.[61–63] However, at least 1 patient with HGA who received a 13-day course of levofloxacin initially had a clinical response only to relapse when the regimen was discontinued, suggesting that fluoroquinolones should not be used.[71]

PROGNOSIS AND LONG-TERM OUTCOME

More than 15,952 patients have been diagnosed with HGA and reported to state and federal health agencies since 1994. Only 8 patients are known from published literature to have died during the active phase of HGA, although a CDC review of national surveillance systems between 2000 and 2007 identified 11 fatalities.[14,21,44,45] Although the case fatality rate for HGA has been estimated at 1.2% among individuals 20 to 39 years of age, the overall case fatality rate is likely between 0.2% and 1.2%.[21] Published case-report series indicate that HGA most often is a mild, self-limited illness that resolves even without antibiotic treatment.[14,15,55,72–74]

Patients who are treated with doxycycline or rifampin typically resolve fever and most of their physical complaints within 24 to 48 hours. A small number of patients who are diagnosed with HGA do not receive any antibiotic therapy or they receive ineffective antibiotic therapy, but nearly all these patients make a complete recovery within 60 days.[14] PCR analysis of serial blood samples collected from untreated patients during convalescence indicates that bacteremia can persist for up to 30 days.[29,75–77] There are no published reports of patients with active clinical illness persisting beyond 2 months, although a single longitudinal study in Wisconsin reported significantly more recurrent or continuous fevers, chills, fatigue, and sweats within 1 year after infection.[73] Thus, the long-term prognosis seems to be favorable and patients are expected to make a complete recovery. There is currently no published clinical evidence to suggest that untreated HGA evolves into a chronic illness in humans, because persistently increased antibody titers should be interpreted as evidence of past infection rather than proof of an ongoing unresolved infectious process.

IMMUNITY AND REINFECTION

Most patients acquire HGA in the geographic region where they live, work, or recreate.[14–16,21,72,73] It is therefore reasonable to assume that those individuals remain at risk for future bites by infected *Ixodes* ticks and potential HGA reinfection. Nevertheless, conclusive evidence of *A phagocytophilum* infection occurring more than once is exceedingly rare.[78] Passive administration of A phagocytophilum antibodies partially protects laboratory animals in murine models of HGA against infection; thus, it is likely that patients who develop high antibody titers to A phagocytophilum are equally protected against reinfection after subsequent tick bites. Serum A phagocytophilum antibody titers remain increased for a median of 12 to 18 months after HGA has resolved.[38] However, some infected patients maintain increased A phagocytophilum antibody titers for as long as 3 years after infection.[16,25,55] Whether previous infection of humans leads to immunologic memory and a subsequent anamnestic protective immune response on rechallenge with A phagocytophilum is unknown.

Horses that are convalescent from A phagocytophilum infection develop immunity and resistance to experimental challenge 8 weeks after infection.[79] However, laboratory mice that were actively immunized with lysates of purified A phagocytophilum were only partially protected against challenges with A phagocytophilum.[80] The incomplete protection by both immunization with heat-inactivated bacteria and passive antibody administration suggests that protective immunity requires more than the presence of antibodies.

PREVENTION

Avoidance of tick bites and prompt removal of attached ticks remains the best disease prevention strategy. Individuals who are exposed in tick habitats should wear protective clothing, including long-sleeved shirts, long-legged pants, socks wrapped outside the pant legs, and closed-toed shoes to make it harder for ticks to reach bare skin and attach (bite). Light-colored pants could make it easier to see and remove crawling ticks. Tick repellents such as DEET (N,N-diethyl-m-toluamide) are available for application to exposed skin and clothing, and alternative repellents such as picaridin are becoming more readily available. These agents should be considered for use by individuals whose occupation or recreation exposes them to tick habitats where the risk of being bitten is high. Permethrin cannot be applied directly to skin, but can be applied to clothing before the clothing is worn and is considered an excellent choice for significant exposure risks. No vaccines that prevent HGA or veterinary granulocytic anaplasmosis are currently available.

Persons who spend time in tick-endemic areas should inspect themselves frequently for ticks. All attached ticks should be removed by gently grasping the tick with tweezers or forceps close to the skin and slowly pulling straight out with constant traction. Routine disinfection of the bite wound with isopropyl alcohol or tincture of iodine reduces the risk of contamination of the bite site with skin bacteria. Studies have shown that a period of 4 to 24 hours or more may be necessary before A phagocytophilum becomes biologically activated and successful transmission of infective organisms from the tick to the host takes place.[81] Thus, the longer an infected tick is permitted to feed, the more likely it is that the bite will result in infection. Therefore, prompt and complete removal of attached ticks is indicated to minimize the risk of infection.

The potential value of prophylactic doxycycline administration has never been tested in prospective, randomized trials.

SUMMARY

Patients who present with nonspecific fever after exposure to ticks should be evaluated by clinical examination and routine laboratory testing to determine whether the illness is potentially a tick-borne infection. Laboratory abnormalities such as leukopenia with relative granulocytosis and a left shift, thrombocytopenia, and mild increases in serum hepatic transaminase activities warrant consideration for treatment with doxycycline. These patients should also undergo specific laboratory testing to confirm the diagnosis of HGA.

Sensitive and specific laboratory tests that provide rapid diagnostic confirmation are generally not available in the acute care setting.[11,41] Thus, patients with suspected HGA should begin empiric antibiotic treatment as soon as blood samples have been collected for confirmatory laboratory testing. Acute phase serum samples should be paired with convalescent serum to detect seroconversion in those instances, especially when blood-smear microscopy, PCR, or cell culture testing are either unavailable or inconclusive.

REFERENCES

1. Ricketts HT. The study of "Rocky Mountain spotted fever" (tick fever) by means of animal inoculations. J Am Med Assoc 1906;47:1–10.
2. Pritt BS, McFadden JD, Stromdahl E, et al. Emergence of a novel *Ehrlichia* sp. agent pathogenic for humans in the Midwestern United States. 6th International Meeting on Rickettsiae and Rickettsial Diseases. Heraklion (Greece): Hellenic Society for Infectious Diseases; 2011. p. 67; Abstract no. P075.
3. Platonov AE, Karan LS, Kolyasnikova NM, et al. Humans infected with relapsing fever spirochete *Borrelia miyamotoi*, Russia. Emerg Infect Dis 2011;17:1816–23.
4. Steere AC, Malawista SE, Snydman DR, et al. Lyme arthritis: an epidemic of oligoarticular arthritis in children and adults in three Connecticut communities. Arthritis Rheum 1977;20:7–17.
5. Maeda K, Markowitz N, Hawley RC, et al. Human infection with *Ehrlichia canis*, a leukocytic rickettsia. N Engl J Med 1987;316:853–6.
6. Healy GR, Speilman A, Gleason N. Human babesiosis: reservoir in infection on Nantucket Island. Science 1976;192:479–80.
7. Buller RS, Arens M, Hmiel SP, et al. *Ehrlichia ewingii*, a newly recognized agent of human ehrlichiosis. N Engl J Med 1999;341:148–55.
8. Bakken JS, Dumler JS, Chen SM, et al. Human granulocytic ehrlichiosis in the upper Midwest United States. A new species emerging? JAMA 1994; 272:212–8.
9. Burgdorfer W. Arthropod-borne spirochetoses: a historical perspective. Eur J Clin Microbiol Infect Dis 2001;20:1–5.
10. McMullan LK, Folk SM, Kelly AJ, et al. A new phlebovirus associated with severe febrile illness in Missouri. N Engl J Med 2012;367:834–41.
11. Chapman AS, Bakken JS, Folk SM, et al. Diagnosis and management of tick-borne rickettsial diseases: Rocky Mountain spotted fever, ehrlichioses, and anaplasmosis–United States: a practical guide for physicians and other healthcare and public health professionals. MMWR Recomm Rep 2006;55:1–27.
12. Wormser GP, Dattwyler RJ, Shapiro ED, et al. The clinical assessment, treatment, and prevention of Lyme disease, human granulocytic anaplasmosis, and babesiosis: clinical practice guidelines by the Infectious Diseases Society of America. Clin Infect Dis 2006;43:1089–134.
13. Goodman JL, Nelson C, Vitale B, et al. Direct cultivation of the causative agent of human granulocytic ehrlichiosis. N Engl J Med 1996;334:209–15.
14. Bakken JS, Krueth J, Wilson-Nordskog C, et al. Clinical and laboratory characteristics of human granulocytic ehrlichiosis. JAMA 1996;275:199–205.
15. Aguero-Rosenfeld ME, Horowitz HW, Wormser GP, et al. Human granulocytic ehrlichiosis: a case series from a medical center in New York State. Ann Intern Med 1996;125:904–8.

16. Horowitz HW, Aguero-Rosenfeld ME, McKenna DF, et al. Clinical and laboratory spectrum of culture-proven human granulocytic ehrlichiosis: comparison with culture-negative cases. Clin Infect Dis 1998;27:1314–7.

17. Steere AC. Lyme disease. N Engl J Med 2001;345:115–25.

18. Krause PJ. Babesiosis. Med Clin North Am 2002;86:361–73.

19. Pritt BS, Sloan LM, Johnson DK, et al. Emergence of a new pathogenic *Ehrlichia* species, Wisconsin and Minnesota, 2009. N Engl J Med 2011;365:422–9.

20. McLean DM, Donohue WL. Powassan virus: isolation of virus from a fatal case of encephalitis. Can Med Assoc J 1959;80:708–11.

21. Dahlgren FS, Mandel EJ, Krebs JW, et al. Increasing incidence of *Ehrlichia chaffeensis* and *Anaplasma phagocytophilum* in the United States, 2000-2007. Am J Trop Med Hyg 2011;85:124–31.

22. Diuk-Wasser MA, Hoen AG, Cislo P, et al. Human risk of infection with *Borrelia burgdorferi*, the Lyme disease agent, in eastern United States. Am J Trop Med Hyg 2012;86:320–7.

23. Koffi JK, Leighton PA, Pelcat Y, et al. Passive surveillance for *I. scapularis* ticks: enhanced analysis for early detection of emerging Lyme disease risk. J Med Entomol 2012;49:400–9.

24. Hao Q, Geng Z, Hou XX, et al. Seroepidemiological investigation of Lyme disease and human granulocytic anaplasmosis among people living in forest areas of eight provinces in China. Biomed Environ Sci 2013;26:185–9.

25. Aguero-Rosenfeld ME, Donnarumma L, Zentmaier L, et al. Seroprevalence of antibodies that react with *Anaplasma phagocytophila*, the agent of human granulocytic ehrlichiosis, in different populations in Westchester County, New York. J Clin Microbiol 2002;40:2612–5.

26. Bakken JS, Goellner P, Van Etten M, et al. Seroprevalence of human granulocytic ehrlichiosis among permanent residents of northwestern Wisconsin. Clin Infect Dis 1998;27:1491–6.

27. Belongia EA, Gale CM, Reed KD, et al. Population-based incidence of human granulocytic ehrlichiosis in northwestern Wisconsin, 1997-1999. J Infect Dis 2001;184:1470–4.

28. Horowitz HW, Kilchevsky E, Haber S, et al. Perinatal transmission of the agent of human granulocytic ehrlichiosis. N Engl J Med 1998;339:375–8.

29. Bakken JS, Krueth JK, Lund T, et al. Exposure to deer blood may be a cause of human granulocytic ehrlichiosis. Clin Infect Dis 1996;23:198.

30. Zhang L, Liu Y, Ni D, et al. Nosocomial transmission of human granulocytic anaplasmosis in China. JAMA 2008;300:2263–70.

31. Kalantarpour F, Chowdhury I, Wormser GP, et al. Survival of the human granulocytic ehrlichiosis agent under refrigeration conditions. J Clin Microbiol 2000;38:2398–9.

32. Leiby DA, Chung AP, Cable RG, et al. Relationship between tick bites and the seroprevalence of *Babesia microti* and *Anaplasma phagocytophila* (previously *Ehrlichia* sp.) in blood donors. Transfusion 2002;42:1585–91.

33. Townsend RL, Moritz ED, Fialkow LB, et al. Probable transfusion-transmission of *Anaplasma phagocytophilum* by leukoreduced platelets. Transfusion 2014;54(11):2828–32.

34. Telford SR 3rd, Dawson JE, Katavolos P, et al. Perpetuation of the agent of human granulocytic ehrlichiosis in a deer tick-rodent cycle. Proc Natl Acad Sci U S A 1996;93:6209–14.

35. Varde S, Beckley J, Schwartz I. Prevalence of tick-borne pathogens in *Ixodes scapularis* in a rural New Jersey County. Emerg Infect Dis 1998;4:97–9.

36. Anderson JF. The natural history of ticks. Med Clin North Am 2002;86:205–18.
37. Stafford KC 3rd, Massung RF, Magnarelli LA, et al. Infection with agents of human granulocytic ehrlichiosis, Lyme disease, and babesiosis in wild white-footed mice (*Peromyscus leucopus*) in Connecticut. J Clin Microbiol 1999;37:2887–92.
38. Mitchell PD, Reed KD, Hofkes JM. Immunoserologic evidence of coinfection with *Borrelia burgdorferi*, *Babesia microti*, and human granulocytic *Ehrlichia* species in residents of Wisconsin and Minnesota. J Clin Microbiol 1996;34:724–7.
39. Dumler JS, Dotevall L, Gustafson R, et al. A population-based seroepidemiologic study of human granulocytic ehrlichiosis and Lyme borreliosis on the west coast of Sweden. J Infect Dis 1997;175:720–2.
40. De Martino SJ, Carlyon JA, Fikrig E. Coinfection with *Borrelia burgdorferi* and the agent of human granulocytic ehrlichiosis. N Engl J Med 2001;345:150–1.
41. Bakken JS, Dumler JS. Clinical diagnosis and treatment of human granulocytotropic anaplasmosis. Ann N Y Acad Sci 2006;1078:236–47.
42. Bakken JS, Dumler JS. Human granulocytic ehrlichiosis. Clin Infect Dis 2000;31:554–60.
43. Lee FS, Chu FK, Tackley M, et al. Human granulocytic ehrlichiosis presenting as facial diplegia in a 42-year-old woman. Clin Infect Dis 2000;31:1288–91.
44. Hardalo CJ, Quagliarello V, Dumler JS. Human granulocytic ehrlichiosis in Connecticut: report of a fatal case. Clin Infect Dis 1995;21:910–4.
45. Jahangir A, Kolbert C, Edwards W, et al. Fatal pancarditis associated with human granulocytic ehrlichiosis in a 44-year-old man. Clin Infect Dis 1998;27:1424–7.
46. Bakken JS, Erlemeyer SA, Kanoff RJ, et al. Demyelinating polyneuropathy associated with human granulocytic ehrlichiosis. Clin Infect Dis 1998;27:1323–4.
47. Horowitz HW, Marks SJ, Weintraub M, et al. Brachial plexopathy associated with human granulocytic ehrlichiosis. Neurology 1996;46:1026–9.
48. Lepidi H, Bunnell JE, Martin ME, et al. Comparative pathology, and immunohistology associated with clinical illness after *Ehrlichia phagocytophila*-group infections. Am J Trop Med Hyg 2000;62:29–37.
49. Bakken JS, Aguero-Rosenfeld ME, Tilden RL, et al. Serial measurements of hematologic counts during the active phase of human granulocytic ehrlichiosis. Clin Infect Dis 2001;32:862–70.
50. Rand JV, Tarasen AJ, Kumar J, et al. Intracytoplasmic granulocytic morulae counts on confirmed cases of ehrlichiosis/anaplasmosis in the Northeast. Am J Clin Pathol 2014;141:683–6.
51. Dumler JS, Madigan JE, Pusterla N, et al. Ehrlichioses in humans: epidemiology, clinical presentation, diagnosis, and treatment. Clin Infect Dis 2007;45(Suppl 1):S45–51.
52. Massung RF, Slater KG. Comparison of PCR assays for detection of the agent of human granulocytic ehrlichiosis, *Anaplasma phagocytophilum*. J Clin Microbiol 2003;41:717–22.
53. Dumler JS, Choi KS, Garcia-Garcia JC, et al. Human granulocytic anaplasmosis and *Anaplasma phagocytophilum*. Emerg Infect Dis 2005;11:1828–34.
54. Aguero-Rosenfeld ME. Diagnosis of human granulocytic ehrlichiosis: state of the art. Vector Borne Zoonotic Dis 2002;2:233–9.
55. Bakken JS, Haller I, Riddell D, et al. The serological response of patients infected with the agent of human granulocytic ehrlichiosis. Clin Infect Dis 2002;34:22–7.
56. Belongia EA, Reed KD, Mitchell PD, et al. Tickborne infections as a cause of nonspecific febrile illness in Wisconsin. Clin Infect Dis 2001;32:1434–9.
57. Walls JJ, Aguero-Rosenfeld M, Bakken JS, et al. Inter- and intralaboratory comparison of *Ehrlichia equi* and human granulocytic ehrlichiosis (HGE) agent strains

for serodiagnosis of HGE by the immunofluorescent-antibody test. J Clin Microbiol 1999;37:2968–73.

58. ICD10Data.com. 2014. Available at: http://www.icd10data.com/ICD10CM/Codes/A00-B99/A75-A79/A77-/A77.49.Accessed September 19, 2014.

59. Steere AC, McHugh G, Damle N, et al. Prospective study of serologic tests for Lyme disease. Clin Infect Dis 2008;47:188–95.

60. Wormser GP, Aguero-Rosenfeld ME, Cox ME, et al. Differences and similarities between culture-confirmed human granulocytic anaplasmosis and early Lyme disease. J Clin Microbiol 2013;51:954–8.

61. Horowitz HW, Hsieh TC, Aguero-Rosenfeld ME, et al. Antimicrobial susceptibility of *Ehrlichia phagocytophila*. Antimicrob Agents Chemother 2001;45:786–8.

62. Klein MB, Nelson CM, Goodman JL. Antibiotic susceptibility of the newly cultivated agent of human granulocytic ehrlichiosis: promising activity of quinolones and rifamycins. Antimicrob Agents Chemother 1997;41:76–9.

63. Maurin M, Bakken JS, Dumler JS. Antibiotic susceptibilities of *Anaplasma* (*Ehrlichia*) *phagocytophilum* strains from various geographic areas in the United States. Antimicrob Agents Chemother 2003;47:413–5.

64. Branger S, Rolain JM, Raoult D. Evaluation of antibiotic susceptibilities of *Ehrlichia canis*, *Ehrlichia chaffeensis*, and *Anaplasma phagocytophilum* by real-time PCR. Antimicrob Agents Chemother 2004;48:4822–8.

65. Bakken JS, Dumler JS. *Ehrlichia* and *Anaplasma* species. In: Yu V, Weber R, Raoult D, editors. Antimicrobial therapy and vaccine. 2nd edition. New York: Apple Trees Production; 2002. p. 875–82.

66. Committee on Infectious Diseases American Academy of Pediatrics. *Ehrlichia* and *Anaplasma* infections (human ehrlichiosis and anaplasmosis). In: Pickering LK, Baker CJ, Kimberlin DW, et al, editors. Red Book®: 2012 report of the Committee on Infectious Diseases. 29th edition. Elk Grove Village (IL): American Academy of Pediatrics; 2012. p. 312–5.

67. Volovitz B, Shkap R, Amir J, et al. Absence of tooth staining with doxycycline treatment in young children. Clin Pediatr (Phila) 2007;46:121–6.

68. Buitrago MI, Ijdo JW, Rinaudo P, et al. Human granulocytic ehrlichiosis during pregnancy treated successfully with rifampin. Clin Infect Dis 1998;27:213–5.

69. Elston DM. Perinatal transmission of human granulocytic ehrlichiosis. N Engl J Med 1998;339:1941–2.

70. Krause PJ, Corrow CL, Bakken JS. Successful treatment of human granulocytic ehrlichiosis in children using rifampin. Pediatrics 2003;112:e252–3.

71. Wormser GP, Filozov A, Telford SR 3rd, et al. Dissociation between inhibition and killing by levofloxacin in human granulocytic anaplasmosis. Vector Borne Zoonotic Dis 2006;6:388–94.

72. Belongia EA, Reed KD, Mitchell PD, et al. Clinical and epidemiological features of early Lyme disease and human granulocytic ehrlichiosis in Wisconsin. Clin Infect Dis 1999;29:1472–7.

73. Ramsey AH, Belongia EA, Gale CM, et al. Outcomes of treated human granulocytic ehrlichiosis cases. Emerg Infect Dis 2002;8:398–401.

74. Wallace BJ, Brady G, Ackman DM, et al. Human granulocytic ehrlichiosis in New York. Arch Intern Med 1998;158:769–73.

75. Bjoersdorff A, Berglund J, Kristiansen BE, et al. Varying clinical picture and course of human granulocytic ehrlichiosis. Twelve Scandinavian cases of the new tick-borne zoonosis are presented. Lakartidningen 1999;96:4200–4 [in Swedish].

76. Schotthoefer AM, Meece JK, Ivacic LC, et al. Comparison of a real-time PCR method with serology and blood smear analysis for diagnosis of human anaplasmosis: importance of infection time course for optimal test utilization. J Clin Microbiol 2013;51:2147–53.

77. Dumler JS, Bakken JS. Human granulocytic ehrlichiosis in Wisconsin and Minnesota: a frequent infection with the potential for persistence. J Infect Dis 1996;173: 1027–30.

78. Horowitz HW, Aguero-Rosenfeld M, Dumler JS, et al. Reinfection with the agent of human granulocytic ehrlichiosis. Ann Intern Med 1998;129:461–3.

79. Barlough JE, Madigan JE, DeRock E, et al. Protection against *Ehrlichia equi* is conferred by prior infection with the human granulocytotropic *Ehrlichia* (HGE agent). J Clin Microbiol 1995;33:3333–4.

80. Sun W, IJdo JW, Telford SR 3rd, et al. Immunization against the agent of human granulocytic ehrlichiosis in a murine model. J Clin Invest 1997;100:3014–8.

81. Katavolos P, Armstrong PM, Dawson JE, et al. Duration of tick attachment required for transmission of granulocytic ehrlichiosis. J Infect Dis 1998;177: 1422–5.

Babesiosis

Edouard G. Vannier, PhD[a], Maria A. Diuk-Wasser, PhD[b],
Choukri Ben Mamoun, PhD[c], Peter J. Krause, MD[d,e],*

KEYWORDS

- Babesiosis • *Babesia microti* • Protozoan • Apicomplexa • Erythrocyte • Tick
- Transfusion

KEY POINTS

- Human babesiosis is an emerging infectious disease caused by hemoprotozoan parasites that are transmitted by tick vectors and less frequently through blood transfusion or transplacentally.
- *Babesia microti*, the most frequent cause of human babesiosis, is endemic in the northeastern and upper midwestern United States and is sporadic throughout the rest of the world.
- The clinical presentation most commonly consists of a viral-like illness but ranges from asymptomatic infection to severe illness that may result in complications or death.
- Diagnosis is confirmed by identification of babesia organisms on blood smear, detection of babesia DNA by PCR, or a four-fold rise in babesia antibody titers in acute and convalescent sera.
- Treatment with atovaquone plus azithromycin is used for mild to moderate babesiosis, whereas clindamycin plus quinine is recommended for severe disease.

INTRODUCTION

Babesiosis is caused by intraerythrocytic protozoan parasites that are transmitted by ticks, or less commonly through blood transfusion or transplacentally. The microorganisms that are now recognized as babesia were first described by Victor Babes

The authors were supported by grants from the Gordon and Llura Gund Foundation (Drs. Krause and Vannier) and the National Institutes of Health (R01 AG019781 to Dr. Vannier, R01 GM105246 to Dr. Diuk-Wasser and R21 AI09486 to Drs. Ben Mamoun and Krause).
^a Division of Geographic Medicine and Infectious Diseases, Tufts Medical Center, Tufts University School of Medicine, 800 Washington Street Box #041, Boston, MA 02111, USA; ^b Department of Ecology, Evolution, and Environmental Biology, Columbia University, 1200 Amsterdam Avenue, New York, NY 10027, USA; ^c Department of Internal Medicine, Yale School of Medicine, 15 York Street, New Haven, CT 06520, USA; ^d Department of Epidemiology of Microbial Diseases, Yale School of Public Health, 60 College Street, New Haven, CT 06520, USA; ^e Departments of Internal Medicine and Pediatrics, Yale School of Medicine, 15 York Street, New Haven, CT 06520, USA
* Corresponding author. Department of Epidemiology of Microbial Diseases, Yale School of Public Health, 60 College Street, New Haven, CT 06520.
E-mail address: peter.krause@yale.edu

Infect Dis Clin N Am 29 (2015) 357–370
http://dx.doi.org/10.1016/j.idc.2015.02.008
0891-5520/15/$ – see front matter © 2015 Elsevier Inc. All rights reserved.

id.theclinics.com

in 1888 when he investigated the cause of hemoglobinuria in febrile cattle. Five years later, Smith and Kilbourne identified a tick as the vector for *Babesia bigemina* that caused Texas cattle fever, thereby establishing for the first time transmission of an infectious agent by an arthropod vector. Human babesiosis was first recognized in a splenectomized patient in Europe but most cases have been reported from the northeastern and upper midwestern United States in people with an intact spleen and no history of immune impairment.[1–3] Cases also are reported in Asia, Africa, Australia, Europe, and South America.[2] Babesiosis shares many clinical features with malaria and can be fatal, particularly in the elderly and the immunocompromised.

EPIDEMIOLOGY
The Pathogens

Babesia species belong to the phylum Apicomplexa, which is comprised of several important human pathogens, such as species of Plasmodium, Toxoplasma, and Cryptosporidium. Of the large number of babesia species that infect wild and domestic animals, only a few are known to cause disease in humans, including *Babesia microti* and *B microti*–like organisms, *Babesia duncani* and *B duncani*-type organisms, *Babesia divergens* and *B divergens*–like organisms, and *Babesia venatorum*.[2,4] The genome of *B microti* recently has been sequenced.[5,6] Phylogenetic analyses indicate that the *B microti* group is distant from all other species of Babesidae and Theileridae and should constitute a new genus in the Apicomplexa phylum.[5–9] *B microti* has the smallest genome among all Apicomplexan parasites sequenced to date with approximately 3500 genes. In addition to the four nuclear chromosomes, the parasite harbors two organellar genomes, one in the mitochrondria and one in the apicoplast. Sequencing of the *B microti* genome has helped gain further understanding about the biology and phylogenetics of the parasite and has identified several targets for the development of novel therapies for human babesiosis.

Transmission

Ixodes ticks are the primary mode of transmission of babesia species to vertebrates, including humans (**Fig. 1**). Babesia species are maintained in a wide range of vertebrate reservoirs; humans are incidental and terminal hosts. The primary reservoir for *B microti* in the northeastern and upper midwestern United States is the white-footed mouse (*Peromyscus leucopus*), but the parasite also has been found in other hosts.[4] The primary vector is *Ixodes scapularis*, which also transmits *Borrelia burgdorferi* (the etiologic agent of Lyme disease), *Anaplasma phagocytophilum*, *Borrelia miyamotoi*, *Ehrlichia muris*–like agent, and Powassan virus.[4,10,11] Humans can be infected with two or more of these pathogens. The prevalence of *B microti* infection in nymphal *I scapularis* ticks ranges from 1% in newly endemic areas to 20% in some well-established endemic areas.[11] Initially identified on the coastal islands of southern New England, *B microti* has spread north, west, and south to encompass much of the northeastern United States. This geographic expansion mimics that of Lyme disease but has proceeded more slowly. The reported incidence of human babesiosis is lower than that of Lyme disease because of a more restricted geographic range, lower tick infection rate, greater proportion of asymptomatic infection, insufficient physician awareness, and greater difficulty in diagnosis.[2,11] Carefully designed epidemiologic studies have shown that differences in the incidence of babesiosis and Lyme disease are small at certain sites that have long been endemic for both diseases.[11,12]

Each of the three active stages in the life cycle of *I scapularis* (larva, nymph, and adult) takes a blood meal from a vertebrate host to mature to the next stage

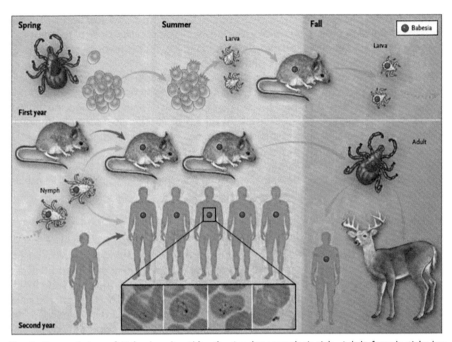

Fig. 1. Transmission of *Babesia microti* by the *Ixodes scapularis* tick. Adult female ticks lay eggs in the spring (*first year, top left*).[4] Larvae hatch in the early summer and become infected with *B microti* (*red circle*) as they take a blood meal from infected white-footed mice (*Peromyscus leucopus*) in late summer. White-footed mice are the primary reservoir host, but other small rodents may carry *B microti*. Larvae molt to nymphs the following spring (*second year, bottom left*). When infected nymphs feed on mice or humans in late spring or early summer, these hosts may become infected. Humans are incidental hosts. In the fall, nymphs molt to adults that feed on white-tailed deer (*Odocoileus virginianus*) but rarely on humans. White-tailed deer do not become infected with *B microti* but amplify the tick population by providing a blood meal for adult ticks. The following spring, adult female ticks lay eggs and the cycle is repeated. *B microti* are obligate parasites of erythrocytes and typically are visualized on a Giemsa-stained thin blood smear (see inset).[2,3] The inset panels from left to right show a ring form with a nonstaining vacuole surrounded by cytoplasm (*blue*) and a small nucleus (*purple*), an ameboid form, a tetrad (also referred to as Maltese Cross), and an extracellular form. (*From* Vannier E, Krause PJ. Human babesiosis. N Engl J Med 2012;366:2399; with permission.)

(see **Fig. 1**).[2,4] The tick transmission cycle begins in late summer when newly hatched larvae ingest the parasite during a blood meal obtained from an infected host. *B microti* eventually cross the tick gut epithelium to reach the hemolymph and travel to the salivary glands. The parasites remain dormant sporoblasts when larvae molt into nymphs. On attachment of a *B microti*–infected nymphal tick to a vertebrate host, sporozoites are produced and released into the dermis of the host within tick saliva. Nymphs transmit *B microti* sporozoites to vertebrate hosts in late spring and early summer of the following year.[4] Once fed, nymphs molt into adults in late summer and early fall. Adults feed on the white-tailed deer (*Odocoileus virginianus*), which is an important host for survival of the adult tick but is not a reservoir for *B microti*.[4] Larvae, nymphs, and adults all feed on humans, but the nymph is the primary vector because of its summer questing activity and its small size. *B microti* transmission from *I scapularis* to vertebrate hosts requires 36 to 72 hours because sporozoites are not readily available in the salivary glands and are generated following activation of dormant sporoblasts on tick exposure to warm blooded hosts.[13] The continuous expansion of the deer population is thought to be a major factor in the increased density of *I scapularis* and increased incidence of human babesiosis.[4]

Babesiosis also may be acquired through blood transfusion and transplacental transmission. More than 170 transfusion-transmitted cases have been reported.[14,15] *B microti* is the most common transfusion-transmitted pathogen reported in the United States. Although most cases occur during or shortly after summer in highly endemic areas, transfusion-transmitted babesiosis occurs year round and in nonendemic areas. About a fifth of the cases acquired through blood transfusion have had a fatal outcome.[14,15] Most cases of babesiosis in neonates have been acquired through blood transfusion, whereas at least one case has been acquired by transplacental transmission.[2,16,17]

Human Epidemiology

The incidence of human babesiosis has exponentially increased in the United States over the past five decades.[2,3,12,18–20] Most cases occur in seven states, five of which are located in the Northeast (MA, CT, RI, NY, and NJ) and two in the upper Midwest (MN and WI). The geographic range of human babesiosis has expanded beyond these highly endemic areas, and cases of human babesiosis caused by *B microti* are now reported all along the northeastern seaboard and inland, ranging from Maine to Maryland (**Fig. 2**).[2,18–21] Most cases of human babesiosis occur in the summer and in areas where the tick vector, vertebrate reservoirs, and deer are in close proximity to humans. At some sites and in certain years of high transmission, babesiosis may impose a significant public health burden.[12] Cases caused by *B duncani* or *B duncani*–type organisms have been sporadic on the Pacific Coast from northern California to Washington State. Three cases caused by *B divergens*–like organisms have been documented in Missouri, Kentucky, and Washington State.

Cases of human babesiosis have been reported throughout the world. *B divergens* is the most common cause of babesiosis in Europe, whereas a few cases of *B microti* and *B venatorum* infections also have been described. Human infection with *B venatorum* is endemic in China, where *B divergens* and *B microti* also have been reported.[22,23] Human babesiosis has been reported elsewhere in Asia, as well as in Africa, Australia, and South America.[2]

CLINICAL MANIFESTATIONS
Asymptomatic Infection

Asymptomatic *B microti* infection has been recorded in about a fifth of adults and half of children in a decade-long cohort study on Block Island, Rhode Island, a highly endemic area.[12] Serosurveys in other highly endemic areas have confirmed the high prevalence of asymptomatic infection as shown by the disparity between seroprevalence rates and the number of reported cases of babesiosis.[12,15,19] In New England, seroprevalence has varied between 0.5% and 16%.[15,19]

Mild to Moderate Disease

Following an incubation period of about 1 to 4 weeks after a tick bite or 1 to 9 weeks (but up to 6 months) following transfusion of contaminated blood products, a gradual onset of malaise and fatigue is accompanied by fever and one or more of the following: chills, sweats, anorexia, headache, myalgia, nausea, nonproductive cough, and arthralgia (**Table 1**).[18,20–29] Also reported are emotional liability and depression,

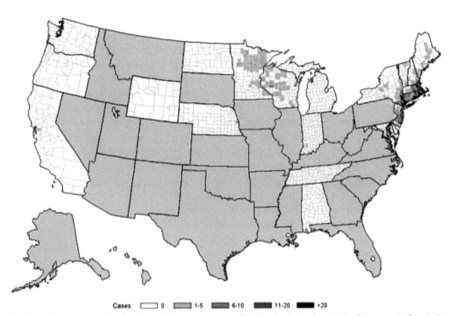

Cases [ ] 0 ░░ 1-5 ▓▓ 6-10 ■■ 11-20 ■■ >20

Fig. 2. Geographic distribution of human cases of babesiosis in the United States. Babesiosis became a nationally notifiable condition in January 2011. As of 2012, babesiosis is reportable in 22 states and the District of Columbia. The figure shows the incidence of babesiosis (number of cases per 100,000 persons) by county of residence in 2012. Human babesiosis caused by *Babesia microti* has long been reported from the Northeast, particularly from Massachusetts to New Jersey, and recently became endemic in northern New England (Maine and New Hampshire) and in the northern Mid-Atlantic States (from Pennsylvania to Maryland). *B microti* also causes disease in the upper Midwest, particularly in Wisconsin and Minnesota. *B duncani* has been the etiologic agent along the northwest Pacific Coast. Cases of *B divergens*–like infection have been reported from Washington State, Kentucky, and Missouri. (*Adapted from* Centers for Disease Control and Prevention. Available at: http://www.cdc.gov/parasites/babesiosis/data-statistics.html.)

Table 1 Symptoms of babesiosis			
Symptoms	Outpatients (%) (N = 41)	Inpatients (%) (N = 249)	All Patients (%) (N = 290)
Fever	88	89	89
Fatigue	85	82	82
Chills	63	68	67
Sweats	73	58	60
Anorexia	56	53	53
Headache	68	44	47
Myalgia	66	39	43
Nausea	32	44	42
Cough	34	27	28
Arthralgia	46	22	25

Outpatient cases are from Ruebush et al,[25] Krause et al,[26] and Krause et al.[27] Inpatient cases are from White et al,[20] Krause et al,[24] Hatcher et al,[28] and Joseph et al.[18]

hyperesthesia, sore throat, abdominal pain, vomiting, conjunctival injection, photophobia, and weight loss.

Fever is the salient feature on physical examination, but splenomegaly and hepatomegaly occasionally are noted. Less common are mild pharyngeal erythema, jaundice, and retinopathy with splinter hemorrhages and retinal infarcts.[18,20,25–28] Rash seldom is noted and if present should raise the possibility of concurrent Lyme disease. Laboratory abnormalities that reflect the hemolytic anemia caused by invasion and lysis of red blood cells by babesia organisms include low hemoglobin, low hematocrit, and elevated lactic dehydrogenase.[18,20,25,27,28] Serum liver enzyme concentrations often are elevated. The leukocyte count is variable. Thrombocytopenia is common.[20] Elevated serum levels of blood urea nitrogen and creatinine may occur, especially in severe illness and often are accompanied by proteinuria. Symptoms usually resolve in a week or two but anemia and fatigue may persist for several months.[25,30] Parasitemia (as measured by parasite DNA) has been detected for more than a year, even after resolution of symptoms and completion of antibiotic therapy.[30]

Severe Disease

Severe babesiosis requires hospital admission and usually occurs in patients who are older than 50 years, are immunocompromised, have comorbidities, or experience B divergens infection. Complications include adult respiratory distress syndrome, pulmonary edema, disseminated intravascular coagulation, congestive heart failure, renal failure, coma, splenic rupture, or a prolonged relapsing course of illness despite standard antibiotic therapy.[18,20,28,29,31] Death occurs in up to a tenth of patients hospitalized for B microti infection.[20,28] The fatality rate is even higher among those who are immunocompromised or acquire the infection through blood transfusion.[2,3,14,15,28,31] Concurrent infection with B microti and one or several tick-transmitted pathogens can occur and may increase the number and duration of acute symptoms.[26,32]

PATHOGENESIS
Red Blood Cell Invasion and Lysis

After attachment and entry into the erythrocyte, babesia organisms mature into trophozoites that eventually undergo asexual budding to yield two or four daughter cells known as merozoites.[33] Released into the bloodstream, free merozoites quickly invade nearby red blood cells to ensure persistence of the infection in the host.

Erythrocyte lysis is associated with many of the clinical manifestations and complications of babesiosis, including fever, anemia, jaundice, hemoglobinemia, hemoglobinuria, and renal insufficiency. The absence of synchrony in asexual reproduction of the parasite may explain the lack of massive hemolysis associated with babesiosis and therefore the milder clinical presentation of babesiosis when compared with malaria.

Host Immune Response

The pathogenesis of babesia infection is closely linked to the host response, and studies of babesiosis in animal models suggest that disease results from the excessive production of proinflammatory cytokines.[34–38] The release of proinflammatory cytokines may be initiated by contact of immune cells with the glycosylphosphatidylinositol anchors of babesia proteins expressed at the surface of the parasite or the surface of infected red blood cells. Proinflammatory cytokines subsequently stimulate production of downstream mediators, such as nitric oxide, which may kill parasites, but also cause cellular damage when produced in excess. Obstruction of blood vessels caused by adherence of parasitized erythrocytes to vascular endothelium with ensuing tissue ischemia and necrosis has been hypothesized to contribute to pathology.[35] Although cytoadherence occurs in cattle infected with *Babesia bovis*, it has not been observed in human babesiosis.[39]

The immune response in babesiosis involves macrophages and their products, such as tumor necrosis factor-α and interleukin-12; B lymphocytes and antibody secretion; T lymphocytes and cytokine production, such as interferon-γ; and complement factors.[2,34–37,40] Many fatal cases of human babesiosis occur in splenectomized individuals, although asplenia does not always result in death or even severe illness. The spleen plays a critical role in protection against *Babesia* spp. because resident phagocytes and histiocytes ingest and clear infected red blood cells. Given that anemia often is more severe than predicted by parasitemia, uninfected red blood cells likely are removed. Whether caused by hemolysis of infected red blood cells or by nonspecific removal of uninfected red blood cells, the anemia of babesiosis elicits stress-induced erythropoiesis and reticulocytosis. The splenic immune response and extramedullary erythropoiesis explain why patients who experience high-grade parasitemia tend to present with splenomegaly.

Aging is an important risk factor for severe babesiosis. Most clinically apparent cases are reported in adults, although seroprevalence studies indicate that children are equally exposed to *Babesia* infected ticks. Most severe cases of babesiosis occur in people older than 50 years of age even if otherwise healthy.[20] Almost all of the pediatric cases reported have been in neonates and caused by transfusion of blood products.[29,41] Data from a murine model of human babesiosis suggest that resistance to *B microti* infection conferred by the adaptive immune system is genetically determined and altered by aging.[41,42] Sterile immunity may be slow to develop because parasite DNA (a marker of parasitemia) persists for months to years after recovery from acute illness.[30]

DIAGNOSIS
Clinical Diagnosis

The diagnosis of babesiosis is based on epidemiologic and medical history, physical examination, and confirmatory laboratory tests (**Fig. 3**).[2] A diagnosis of babesiosis should be considered when a patient has a history of travel to or residence in a babesia endemic area or has received a blood transfusion in the previous 6 months and presents with symptoms that are consistent with babesiosis. A history of tick exposure is useful but may be absent because the bite often is unnoticed.

Laboratory Diagnosis

The diagnosis of babesiosis is confirmed by laboratory testing, most commonly by identification of the organism on Giemsa- or Wright-stained thin blood smears (see **Fig. 1**).[2,3,43] Trophozoites of *Babesia* spp. are round, oval, or pear-shaped and have blue cytoplasm with red chromatin. Ring forms are most common and may resemble the rings of early stage *Plasmodium falciparum* trophozoites. Babesia are distinguished from plasmodia by the absence of hemozoin deposit in the ring form, the lack of banana-shaped gametocytes, and the presence of tetrads (Maltese cross).[2] Multiple thin blood smears should be examined in the early stage of the illness, because parasitemia often is low at presentation.

Polymerase chain reaction (PCR) is a more sensitive diagnostic test than blood smear and provides a molecular characterization of the *Babesia* species.[43] The advent of real-time PCR has considerably lowered the limit of detection.[44–46] End point *B microti* PCR has been widely available for about two decades, whereas real-time

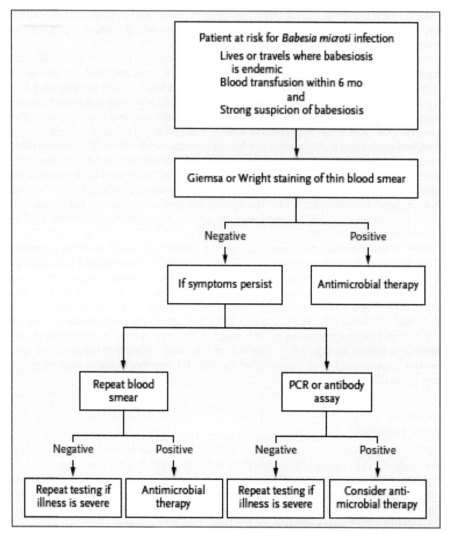

Fig. 3. Algorithm for diagnosis of human babesiosis caused by *Babesia microti*. The laboratory diagnosis of babesiosis should only be initiated for patients who are at risk of infection and for whom there is strong suspicion of infection.[2,10] Laboratory testing is required for definitive diagnosis of babesiosis. PCR signifies polymerase chain reaction. (*From* Vannier E, Krause PJ. Human babesiosis. N Engl J Med 2012;366:2403; with permission.)

B microti PCR has been developed more recently and is now available from several commercial diagnostic laboratories. The diagnosis also can be confirmed and the organism amplified for genetic sequencing by injecting patient blood into small laboratory animals, although this approach is less sensitive and more time-consuming and costly than PCR.[43]

Serology is useful for supporting or confirming the diagnosis. A four-fold rise in babesia IgG titer in acute and convalescent sera confirms recent infection, whereas a single positive antibody titer is not confirmatory because it cannot distinguish recent from past infection. The indirect immunofluorescence assay is the most common babesia serologic test. Others include enzyme-linked immunosorbent assay and Western blot.[47,48] The antigen used in babesia antibody testing should be specific for the *Babesia* species that is locally prevalent. For example, *B duncani* antibody testing would not be informative in areas where *B microti* is endemic and *B duncani* absent. Furthermore, the antibody titer that defines the threshold for a positive serology often differs from one *Babesia* species antibody assay to another and occasionally from one laboratory to another for the same *Babesia* species. Babesia antibody testing is of limited use in fulminant infection, such as *B divergens* illness, because initial antibody testing often is negative. During the acute phase of the illness, *B microti* IgG titers usually exceed 1:1024, but typically decline to 1:64 or less within 8 to 12 months.[30] A positive serology for *B divergens* does not exclude *B venatorum* infection because sera from *B venatorum* infected patients react with *B divergens* antigen. Cases of *B duncani* infection have been too few to validate the immunofluorescence assay for this pathogen.

TREATMENT
Asymptomatic Infection

A 1-week course of atovaquone plus azithromycin should be considered for any person identified with asymptomatic babesial infection (as determined by blood smear or PCR) for longer than 3 months.[24,49,50] People who have a positive serology but in whom parasites cannot be detected by blood smears and by PCR should not be treated, because they likely have resolved the infection.

Mild to Moderate Disease

The recommended treatment of mild to moderate babesiosis consists of atovaquone plus azithromycin for 7 to 10 days (**Table 2**).[24,50] This regimen was compared with clindamycin plus quinine in the only prospective trial of antibabesial therapy in humans.[24]

Table 2
Treatment of human babesiosis

Antimicrobials	Dose	Frequency
Atovaquone plus azithromycin		
Atovaquone	Adult: 750 mg	Every 12 h
	Child: 20 mg/kg	Every 12 h (maximum 750 mg/dose)
Azithromycin	Adult: 500–1000 mg	On Day 1
	250–1000 mg	On subsequent days
	Child: 10 mg/kg	On Day 1 (maximum 500 mg/dose)
	5 mg/kg	On subsequent days (maximum 250 mg/dose)
Clindamycin plus quinine		
Clindamycin	Adult: 600 mg	Every 8 h
	Child: 7–10 mg/kg	Every 6–8 h (maximum 600 mg/dose)
	Intravenous administration	
	Adult: 300–600 mg	Every 6 h
	Child: 7–10 mg/kg	Every 6–8 h (maximum 600 mg/dose)
Quinine	Adult: 650 mg	Every 6–8 h
	Child: 8 mg/kg	Every 8 h (maximum 650 mg/dose)

All antibiotics are administered by mouth unless otherwise specified. All doses administered for 7 to 10 days except for persistent relapsing infection (see text). Partial or complete exchange transfusion should be considered for treatment of severe cases of babesiosis. Exchange transfusion is recommended for any patient who is infected with *Babesia divergens*.

Both drug combinations were equally effective in clearing symptoms and parasitemia. Adverse effects were reported in 15% of subjects who received atovaquone plus azithromycin compared with 72% of subjects who received clindamycin plus quinine. Drug reactions were so severe that treatment had to be stopped or drug dosage decreased in approximately one-third of subjects who took clindamycin plus quinine but in only 2% of subjects who received atovaquone plus azithromycin. Although rare cases of resistance to atovaquone plus azithromycin have been reported, this combination has been proved effective in most children and adults.[24,50]

Severe Disease

Severe disease typically develops in patients who have one or more of the following risk factors: age greater than 50 years, splenectomy, malignancy, HIV infection, or immunosuppressive therapy. Clindamycin plus quinine is the treatment of choice for these patients because of cumulative experience with this combination for severe disease.[29,50] Oral quinine can be replaced with intravenous quinidine, but a patient treated with intravenous quinine or quinidine must be closely monitored in a hospital setting for possible QT prolongation.

Persistent or relapsing babesiosis despite a standard course of antimicrobial therapy has occurred in patients who present with two or more of the risk factors listed previously. In these patients, resolution of infection may require at least 6 weeks of antimicrobial therapy, including 2 weeks after babesia parasites are no longer detected on blood smears.[31] In addition to clindamycin plus quinine, several antibiotic combinations have been reported to be effective in a few highly immunocompromised patients. These alternative regimens have consisted of atovaquone-proguanil; atovaquone, clindamycin plus doxycycline; atovaquone, azithromycin plus doxycycline; artemisinin, atovaquone plus doxycycline; atovaquone, azithromycin plus clindamycin; and azithromycin plus quinine.[31] Close clinical follow-up with repeat blood smears, babesia PCR, and complete blood counts should be performed immediately if symptoms recur.

Partial or complete red blood cell exchange transfusion is recommended for patients with parasitemia greater than or equal to 10%; severe anemia (hemoglobin <10 g/dL); or pulmonary, liver, or renal impairment. Exchange transfusion rapidly decreases parasitemia, corrects anemia, and removes toxic by-products of babesia infections.[2,51] Immediate exchange transfusion and treatment with clindamycin plus quinine is recommended for any patient infected with *B divergens* because the illness often is fulminant. A combination of intravenous pentamidine plus oral trimethoprim-sulfamethoxazole was effective in treating a case of *B divergens* infection.[52]

PREVENTION

Babesiosis can be prevented by avoiding areas where ticks, deer, and mice are known to thrive. It is especially important for asplenic individuals and other immunocompromised patients who are at risk of severe babesiosis, and who live or travel in endemic areas, to avoid tall grass, brush, and forested areas where *I scapularis* ticks may abound. Use of protective clothing that is sprayed or impregnated with diethyltoluamide (DEET), dimethyl phthalate, or permethrin is recommended for individuals who travel into the foliage of endemic areas.[53,54] A search for ticks should be carried out and the ticks removed as soon as possible.[54,55] Embedded ticks are best removed by use of tweezers to grasp the mouth parts without squeezing the body of the tick.

Landscape-management approaches, such as keeping grass mowed, clearing leaf litter, and spraying property with acaricides where tick density is high may help reduce the risk of infection. The risk of Lyme disease and presumably other tick-borne diseases can be decreased by limiting the amount of edge between lawn and shrub on private properties.[53,54,56] Acaricide application to deer using a four-poster device decreases the number of *I scapularis* ticks.[57] Reduction in the number of deer on several islands has decreased the number of *I scapularis* ticks and the incidence of Lyme disease.[58,59]

Prospective blood donors who have had a history of babesiosis are permanently deferred from donating. There is no Food and Drug Administration approved test for screening of the blood supply for *B microti*, but some states in highly endemic regions have instituted screening that combines serology and PCR.[15,60–62]

Although *B bovis* and *B bigemina* vaccines are available for use in cattle, no human babesiosis vaccine has been developed.

SUMMARY

Babesiosis is a worldwide tick-borne zoonosis caused by hemoprotozoan parasites of the genus *Babesia*. *B microti* is the main etiologic agent of human babesiosis and is endemic in the northeastern and the upper Midwestern United States. The geographic expansion of babesiosis has followed that of Lyme disease, but has remained more restricted. The emergence of human babesiosis poses a serious health threat in highly endemic areas. Fever is the salient feature of babesiosis and often is accompanied by a series of nonspecific symptoms, explaining why diagnosis may be delayed or missed. The diagnosis is confirmed by identification of babesia organisms on Giemsa-stained blood smears, detection of babesia DNA by PCR, or a four-fold rise in antibabesia antibody titers in acute and convalescent sera. The disease may be severe or fatal, particularly in patients who are otherwise healthy but older than 50 years of age, and in patients who are immunocompromised regardless of age. Most patients have complete recovery following a standard 7- to 10-day course of antimicrobial therapy.

REFERENCES

1. Skrabalo A, Deanovic A. Piroplasmosis in man: report on a case. Doc Med Geogr Trop 1957;9:11–6.
2. Vannier E, Krause PJ. Human babesiosis. N Engl J Med 2012;366:2397–407.
3. Hunfeld KP, Hildebrandt A, Gray JS. Babesiosis: recent insights into an ancient disease. Int J Parasitol 2008;38:1219–37.
4. Spielman A, Wilson ML, Levine JF, et al. Ecology of Ixodes dammini borne human babesiosis and Lyme disease. Annu Rev Entomol 1985;30:439–60.
5. Cornillot E, Hadj-Kaddour K, Dassouli A, et al. Sequencing of the smallest Apicomplexan genome from the human pathogen Babesia microti. Nucleic Acids Res 2012;1–13.
6. Cornillot E, Dassouli A, Garg A, et al. Whole genome mapping and re-organization of the nuclear and mitochondrial genomes of Babesia microti isolates. PLoS One 2013;8.
7. Goethert HK, Telford SR 3rd. What is Babesia microti? Parasitology 2003;127: 301–9.
8. Nakajima R, Tsuji M, Oda K, et al. Babesia microti-group parasites compared phylogenetically by complete sequencing of the CCTeta gene in 36 isolates. J Vet Med Sci 2009;71:55.

9. Fujisawa K, Nakajima R, Jinnai M, et al. Intron sequences from the CCT7 gene exhibit diverse evolutionary histories among the four lineages within the Babesia microti-group, a genetically related species complex that includes human pathogens. Jpn J Infect Dis 2011;64:403–10.

10. Dunn J, Krause PJ, Davis S, et al. Borrelia burgdorferi promotes the establishment of Babesia microti in the northeastern United States. PLoS One 2014; 9(12):e115494.

11. Diuk-Wasser M, Liu L, Steeves T, et al. Monitoring human babesiosis emergence through vector surveillance New England USA. Emerg Infect Dis 2014; 20:225–31.

12. Krause PJ, McKay K, Gadbaw J, et al. Increasing health burden of human babesiosis in endemic sites. Am J Trop Med Hyg 2003;68:431–6.

13. Piesman J, Spielman A. Human babesiosis on Nantucket Island: Prevalence of Babesia microti in ticks. Am J Trop Med Hyg 1980;29:742–6.

14. Herwaldt BL, Linden JV, Bosserman E, et al. Transfusion-associated babesiosis in the United States: a description of cases. Ann Intern Med 2011;155:509–19.

15. Leiby DA. Transfusion-transmitted Babesia spp.: bull's-eye on Babesia microti. Clin Microbiol Rev 2011;24:14–28.

16. Cornett JK, Malhotra A, Hart D. Vertical transmission of babesiosis from a pregnant, splenectomized mother to her neonate. Infect Dis Clin Practice 2012;20: 408–10.

17. Joseph JT, Purtill K, Wong SJ, et al. Vertical transmission of Babesia microti, United States. Emerg Infect Dis 2012;18:1318–21.

18. Joseph JT, Roy SS, Shams N, et al. Babesiosis in lower Hudson Valley, New York, USA. Emerg Infect Dis 2011;17:843–7.

19. Krause PJ, Telford SR, Ryan R, et al. Geographical and temporal distribution of babesial infection in Connecticut. J Clin Microbiol 1991;29:1–4.

20. White DJ, Talarico J, Chang HG, et al. Human babesiosis in New York State: Review of 139 hospitalized cases and analysis of prognostic factors. Arch Intern Med 1998;158:2149–54.

21. Herwaldt BL, Montgomery S, Woodhall D, Bosserman EA. Babesiosis surveillance – 18 States, 2011. MMWR Morb Mortal Wkly Rep 2012;61:505–9.

22. Jiang JF, Zheng YC, Jiang RR, et al. Epidemiological, clinical, and laboratory characteristics of 48 cases of "Babesia venatorum" infection in China: a descriptive study. Lancet Infect Dis 2014 [pii:S1473-3099(14) 71046–1].

23. Vannier E, Krause PJ. Babesiosis in China, an emerging threat. Lancet Infect Dis 2014. http://dx.doi.org/10.1016/S1473-3099(14)71062-X.

24. Krause PJ, Lepore T, Sikand VJ, et al. Atovaquone and azithromycin for the treatment of human babesiosis. N Engl J Med 2000;343:1454–8.

25. Ruebush TK 2nd, Cassaday PB, Marsh HJ, et al. Human babesiosis on Nantucket Island: clinical features. Ann Intern Med 1977;86:6–9.

26. Krause PJ, Telford SR 3rd, Spielman A, et al. Concurrent Lyme disease and babesiosis. Evidence for increased severity and duration of illness. JAMA 1996;275: 1657–60.

27. Krause PJ, McKay K, Thompson CA, et al. Disease-specific diagnosis of coinfecting tickborne zoonoses: babesiosis, human granulocytic ehrlichiosis, and Lyme disease. Clin Infect Dis 2002;34:1184–91.

28. Hatcher JC, Greenberg PD, Antique J, et al. Severe babesiosis in Long Island: Review of 34 cases and their complications. Clin Infect Dis 2001;32:1117–25.

29. Wittner M, Rowin KS, Tanowitz HB, et al. Successful chemotherapy of transfusion babesiosis. Ann Intern Med 1982;96:601–4.

30. Krause PJ, Spielman A, Telford S, et al. Persistent parasitemia after acute babesiosis. N Engl J Med 1998;339:160–5.
31. Krause PJ, Gewurz BE, Hill D, et al. Persistent and relapsing babesiosis in immunocompromised patients. Clin Infect Dis 2008;46:370–6.
32. Thompson C, Spielman A, Krause PJ. Coinfecting deer associated zoonoses: Lyme disease, babesiosis, and ehrlichiosis. Clin Infect Dis 2001;33:676–85.
33. Lobo CA, Rodriguez M, Cursino-Santos JR. Babesia and red cell invasion. Curr Opin Hematol 2012;19:170–5.
34. Clark IA, Jacobson LS. Do babesiosis and malaria share a common disease process? Ann Trop Med Parasitol 1998;92:483–8.
35. Krause PJ, Daily J, Telford SR, et al. Shared features in the pathobiology of babesiosis and malaria. Trends Parasitol 2007;23:605–10.
36. Shaio MF, Lin PR. A case study of cytokine profiles in acute human babesiosis. Am J Trop Med Hyg 1998;58:335–7.
37. Igarashi I, Waki S, Ito M, et al. Role of CD4+ T cells in the control of primary infection with Babesia microti in mice. J Protozool Res 1994;4:164–71.
38. Hemmer RM, Ferrick DA, Conrad PA. Up-regulation of tumor necrosis factor-alpha and interferon-gamma expression in the spleen and lungs of mice infected with the human Babesia isolate WA1. Parasitol Res 2000;86:121–8.
39. Clark IA, Budd AC, Hsue G, et al. Absence of erythrocyte sequestration in a case of babesiosis in a splenectomized human patient. Malar J 2006;5:69.
40. Terkawi MA, Cao S, Herbas MS, et al. Macrophage is the determinant of resistance to and outcome of non-lethal Babesia microti infection in mice. Infect Immun 2014. [Epub ahead of print].
41. Krause PJ, Telford SR, Pollack RJ, et al. Babesiosis: an underdiagnosed disease of children. Pediatrics 1992;89:1045–8.
42. Vannier E, Borggraefe I, Telford SR, et al. Age-associated decline in resistance to Babesia microti is genetically determined. J Infect Dis 2004;189:1721–8.
43. Krause PJ, Telford SR, Spielman A, et al. Comparison of PCR with blood smear and inoculation of small animals for diagnosis of Babesia microti parasitemia. J Clin Microbiol 1996;34:2791–4.
44. Teal AE, Habura A, Ennis J, et al. A new real-time PCR assay for improved detection of the parasite Babesia microti. J Clin Microbiol 2012;50:903–8.
45. Rollend L, Bent SJ, Krause PJ, et al. Quantitative PCR for detection of Babesia microti in Ixodes scapularis ticks and in human blood. Vector Borne Zoonotic Dis 2013;13:784–90.
46. Bloch EM, Lee TH, Krause PJ, et al. Development of a real-time PCR assay for sensitive detection and quantitation of Babesia microti infection. Transfusion 2013;53:2299–306.
47. Krause PJ, Telford S, Ryan R, et al. Diagnosis of babesiosis: evaluation of a serologic test for the detection of Babesia microti antibody. J Infect Dis 1994;169:923–6.
48. Levin AE, Williamson PC, Erwin JL, et al. Determination of Babesia microti seroprevalence in blood donor populations using an investigational enzyme immunoassay. Transfusion 2014;54:2237–44.
49. Kjemtrup AM, Conrad PA. Human babesiosis: an emerging tick-borne disease. Int J Parasitol 2000;30:1323–37.
50. Wormser GP, Dattwyler RJ, Shapiro ED, et al. The clinical assessment, treatment, and prevention of Lyme disease, human granulocytic anaplasmosis, and babesiosis: Clinical practice guidelines by the Infectious Diseases Society of America. Clin Infect Dis 2006;43:1089–94.

51. Spaete J, Patrozou E, Rich JD, et al. Red cell exchange transfusion for babesiosis in RhodeIsland. J Clin Apher 2009;24:97–105.
52. Raoult D, Soulayrol L, Toga B, Dumon H, Casanova P. Babesiosis, pentamidine, and cotrimoxazole. Ann Intern Med 1987;107:944.
53. Finch C, Al-Damluji MS, Krause PJ, et al. Integrated assessment of behavioral and environmental risk factors for Lyme disease infection on Block Island, Rhode Island. PLoS One 2014;9:e84758.
54. Stafford KC 3rd. Tick management handbook: an integrated guide for homeowners, pest control operators, and public health officials for the prevention of tick-associated disease. New Haven (CT): The Connecticut Agricultural Experimental Station; 2007. p. 1–77.
55. Connally NP, Durante AJ, Yousey-Hindes KM, et al. Peridomestic Lyme disease prevention: results of a population-based case-control study. Am J Prev Med 2009;37:201–6.
56. Dister SW, Fish D, Bros SM, et al. Landscape characterization of peridomestic risk for Lyme disease using satellite imagery. Am J Trop Med Hyg 1997;57:687–92.
57. Fish D, Childs JE. Community-based prevention of Lyme disease and other tick-borne diseases through topical application of acaricide to white-tailed deer: background and rationale. Vector Borne Zoonotic Dis 2009;9:357–64.
58. Wilson ML, Telford SR, Piesman J, Spielman A. Reduced abundance of immature Ixodes dammini (Acari: Ixodidae) following elimination of deer. J Med Entomol 1988;25:224–8.
59. Kilpatrick HJ, Labonte AM, Stafford K. The relationship between deer density, tick abundance, and human cases of Lyme disease in a residential community. J Med Entomol 2014;51:777–84.
60. Young C, Chawla A, Berardi V, et al. Preventing transfusion transmitted babesiosis: Preliminary experience of the first laboratory-based blood donor screening program. Transfusion 2012;52:1523–9.
61. Goodell A, Bloch EM, Krause PJ, et al. Costs, consequences, and cost-effectiveness of strategies for Babesia microti blood donor screening strategies the US blood supply. Transfusion 2014;54:2245–57.
62. Johnson ST, Cable RG, Leiby DA. Lookback investigations of Babesia microti-seropositive blood donors: seven-year experience in a Babesia-endemic area. Transfusion 2012;52:1509–16.

Update and Commentary on Four Emerging Tick-Borne Infections

Ehrlichia muris–like Agent, Borrelia miyamotoi, Deer Tick Virus, Heartland Virus, and Whether Ticks Play a Role in Transmission of Bartonella henselae

Gary P. Wormser, MD[a],*, Bobbi Pritt, MD, MSc, DTM&H[b]

KEYWORDS

- Tick-transmitted infections • *Ehrlichia* • *Borrelia* • Deer tick virus • Powassan virus
- Heartland virus • *Bartonella*

KEY POINTS

- Emerging tick-transmitted infections in the United States include infections due to *Ehrlichia muris*–like agent, *Borrelia miyamotoi* sensu lato, deer tick virus, and Heartland virus.
- Too few cases have been reported to characterize accurately or completely the range of possible clinical and laboratory manifestations of these infections.
- There is a need for the development of sensitive and specific serologic and molecular assays for these infections that are easily accessible to clinicians.

Disclosures: Dr G.P. Wormser reports receiving research grants from Immunetics, Inc, RareCyte, Inc, Institute for Systems Biology and bioMérieux SA. He owns equity in Abbott; has been an expert witness in malpractice cases involving Lyme disease; is an unpaid board member of the American Lyme Disease Foundation; has been an expert witness regarding Lyme disease in a disciplinary action for the Missouri Board of Registration for the Healing Arts; and was a consultant to Baxter for Lyme disease vaccine development. Dr B. Pritt reports receiving a research grant from the Minnesota Partnership for Biotechnology and Medical Genomics for malaria research. She is an unpaid board member for the College of American Pathologists Microbiology Resource Committee and receives a reviewer's stipend from the *Journal of Clinical Microbiology*.
[a] Division of Infectious Diseases, New York Medical College, 40 Sunshine Cottage Road, Skyline Office #2N-C20, Valhalla, NY 10595, USA; [b] Division of Clinical Microbiology, Department of Pathology and Laboratory Medicine, Mayo Clinic, 200 1st Street, SW, Rochester, MN 55905, USA
* Corresponding author.
E-mail address: gwormser@nymc.edu

Infect Dis Clin N Am 29 (2015) 371–381
http://dx.doi.org/10.1016/j.idc.2015.02.009
0891-5520/15/$ – see front matter © 2015 Elsevier Inc. All rights reserved.

INTRODUCTION

Besides Lyme disease, there are 5 other known *Ixodes scapularis* transmitted infections in the United States: babesiosis, human granulocytic anaplasmosis, deer tick virus infection, *Ehrlichia muris*–like agent infection (also referred to as *Ehrlichia* sp Wisconsin), and *Borrelia miyamotoi* sensu lato infection. This review provides current information on the epidemiology, clinical and laboratory features, and treatment of the newest, least common, and least well-understood members of this group of infections: infection due to *E muris*–like agent, deer tick virus infection, and *B miyamotoi* sensu lato infection (**Table 1**). Heartland virus infections (for which a vector has not been definitely established) is also discussed and the evidence that *Bartonella henselae* is a tick-borne pathogen is critically reviewed.

EHRLICHIA MURIS–LIKE AGENT

Ehrlichiae are obligate intracellular gram-negative bacteria that infect leukocytes and cause a febrile illness in humans. Ehrlichiosis in the United States is due primarily to *Ehrlichia chaffeensis*, and less commonly, to *Ehrlichia ewingii*, which are both transmitted by *Amblyomma americanum*, the Lone Star tick. In 2009, a third cause of human ehrlichiosis was identified in patients from the upper Midwest, with the first cases reported in the medical literature in 2011.[1] The formal taxonomic disposition of this agent is currently unclear, but studies have demonstrated a 95% to 98% sequence homology between this organism and *E muris* when examining multiple genes (*groEL*, 16S, *gltA*, *fbpA*, *nadA*, and *dsb*),[2] and the organism is commonly referred to as the *E muris*-like (EML) agent. *E muris* is currently recognized to exist in Eastern Europe and parts of Asia, where it is found in ticks of the *Ixodes persulcatus* complex and in rodents and deer.[3–5]

The first published report of clinical illness associated with this infection described 4 patients from Wisconsin and Minnesota.[1] In total from 2009 to 2013, 67 patients have been identified by testing EDTA whole-blood samples using a polymerase chain reaction (PCR) assay targeting the *groEL* gene.[6] All of the patients were from the upper Midwestern United States and reported probable tick exposure in Wisconsin or Minnesota. The 67 patients included 42 men and 25 women. All of the patients were adults or adolescents whose ages ranged from 15 to 94 years (mean age, 61 years). Patients presented commonly with fever (89%), fatigue (81%), headache (69%), and myalgia (63%), while laboratory findings included lymphopenia (66%) and thrombocytopenia (58%). Elevated liver enzyme levels have been noted but the frequency is uncertain from the available data. Twelve (50%) of the 24 patients whose immune status was known were immunocompromised because of receipt of immunosuppressive therapies. Thirteen patients were hospitalized for a median duration of 7 days.[6] Nevertheless, all patients recovered, with 66 of the 67 receiving doxycycline. Patients seemed to respond to doxycycline as would be expected from experience with the treatment of human monocytic ehrlichiosis and human granulocytic anaplasmosis.

The diagnosis has been most conclusively established by PCR detection of pathogen DNA in blood samples, although seroreactivity with *E chaffeensis*, but not with *Anaplasma phagocytophilum*, has been noted.[1] The cell type that is infected by this microorganism in humans is unknown, and intracellular inclusions (morulae) have not yet been identified in peripheral blood smears of patients with this infection.

As of 2012, the EML agent has been detected by PCR targeting the *groEL* gene in at least 34 (2.5%) of 1384 *I scapularis* ticks from Wisconsin or Minnesota collected from 2007 to 2010 but has not been found in ticks outside of this geographic area, including 1547 *I scapularis* and 6563 *A americanum* ticks that were tested.[1,7] Indeed,

Table 1
Four emerging tick-borne infections

Infection	Year First Reported in Patients	Class of Etiologic Agent	Probable Vector	Clinical Features	Laboratory Features	Treatment	Comments
E muris–like agent	2011	Bacteria	I scapularis	Fever, fatigue, headache, myalgia	Cytopenia ↑ LFTs	Doxycycline	So far, >65 cases, all with tick exposure in Wisconsin and Minnesota
B miyamotoi sensu lato	2011	Bacteria	Ixodes spp ticks that transmit B burgdorferi	Fever, fatigue, headache, myalgia, meningoencephalitis	↑ LFTs	Same antibiotics as for Lyme disease	Unclear if opportunistic infection in the US
Deer tick virus	1997	Virus	I scapularis	Fever, weakness, lethargy associated with meningoencephalitis	Cerebrospinal fluid pleocytosis; no cytopenia or ↑ LFTs	Supportive care	Four proven neuroinvasive infections, but others may have occurred and were diagnosed as Powassan virus
Heartland virus	2012	Virus	A americanum	Fever, fatigue, anorexia, headache, nausea, myalgia, arthralgia	Cytopenia ↑ LFTs	Supportive care	Eight total cases; 7 in Missouri and 1 in Tennessee

Abbreviation: LFTs, liver enzyme levels in this context.

E muris or a closely related species of ehrlichia was present in ticks from Wisconsin collected in the 1990s.[8] Efforts to prevent *I scapularis* tick bites should reduce or eliminate cases.

Commentary

The EML agent is the only *I scapularis* transmitted pathogen not found in *I scapularis* ticks from the eastern United States and to date all human infections appear to be associated with tick exposure in Wisconsin or Minnesota. Although the clinical and the laboratory features described to date are similar to infections caused by *A phagocytophilum*, the spectrum of infection due to the EML agent cannot be fully appreciated with so few documented cases, many of whom were undoubtedly tested because of the presumption that fever with headache and cytopenia suggest this kind of infection. How many patients with illnesses without fever, headache, or cytopenia that may have been tested by a PCR assay capable of detecting the EML agent is unknown. Also, it is unclear whether subclinical or even asymptomatic infections may occur. Testing is currently limited to select reference and public health laboratories in the Upper Midwest.

BORRELIA MIYAMOTOI

B miyamotoi sensu lato is a relapsing fever borrelia[9,10] that is present in approximately 2% (with a range of up to 10.5% in certain geographic locations) of *Ixodes* species ticks that are known to transmit *Borrelia burgdorferi* in the United States[11,12] and has also been detected in all of the *Ixodes* tick species that transmit Lyme borrelia in Europe and in parts of Asia.[13–16] In general, the rate of tick infection is about one-tenth that of *B burgdorferi* in the same *Ixodes* tick populations in a particular geographic area.[17] The term "sensu lato" is used to denote that strains of *B miyamotoi* present in one geographic area are not necessarily identical to those present in another geographic area.[9,11] *B miyamotoi* was first discovered and cultivated in vitro in Japan[13] (this isolate is sometimes referred to as *B miyamotoi* sensu stricto), whereas the US strain (or strains) had not been successfully cultivated in vitro until 2014, when a novel culture medium was successfully used for a single strain.[18] Whether such genetic differences might account for some of the discrepant clinical and laboratory features of infection found in patients from different geographic areas, as described below, is unknown.

The first report of human infection due to *B miyamotoi* sensu lato was from Russia in 2011.[15] By PCR methodology, 51 patients were found to be positive on a blood sample, and detailed clinical information was provided for 46 of these patients. Characteristic clinical features included fever, fatigue, headache, and myalgia. The median age was 54 years (range, 21–77 years) and 52% were men. A relapsing fever course was atypical and only observed in 11% of the 46 patients. Four patients had an erythema migrans skin lesion. Elevated liver enzyme levels were found in 68%; none of the patients had cytopenia. Of the 51 patients with a positive PCR for *B miyamotoi* sensu lato in a blood sample, 48 were seropositive for immunoglobulin (Ig) M antibodies to *B burgdorferi* sensu lato. A Jarisch-Herxheimer reaction was observed with initiation of antibiotic treatment in 15% of the 46 patients. In this case series, all 46 patients had had a recognized tick bite preceding their illness (a prerequisite for inclusion in this study); the mean time from tick bite to onset of symptoms was 15 days.[15]

A detailed clinical description has been reported for only 3 cases of *B miyamotoi* sensu lato in the United States[17,19] and for only one in Europe.[16] One patient was

61 years old and acquired this infection in Massachusetts; 2 others, aged 80 and 87 years, lived in New Jersey, and one patient, aged 70 years, acquired the infection in the Netherlands. Two of the 4 cases were highly immunocompromised and presented with a chronic meningoencephalitis in which B miyamotoi sensu lato could be detected by PCR and by microscopy in cerebrospinal fluid.[16,17] The 2 others presented with fever plus leukopenia and thrombocytopenia and had elevated liver enzyme levels.[19]

Two additional cases of B miyamotoi sensu lato infection have been reported from Japan.[14] In both patients with this infection, B miyamotoi sensu lato DNA was detected in serum samples and one of the cases showed seroconversion for antibody to the glycerophosphodiester phosphodiesterase (GlpQ) protein of B miyamotoi sensu lato. One of the patients was a 72-year-old woman who had fever and an erythema migrans skin lesion. Leukopenia was present in this patient, but the platelet count was normal. Symptoms were said to have improved rapidly on minocycline therapy. The second patient was a 37-year-old man who also had fever and an erythema migrans skin lesion. Symptoms were said to have improved rapidly on ceftriaxone therapy. In both cases, serum samples showed reactivity with B burgdorferi sensu lato antigens.

In a study from the United States, frozen stored sera that were collected between 1991 and 2012 from donors in New England or in New York State were tested by both an IgG enzyme-linked immunoassay and separate IgG and IgM Western blots for antibody to a recombinant GlpQ protein.[11,20] GlpQ protein is present in B miyamotoi sensu lato (and some other microorganisms), but not in B burgdorferi. IgG seropositivity rates of 3.9% on 639 healthy individuals, 9.8% on 194 patients with Lyme disease, and 3.6% on 221 patients with a summertime viral-like illness were found. Seropositivity was significantly more frequently observed with sera from Lyme disease patients compared with either of the other groups ($P<.05$).

Treatment of B miyamotoi sensu lato infection with antibiotics effective against other relapsing borrelial species or against B burgdorferi sensu lato seems to be effective.[14–17,19] Efforts to prevent tick bites should reduce or eliminate cases.

Commentary

Clearly too few cases of B miyamotoi sensu lato infection in the United States and Europe have been described to characterize accurately the clinical or laboratory features of this infection. The fact that all 4 of the published cases in these geographic areas occurred in individuals older than 60 years of age,[16,17,19] 2 of whom were highly immunocompromised, is consistent with the hypothesis that strains of B miyamotoi sensu lato in these regions are opportunistic pathogens. Concerning is the presence of cytopenia in the 2 US patients not known to be immunocompromised,[19] because leukopenia is not characteristic of relapsing fever infection and neither leukopenia nor thrombocytopenia was present in any of the 46 patients reported from Russia.[15] Furthermore, it was emphasized for these 2 patients that there was a delayed response to doxycycline therapy,[19] which would be unexpected for any kind of borrelial infection. These observations collectively raise the question as to whether the diagnosis of B miyamotoi sensu lato was correct or, if it was, whether there may have been an unidentified coinfecting pathogen.

The observation that the GlpQ seropositivity rate was no higher in US patients with a summertime viral-like illness compared with healthy subjects[11] lends support to raising the question of whether the US strains of B miyamotoi sensu lato are opportunistic pathogens. The observation that B miyamotoi sensu lato is present in about 2% of I scapularis ticks[12] does not prove human pathogenicity. Another relapsing fever borrelial species present in hard ticks in the United States is *Borrelia lonestari*. This borrelial species has been found in approximately 2% of *A americanum* ticks, a tick species responsible for thousands of tick bites in humans residing in the Southeastern and South Central regions of the United States. Nevertheless, to date, there has been only one well-documented human infection due to this borrelial species.[21]

In addition, unlike the experience in the Russian case series,[15] most sera from individuals from the United States with antibodies to GlpQ of *B miyamotoi* sensu lato failed to react with Lyme borrelia on either first- or second-tier Lyme disease serologic assays.[11] The numerous disparities discussed above should stimulate more research on *B miyamotoi* sensu lato infections. A first step should be the development of reliable PCR assays for this organism with ready accessibility of testing for researchers as well as for clinicians treating potential cases. At this time, molecular and serology-based assays are principally limited to the research setting.

DEER TICK VIRUS

Deer tick virus, a flavivirus in the tick-borne encephalitis group, is a genetically distinct lineage (subtype) of the Powassan virus[22,23] that may cause neuroinvasive infection in humans. Strains of Powassan virus other than deer tick virus are referred to hereafter as the prototype Powassan virus. Deer tick virus has 84% identity in nucleotides and 94% in amino acids with the prototype Powassan virus.[22] Prototype Powassan virus is a cause of infection in parts of both North America and Russia, whereas deer tick virus is only known to cause infection in North America.

Deer tick virus was originally isolated from *Dermacentor andersoni* ticks[24] but is mainly found in *I scapularis* ticks. Deer tick virus was first isolated from *I scapularis* ticks collected in coastal New England in 1997.[25] Up to 6% of adult *I scapularis* ticks are infected with deer tick virus,[26] whereas prototype Powassan virus has never been found in this tick species.[23,26] Thus, deer tick virus and the prototype Powassan virus have different enzootic cycles.[23,27,28] For the deer tick virus, the tick vector is *I scapularis* and the animal reservoir is presumably the white-footed mouse, whereas for the prototype Powassan virus, the tick vector is *I cookei* and the animal reservoir ground hogs and skunks. *I cookei* is found throughout the United States, east of the Rocky Mountains, but is a much less common cause of tick bites for humans than *I scapularis*.[23] In general, recognized neuroinvasive Powassan virus infections are uncommon.[29] Experimentally, deer tick virus can be transmitted by *I scapularis* ticks within 15 minutes of the tick bite,[30] which contrasts with the delayed transmission of *B burgdorferi*, *Babesia microti*, and *A phagocytophilum*.

The first known human case of deer tick virus infection occurred in 1997,[31] but proof based on genetic sequence data was not available until 2001.[22] To date, there are only 4 published cases of proven deer tick virus infection encephalitis: 1 from Canada,[22,31] 2 from New York State,[28,32] and 1 from Minnesota.[33] However, deer tick virus and the prototype Powassan virus are antigenically identical and therefore cannot be distinguished by serologic testing, which is the most widely used diagnostic modality. Immunofluorescent serologic assays for Powassan virus may also cross-react with other flaviviruses, such as West Nile virus, and thus need to be confirmed by neutralizing antibody assays or by PCR.[23,27,28] The only method to establish the presence of deer tick virus infection specifically is by genotypic analysis of the nucleic acids of the virus, which has been infrequently performed.

Supportive care is the only available treatment for prototype Powassan virus or deer tick virus neuroinvasive infections. Whether corticosteroids might prove beneficial requires further study.[23] Morbidity is high, and mortalities have occurred.[23,28,32] Efforts to prevent *I scapularis* tick bites should reduce or eliminate cases.

Commentary

The changing epidemiology of neuroinvasive Powassan virus infections in the United States suggests the emergence of the deer tick virus subtype of Powassan virus.[27,29] From 1958 to 1998, there were 27 reported cases or 0.7 cases per year, and none of the cases were from Wisconsin or Minnesota, 2 states that currently report numerous *I scapularis*–transmitted infections. From 1999 to 2007, there were 17 cases (1.9 cases per year) of neuroinvasive Powassan virus infections and 17.6% were from Wisconsin or Minnesota. From 2008 to 2013, there were 47 reported cases (7.8 cases per year) and 66.0% were from Wisconsin or Minnesota. One factor likely influencing this changing epidemiology was the introduction of diagnostic testing for Powassan virus by the Minnesota Department of Health. However, these data are consistent with the emergence with the deer tick virus subtype of Powassan virus in the north central region of the United States, as are other data from New York State.[23,27]

Of the 14 cases of Powassan virus encephalitis reported from New York State between 2004 and 2012, 10 (71%) were from counties highly endemic for Lyme disease and where *I cookei* tick bites are rare.[23] In contrast, of the 9 cases of Powassan virus encephalitis in New York State preceding 2004, none originated in counties highly endemic for Lyme disease.[23] Furthermore, of the 10 Powassan virus encephalitis cases diagnosed between 2004 and 2012, 2 were proven to be due to deer tick virus based on genotypic analysis,[28,32] and 2 other cases had concomitant Lyme disease (ie, erythema migrans),[23] making the suspicion of deer tick virus infection extremely plausible. Overall, the paucity of cases of recognized neuroinvasive deer tick virus infections, whether or not they are labeled as Powassan virus infections, raises the question of whether most human infections are not in fact neuroinvasive and perhaps may even be subclinical. Unfortunately, testing for both the prototype Powassan virus and the deer tick virus is currently limited to select research and public health laboratories, including the Centers for Disease Control and Prevention (CDC), and is not easily accessible to clinicians. Efforts to prevent *I scapularis* tick bites should reduce or eliminate cases.

HEARTLAND VIRUS

Heartland virus is in the phlebovirus genus of the Bunyaviridae family. This virus was first reported as a cause of human infection in 2012.[34] Only 8 cases have been identified, all but one of whom resided in and acquired the infection in Missouri[34,35]; the other patient was from Tennessee.[36] All patients were men 50 years of age or older (range, 50 to 80 years). Clinical features have included fever, fatigue, headache, myalgia, arthralgia, anorexia, and diarrhea that began within 14 days of a tick bite. Laboratory features included leukopenia with neutropenia and lymphopenia, thrombocytopenia, and elevated liver enzyme levels. The single fatality was an 80-year-old man from Tennessee who was hospitalized with fever, confusion, and cytopenia and developed multiorgan failure and hemorrhage.[36] The Heartland virus has been detected in nymphal unfed host-seeking *A americanum* ticks from Missouri,[37] and although vector competence has not been determined, this infection is presumed to be transmitted by this tick species. An animal reservoir has not been established.

Diagnosis of Heartland virus infection can be made by detection of viral RNA by reverse-transcriptase PCR in blood or tissue or by demonstrating a 4-fold or greater increase in virus-specific plaque reduction neutralization antibody titers between acute and convalescent serum specimens.[34–36,38] Diagnosis should be considered in a patient with exposure to *A americanum* ticks who presents with fever and cytopenia and who has not responded to empiric doxycycline therapy.[35] When tested, such patients will not have smear or PCR evidence for ehrlichia or anaplasma. Efforts to prevent *A americanum* tick bites should reduce or eliminate cases.

Commentary

Heartland virus is most closely related genetically to the emerging severe fever with thrombocytopenia syndrome virus (SFTSV). SFTSV is known to cause disease in China, Japan, and Korea and is most often acquired by a tick bite from *Haemaphysalis longicornis* and possibly from the bite of the tick *Boophilus microplus*.[39,40] SFTSV causes a potentially fatal hemorrhagic fever characterized by acute onset of fever and respiratory tract or gastrointestinal symptoms associated with leukopenia and thrombocytopenia, along with elevated muscle and liver enzymes. Infection may be complicated by multiorgan failure and neurologic symptoms. Most fatalities have occurred in patients greater than 70 years of age.

Of note, SFTSV can be transmitted from human to human by contact with infected blood or bloody secretions.[39] Although there has been no evidence to date for this route of transmission for the Heartland virus, the potential for human-to-human transmission of this virus should be kept in mind and appropriate precautions taken to prevent this occurrence. In addition, blood from infected animals could potentially be a source of human infection.

To date, testing for Heartland virus is limited to the CDC and select research settings. As with the other emerging tick-borne agents described above, there is a growing need for sensitive organism-specific serologic and molecular assays.

BARTONELLA HENSELAE

Bartonella species are fastidious, hemotropic, intracellular gram-negative bacteria. *B henselae* is thought by some to be transmitted to humans by *I scapularis* tick bites.[41] Whether bartonella infections, in general, and *B henselae*, in particular, are transmitted to humans or animals by ticks, however, has not been established.[41] Evidence does support that ticks commonly feed on bartonella-infected animals,[41,42] that bartonella DNA has been detected by PCR in ticks,[41,42] and that *Ixodes ricinus* is vector competent for transmission of *B birtlesii* in a murine model.[43]

Commentary

Although it would not be surprising to find *Bartonella* species in ticks that have fed on infected animals, a limitation of the available studies is that they primarily relied on PCR testing of ticks to establish the existence of bartonella infection, and questions have been raised by several groups of investigators about both the specificity and the significance of the PCR results obtained.[41,44,45] It is perhaps surprising how few studies have attempted to establish the presence of bartonella infection in ticks by culture. Furthermore, in view of the fact that *I scapularis* ticks will feed on cats, it is remarkable that no study has ever attempted to ascertain vector competence of this tick species for *B henselae* using a feline model (or any other animal system).[46]

There is no convincing clinical or epidemiologic evidence to support the hypothesis that *Ixodes* ticks transmit *B henselae* to humans.[41] Evidence against this hypothesis is that *Ixodes* tick bites are commonly recognized, and if tick bites lead to transmission of *B henselae*, then typical manifestations of cat scratch disease should occur at the bite site and lead to the development of a skin lesion plus regional lymphadenopathy.

However, this sequence of events has not been observed clinically. In addition, most cat scratch disease cases occur in the fall and winter, whereas *I scapularis* ticks transmit infections primarily during the summer months.

The available seroepidemiologic studies also fail to provide convincing evidence for tick transmission of *B henselae*. For example, a tick bite is common among participants of the sport of orienteering in Sweden, but has no predictive value regarding bartonella seropositivity. In this study, 61% of orienteers with bartonella antibodies reported tick bites compared with 60% of those who were seronegative.[47] In a case control study in Connecticut, there was no significant association between having found a tick on the body and cat scratch disease after controlling for exposure to kittens.[48]

SUMMARY

In conclusion, newly described tick-transmitted infections continue to be observed in the United States and elsewhere. More research is needed to define the incidence and understand the clinical and laboratory features of infections due to the EML agent, *B miyamotoi* sensu lato, deer tick virus, and Heartland virus, both as single infections and as possible coinfections in patients also infected with another pathogen transmitted by the same tick bite. There is also a need for easily accessible, sensitive and specific serologic and molecular assays for these infections. Reducing tick exposure and avoiding tick bites whenever possible should be effective prevention measures. Tick transmission of *B henselae* has not been established.

ACKNOWLEDGMENTS

The authors thank Deborah Renois, Lisa Giarratano, and Olga Melnychuk for their assistance.

REFERENCES

1. Pritt BS, Sloan LM, Johnson DK, et al. Emergence of a new pathogenic ehrlichia species, Wisconsin and Minnesota, 2009. N Engl J Med 2011;365:422–9.
2. Allerdice MEJ, Pritt BS, Paskewitz S, et al. Genetic Diversity of the Ehrlichia muris-like (EML) agent in Minnesota and Wisconsin, USA. 26th Meeting of the American Society for Rickettsiology. Portland (ME), June 15–18, 2013.
3. Eremeeva ME, Oliveira A, Moriarity J, et al. Detection and identification of bacterial, agents in Ixodes persulcatus Schulze ticks from the north western region of Russia. Vector Borne Zoonotic Dis 2007;7:426–36.
4. Spitalsko E, Boldis V, Kostanova Z, et al. Incidence of various, tick-borne microorganisms in rodents and ticks of central Slovakia. Acta Virol 2008;52:175–9.
5. Rar VA, Fomenko NV, Dobrotvorsky AK, et al. Tickborne pathogen detection, Western Siberia, Russia. Emerg Infect Dis 2005;11:1708–15.
6. Johnson DK, Neitzel DF, Miller TK, et al. Five years' experience with the novel human Ehrlichia sp. in the Upper Midwestern United States: 2009-2013. American Society of Tropical Medicine and Hygiene 63rd Annual Meeting, Late Breaker Presentation. New Orleans (LA), November 2–6, 2014.
7. Pritt BS, McFadden JD, Stromdah E, et al. Emergence of a novel Ehrlichia sp. agent pathogenic for humans in the Midwestern United States. 6th International Meeting on Rickettsiae and Rickettsial Diseases. Heraklion (Greece), June 5–7, 2011.
8. Telford SA III, Goethert HK, Cunningham JA. Prevalence of Ehrlichia muris in Wisconsin deer ticks collected during the mid-1990s. Open Microbiol J 2011;5: 18–20.

9. Barbour A. Phylogeny of a relapsing fever Borrelia species transmitted by the hard tick Ixodes scapularis. Infect Genet Evol 2014;7:551–8.

10. Hue F, Ghalyanchi A, Barbour AG. Chromosome sequence of Borrelia miyamotoi, an uncultivable tick-borne agent of human infection. Genome Announc 2013;1(5). pii:e00713–13.

11. Krause PJ, Narasimhan S, Wormser GP, et al. Borrelia miyamotoi sensu lato seroreactivity and seroprevalence in the Northeastern United States. Emerg Infect Dis 2014;20:1183–90.

12. Barbour AG, Bunikis J, Travinsky B, et al. Niche partitioning of Borrelia burgdorferi and Borrelia miyamotoi in the same tick vector and mammalian reservoir species. Am J Trop Med Hyg 2009;81:1120–31.

13. Fukunaga M, Takahashi Y, Tsurata Y, et al. Genetic and phenotypic analysis of Borrelia miyamotoi sp. nov., isolated from the ixodid tick Ixodes persulcatus, the vector for Lyme disease in Japan. Int J Syst Bacteriol 1995;45:804–10.

14. Sato K, Takano A, Konnai S, et al. Human infections with Borrelia miyamotoi, Japan. Emerg Infect Dis 2014;20:1391–3.

15. Platonov AE, Karan LS, Kolyasnikova NM, et al. Humans infected with relapsing fever spirochete Borrelia miyamotoi, Russia. Emerg Infect Dis 2011;17:1816–23.

16. Hovius JW, deWever B, Sohne M, et al. A case of meningocephalitis by the relapsing fever spirochete Borrelia miyamotoi in Europe. Lancet 2013;382:658.

17. Gugliotta JL, Goethert HK, Berardi VP, et al. Meningoencephalitis from Borrelia miyamotoi in an immunocompromised patient. N Engl J Med 2013;368:240–5.

18. Wagemakers A, Oei A, Fikrig MM, et al. The relapsing fever spirochete Borrelia miyamotoi is cultivable in a modified Kelly-Pettenkofer medium, and is resistant to complement. Parasit Vectors 2014;7:418.

19. Chowdri HR, Gugliotta JL, Berardi VP, et al. Borrelia miyamotoi infection presenting as human granulocytic anaplasmosis. Ann Intern Med 2013;159:21–7.

20. Krause PJ, Narasimhan S, Wormser GP, et al. Human Borrelia miyamotoi infection in the United States. N Engl J Med 2013;368:291–3.

21. James AM, Liveris D, Wormser GP, et al. Borrelia lonestari infection after a bite by an Ambylomma americanum tick. J Infect Dis 2001;183:1810–4.

22. Kuno G, Artsob H, Karabatsos N, et al. Genomic sequencing of deer tick virus and phylogeny of powassan-related viruses of North America. Am J Trop Med Hyg 2001;65:671–6.

23. El Khoury MY, Camargo JF, White JL, et al. Potential role of deer tick virus in Powassan encephalitis cases in Lyme disease-endemic areas of New York, USA. Emerg Infect Dis 2013;19:1926–33.

24. Thomas LA, Kennedy RC, Eklund CM. Isolation of a virus closely related to Powassan virus from Dermacenter andersoni collected along the North Cache la Poudre River, Colo. Proc Soc Exp Biol Med 1960;104:355–9.

25. Telford SR 3rd, Armstrong PM, Katavolos P, et al. A new tick-borne encephalitis-like virus infecting New England deer ticks Ixodes dammini. Emerg Infect Dis 1997;3:165–70.

26. Dupuis AP II, Peters RJ, Prusinski MA, et al. Isolation of deer tick virus (Powassan virus, lineage II) from Ixodes scapularis and detection of antibody in vertebrate hosts sampled in the Hudson Valley, New York State. Parasit Vectors 2013;6:185.

27. El Khoury MY, Camargo JF, Wormser GP. Changing epidemiology of Powassan encephalitis in North America suggests the emergence of the deer tick virus subtype. Expert Rev Anti Infect Ther 2013;11:983–5.

28. El Khoury MY, Hull RC, Bryant PW, et al. Diagnosis of acute deer tick virus encephalitis. Clin Infect Dis 2013;56:e40–7.

29. Centers for Disease Control and Prevention. Notice to Readers: final 2013 reports of nationally notifiable infectious diseases. MMWR Morb Mortal Wkly Rep 2014; 63:702–11.
30. Ebel GD, Kramer LD. Short report: duration of tick attachment required for transmission of Powassan virus by deer ticks. Am J Trop Med Hyg 2004;71: 268–71.
31. Gholam BI, Puksa S, Provias JP. Powassan encephalitis: a case report with neuropathology and literature review. CMAJ 1999;161:1419–22.
32. Tavakoli NP, Wang H, Dupuis M, et al. Fatal case of deer tick virus encephalitis. N Engl J Med 2009;360:2099–107.
33. Neitzel DF, Lynfield R, Smith K. Powassan virus encephalitis, Minnesota, USA. Emerg Infect Dis 2013;19:686.
34. McMullan LK, Folk SM, Kelly AJ, et al. A new phlebovirus associated with severe febrile illness in Missouri. N Engl J Med 2012;367:834–41.
35. Pastula DM, Turabelidze G, Yates KF, et al. Notes from the field: Heartland virus disease - United States, 2012-2013. MMWR Morb Mortal Wkly Rep 2014;63: 270–1.
36. Muehlenbachs A, Fata CR, Lambert AJ, et al. Heartland virus-associated death in Tennessee. Clin Infect Dis 2014;59:845–50.
37. Savage HM, Godsey MS Jr, Lambert A, et al. First detection of heartland virus (Bunyaviridae: phebovirus) from field collected arthropods. Am J Trop Med Hyg 2013;89:445–52.
38. CDC. Heartland virus. Atlanta (GA): US Department of Health and Human Services, CDC; 2014. Available at: http://www.cdc.gov/ncezid/dvbd/heartland/index.html.
39. Liu Q, He B, Huang SY, et al. Severe fever with thrombocytopenia syndrome, an emerging tick-borne zoonosis. Lancet Infect Dis 2014;14:763–72.
40. Ding F, Zhang W, Wang L, et al. Epidemiologic features of severe fever and thrombocytopenia syndrome in China, 2011-2012. Clin Infect Dis 2013;56: 1682–3.
41. Telford SR III, Wormser GP. Bartonella spp. transmission by ticks not established. Emerg Infect Dis 2010;16:379–84.
42. Billeter SA, Levy MG, Chronel BB, et al. Vector transmission of Bartonella species with emphasis on the potential for tick transmission. Med Vet Entomol 2008;22: 1–15.
43. Reis C, Cote M, Le Rhun D, et al. Vector competence of the tick Ixodes ricinus for transmission of Bartonella birtlesii. PLoS Negl Trop Dis 2011;5(5):e1186.
44. Tijsse-Klasen E, Fonville M, Gassner F, et al. Absence of zoonotic Bartonella species in questing ticks: first detection of Bartonella clarridgeiae and Rickettsia felis in cat fleas in the Netherlands. Parasit Vectors 2011;4:61.
45. Adelson ME, Rao RV, Tilton RC, et al. Prevalence of Borrelia burgdorferi, Bartonella spp., Babesia microti, and Anaplasma phagocytophilum in Ixodes scapularis ticks collected in Northern New Jersey. J Clin Microbiol 2004;42:2799–801.
46. Cotte V, Bonnet S, Le Rhun D, et al. Transmission of Bartonella henselae by Ixodes ricinus. Emerg Infect Dis 2008;14:1074–80.
47. McGill S, Wesslen L, Hjelm E, et al. Serological and epidemiological analysis of the prevalence of Bartonella spp. antibodies in Swedish elite orienteers 1992-93. Scand J Infect Dis 2001;33:423–8.
48. Zangwill KM, Hamilton DH, Perkins BA, et al. Cat scratch disease in Connecticut. Epidemiology, risk factors and evaluation of a new diagnostic test. N Engl J Med 1993;329:8–13.

Index

Note: Page numbers of article titles are in **boldface** type.

Infect Dis Clin N Am 29 (2015) 383–390
http://dx.doi.org/10.1016/S0891-5520(15)00039-2
0891-5520/15/$ – see front matter © 2015 Elsevier Inc. All rights reserved.

id.theclinics.com

Moving?

Make sure your subscription moves with you!

To notify us of your new address, find your **Clinics Account Number** (located on your mailing label above your name), and contact customer service at:

Email: journalscustomerservice-usa@elsevier.com

800-654-2452 (subscribers in the U.S. & Canada)
314-447-8871 (subscribers outside of the U.S. & Canada)

Fax number: 314-447-8029

Elsevier Health Sciences Division
Subscription Customer Service
3251 Riverport Lane
Maryland Heights, MO 63043

*To ensure uninterrupted delivery of your subscription, please notify us at least 4 weeks in advance of move.

Printed and bound by CPI Group (UK) Ltd, Croydon, CR0 4YY

03/10/2024

01040496-0001